£103.50

D1454420

Royal Liverpool University Hospital – Staff Library

Please return or renew, on or before the last date below.
Items may be renewed **twice**, <u>if not reserved for another
user</u>. Renewals may be made in person, by telephone:
0151 706 2248 or email: <u>library.service@rlbuht.nhs.uk</u>.
There is a charge of 10p per day for late items.

Library
Education Centre
Royal Liverpool University Hospital
Prescot Street
L7 8XP

STEM CELLS AND MYOCARDIAL REGENERATION

CONTEMPORARY CARDIOLOGY

CHRISTOPHER P. CANNON, MD
SERIES EDITOR
ANNEMARIE M. ARMANI, MD
EXECUTIVE EDITOR

STEM CELLS
AND MYOCARDIAL
REGENERATION

Edited by

MARC S. PENN, MD, PhD

Bakken Heart Brain Institute
and Coronary Intensive Care Unit,
The Cleveland Clinic Foundation
Cleveland, OH

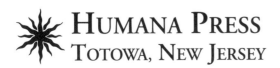

HUMANA PRESS
TOTOWA, NEW JERSEY

Production Editor: Robin B. Weisberg

Cover design by Patricia F. Cleary

Cover illustration: From Figure 1, Chapter 3, "Mesenchymal Stem Cells for Cardiac Therapy," by Mark F. Pittenger

For additional copies, pricing for bulk purchases, and/or information about other Humana titles, contact Humana at the above address or at any of the following numbers: Tel.: 973-256-1699; Fax: 973-256-8341, E-mail: orders@ humanapr.com; or visit our Website: www.humanapress.com

This publication is printed on acid-free paper.⊚
ANSI Z39.48-1984 (American National Standards Institute) Permanence of Paper for Printed Library Materials.

Printed in the United States of America.   10 9 8 7 6 5 4 3 2 1

e-ISBN 1-59745-272-6

Library of Congress Cataloging-in-Publication Data

Stem cells and myocardial regeneration / edited by Marc S. Penn.
   p. ; cm. -- (Contemporary cardiology)
  Includes bibliographical references and index.
  ISBN 1-58829-664-4 (alk. paper)
   1. Stem cells--Therapeutic use. 2. Regeneration (Biology)
 3. Myocardium--Regeneration. 4. Transplantation of organs, tissues,
 etc.   I. Penn, Marc S. II. Series: Contemporary cardiology
(Totowa, N.J. : Unnumbered)
  [DNLM: 1. Myocardium--cytology. 2. Stem Cells--physiology.
 3. Regeneration--physiology.   WG 280 S824 2007]
 QH588.S83S74 2007
 616.1'24060724--dc22   2006006484

DEDICATION

To my *parents* for all the opportunities they afforded me
To my *wife* for her never ending love and support
To my *children* for their inspiration and energy

PREFACE

Over the past 5 years there has been great excitement and controversy in the scientific, financial, and lay literature for the potential of stem cell-based strategies for the prevention and treatment of chronic heart failure (CHF). Not that long ago we believed we were born with a set number of cardiac myocytes and that once damaged there was no hope to replace them. The interest in the field stems from the magnitude of cardiovascular disease in the world. Our ability to treat and help patients survive acute myocardial infarction (MI) has resulted in a near epidemic of CHF. There are more than 5 million Americans who currently carry the diagnosis of CHF. With more than 1 million MIs a year in the United States, there are approx 500,000 new cases of CHF diagnosed each year. The goal of *Stem Cells and Myocardial Regeneration* is to present, in a coherent manner, the current state of knowledge of stem cell-based therapies for cardiac dysfunction, including current findings in both the laboratory and the clinic trials.

The first section of this *Stem Cells and Myocardial Regeneration* focuses on the magnitude of the problem and the successes and failures of what we consider optimal medical therapy. It is on this background that stem cell-based therapy needs to build. The following two sections focus on the basic science behind stem cell-based therapies, first reviewing the different stem cell types of interest, then the critical physiological pathways that need to be understood including chemokines, stem cell differentiation, and mechanisms of arrhythmia.

The focus of *Stem Cells and Myocardial Regeneration* then turns to the clinical issues surrounding stem cell delivery to the heart at the time of MI and in patients with CHF. The book ends with separate reviews of findings of stem cell-based clinical trials of acute MI and CHF.

It is my hope that the reader will take away many things from *Stem Cells and Myocardial Regeneration*. First, I hope the reader sees the excitement that this field offers to the millions of patients at risk of or afflicted with cardiovascular disease. We are truly at the beginning of a great frontier of new medical therapy. Second, I hope the reader realizes that although we have learned a great deal about stem cells and the heart, we are still far from correct or optimal therapy and have much yet to learn. And third, I hope the reader develops a framework with which he or she may be able to put future findings in perspective.

It was a great pleasure to work with my many colleagues who graciously gave their time to bring this project to fruition. Although it would be impossible to delve into all the controversies and nuances of stem cell-based therapies for the heart, I believe readers will find this to be a detailed and fair representation of the current state of knowledge.

Marc S. Penn, MD, PhD

CONTENTS

CONTRIBUTORS

ANTHONY W. ASHTON, MD • *Cardiovascular Research Center, Heart Center, Montefiore Medical Center, Albert Einstein College of Medicine, New York, NY*

ARMAN T. ASKARI, MD • *Department of Cardiovascular Medicine, Cleveland Clinic Foundation, Cleveland, OH*

FERNANDO A. ATIK, MD • *Department of Cardiothoracic Surgery, Cleveland Clinic Foundation, Cleveland, OH*

CESARE BEGHI, MD • *Cardiac Surgery Unit, Università degli Studi di Parma, Parma, Italy*

SHYAM BHAKTA, MD • *Division of Cardiology, Case Western Reserve University, Cleveland, OH*

BRIAN J. BOLWELL, MD • *Bone Marrow Transplant Program, Cleveland Clinic Foundation, Cleveland, OH*

RICHARD O. CANNON III, MD • *Cardiovascular Branch, National Heart Lung and Blood Institute, Bethesda, MD*

MANUEL D. CERQUEIRA, MD • *Department of Molecular and Functional Imaging, Cleveland Clinic Foundation, Cleveland, OH*

DAVID D'ALESSANDRO, MD • *Department of Cardiothoracic Surgery, Heart Center, Montefiore Medical Center, Albert Einstein College of Medicine, New York, NY*

ROBERT DEANS, PhD • *Regenerative Medicine Program, Athersys Inc., Cleveland, OH*

STEPHEN G. ELLIS, MD • *Department of Cardiovascular Medicine, Cleveland Clinic Foundation, Cleveland, OH*

JORGE GENOVESE, MD • *Heart, Lung, and Esophageal Surgery Institute, McGowan Institute of Regenerative Medicine, University of Pittsburgh Medical Center, Pittsburgh, PA*

LIOR GEPSTEIN, MD, PhD • *Department of Cardiology, Technion University, Haifa, Israel*

ALESSANDRO GIACOMELLO, MD, PhD • *Department of Experimental Medicine and Pathology, University of Rome "La Sapienza," Rome, Italy*

MATTHEW HOOK, MD • *Department of Cardiovascular Medicine, Cleveland Clinic Foundation, Cleveland, OH*

DAYI HU, MD • *Cardiology Department, People's Hospital, Peking University, Beijing China*

SILVIU ITESCU, MD • *Department of Transplantation Immunology, Columbia University Medical Center, New York, NY*

WAEL A. JABER, MD • *Department of Cardiovascular Medicine, Cleveland Clinic Foundation, Cleveland, OH*

ANDREA N. LADD, PhD • *Department of Cell Biology, Cleveland Clinic Foundation, Cleveland, OH*

MARY J. LAUGHLIN, MD • *Department of Hematology and Oncology, Case Western Reserve University, Cleveland, OH*

KENNETH R. LAURITA, PhD • *Heart and Vascular Research Center, MetroHealth Campus, Case Western Reserve University, Cleveland, OH*

ROBERTO LORUSSO, MD, PhD • *Experimental Cardiac Surgery Laboratory, Cardiac Surgery Unit, Civic Hospital, Brescia, Italy*

NILADRI MAL, MD • *Department of Cell Biology, Cleveland Clinic Foundation, Cleveland, OH*

EDUARDO MARBÁN, MD, PhD • *Division of Cardiology, Johns Hopkins University School of Medicine, Baltimore, MD*

TIMOTHY MARTENS MD • *Department of Transplantation Immunology, Columbia University Medical Center, New York, NY*

ELISA MESSINA, MD, PhD • *Department of Experimental Medicine and Pathology, University of Rome "La Sapienza," Rome, Italy*

ROBERT E. MICHLER, MD • *Department of Cardiothoracic Surgery, Heart Center, Montefiore Medical Center, Albert Einstein College of Medicine, New York, NY*

WILLIAM R. MILLS, MD • *Heart and Vascular Research Center, MetroHealth Campus, Case Western Reserve University, Cleveland, OH*

JOSÈ L. NAVIA, MD • *Department of Cardiothoracic Surgery, Cleveland Clinic Foundation, Cleveland, OH*

DONALD ORLIC, PhD • *Cardiovascular Branch, National Heart Lung and Blood Institute, National Institutes of Health, Bethesda, MD,*

AMIT N. PATEL, MD, MS • *McGowan Institute of Regenerative Medicine, University of Pittsburgh Medical Center, Pittsburgh, PA*

MARC S. PENN, MD, PhD • *Bakken Heart Brain Institute and Coronary Intensive Care Unit, Cleveland Clinic Foundation, Cleveland, OH*

EMERSON C. PERIN, MD, PhD • *Department of Cardiology, Texas Heart Institute, Houston, TX*

MARK F. PITTENGER, PhD • *Department of Cardiology, Johns Hopkins School of Medicine, Baltimore, MD*

AMY RABER, BS • *Regenerative Medicine Program, Athersys Inc., Cleveland, OH*

FIONA SEE, PhD • *Department of Transplantation Immunology, Columbia University Medical Center, New York, NY*

GUILHERME V. SILVA, MD • *Department of Cardiology, Texas Heart Institute, Houston, TX*

ANTHONY TING, PhD • *Regenerative Medicine Program, Regenerative Medicine Program, Athersys Inc., Cleveland, OH*

ERIC J. TOPOL, MD • *Department of Genetics, Case Western Reserve University, Cleveland, OH*

SAMUEL UNZEK, MD • *Department of Cardiovascular Medicine, Cleveland Clinic Foundation, Cleveland, OH*

WOUTER VAN'T HOF, PhD • *Regenerative Medicine Program, Athersys Inc., Cleveland, OH*

KAI WANG, MD, PhD • *Department of Cardiovascular Medicine, Cleveland Clinic Foundation, Cleveland, OH*

PATRICK WHITLOW, MD • *Department of Cardiovascular Medicine, Cleveland Clinic Foundation, Cleveland, OH*

SHUIXIANG YANG, MD • *Cardiology Department, People's Hospital, Peking University, Beijing, China*

MING ZHANG, MD, PhD • *Department of Cell Biology, Cleveland Clinic Foundation, Cleveland, OH*

COLOR PLATES

Color Plates follow p. 114.

1

The Challenge for Stem Cell Therapy

Overview of the Problem: Heart Attack and Heart Failure

Marc S. Penn, MD, PhD *and Eric J. Topol,* MD

SUMMARY

Ischemic heart disease remains the leading cause of chronic heart failure (CHF). The prevalence of CHF has increased dramatically over the last three decades, with more than 10% of the US population over 65 years of age now carrying the diagnosis. Based on current trends, heart failure is predicted to increase to more than 6 million people in the United States by the year 2030 *(1)*. One cause of the increased prevalence of CHF is our success in the treatment of acute myocardial infarction (MI). Mortality rates of transmural MI in clinical trials has decreased from more than 10% in clinical trials in the late 1980s to less than 5% in recent primary percutaneous coronary intervention trials. These advances, combined with the compelling data that cholesterol-lowering therapy significantly decreases the risk of MI, would lead one to hypothesize that the incidence of CHF should be on the decline. However, we are a population of increasing risk, given the increasing incidence of diabetes, hypertension, obesity, and sedentary lifestyle. Thus, although great advances have been made in the treatment of cardiovascular disease, there is a great need for stem cell therapy to prevent and treat CHF.

Key Words: Acute myocardial infarction; primary percutaneous coronary intervention; statin therapy; chronic heart failure.

One cause of the increased prevalence of chronic heart failure (CHF) is our success in the treatment of acute myocardial infarction (MI). Thrombolytic therapy for acute MI and the more recent growing acceptance and availability of primary percutaneous coronary intervention (PCI) for ST elevation MI have caused the mortality rate of this devastating ischemic event to decrease from more than 10% in clinical trials in the late 1980s *(2)* to less than 5% in recent primary PCI trials *(3)*. The data in Fig. 1 depict 30-day mortality in thrombolytic and primary PCI trials over the last two decades. Because these are all active control arms, the trend toward convergence of the treatment and experimental arms in these trials may suggest that we are reaching a point of limited return with our current treatment strategies.

Similar reductions in mortality have been seen in the patient population that presents with acute non-ST elevation MI, with the mortality rate in contemporary trials

From: *Contemporary Cardiology: Stem Cells and Myocardial Regeneration*
Edited by: M. S. Penn © Humana Press Inc., Totowa, NJ

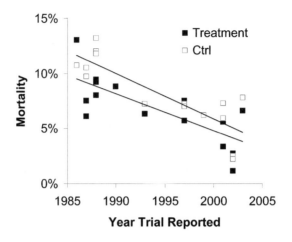

Fig. 1. Graph (top) and listing (bottom) of reported 30-day mortalities in representative trials involving patients with acute myocardial infarction between 1985 and 2003. SK, streptokinase; ASA, aspirin; Tx, treatment arm; Ctrl, control arm. *Note:* Not all trials were placebo-controlled.

being 2.9–4.5% (PURSUIT *[4]*, PRISM-PLUS *[5]*). Aggressive protocols with early angiography and revascularization have been shown to decrease mortality 2.2% in the TACTICS trial *(6)*.

Our understanding of the importance of platelets in the thromobotic process has led to the development of multiple pharmacological strategies that have made mechanical reperfusion safer and improved the outcomes of patients with stable and unstable coronary artery disease *(7)*. These advances, combined with the development of drug-eluting stents, which decrease the rate of restenosis from 40% with angioplasty to 19% with stenting with bare metal stents *(8)* to 4.1% with drug-eluting stents, have significantly advanced our pursuit to restore and maintain myocardial perfusion.

This improved ability to restore and maintain myocardial perfusion combined with the compelling data that cholesterol-lowering therapy significantly decreases the risk of MI would lead one to hypothesize that the incidence of CHF should be on the decline. Figure 2 depicts the decrease in mortality in statin trials over the past decade. These trials are of patients with stable coronary artery disease or at high risk of having coronary disease with follow-up between 4 and 6 years. Since the landmark 4S trial

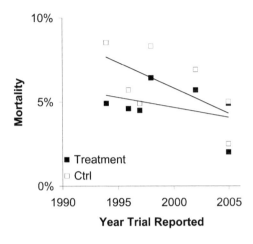

Fig. 2. Graph (top) and listing (bottom) of reported long-term mortality in representative trials studying the effects of cholesterol-lowering therapies in high-risk patients or patients with coronary artery disease. Tx, treatment arm; Ctrl, control arm. *Note:* Not all trials were placebo-controlled. Year, year the trial results were reported; F/U was the average time for follow-up in the study; Number represents the total number of patients in the trial.

published in 1994 *(9)*, mortality has decreased significantly, likely at least in part as a result of the improvement in overall medical management, including the use of antiplatelets and lowering of blood pressure standards *(10)*. One of the main reasons for convergence of the treatment and control curves in Fig. 3 might be the fact that contemporary trials have active control arms because it is no longer ethical to conduct placebo control trials in this population.

So where is the disconnect between all of these advances in our understanding of the disease process, our ability to prevent and treat acute ischemic events, and the increasing incidence of CHF? One problem is the vast increase in the number of people at risk. The population is aging, and the incidence of adult and childhood obesity is dramatically rising. Added to these demographics are the increasing rates of type 2 diabetes, hypertension, hypercholesterolemia, and a general lack of daily activity. Thus, the rate of the increase in the number of patients at risk is outpacing our ability to decrease the likelihood of an event.

Another major contributor to the disconnect is based on the old adage: "time is muscle." The median time from symptom onset to initating reperfusion therapy is more than 3 hours—unchanged from a decade ago. Patients are surviving large acute ischemic events that may have been lethal in earlier years, but now have to live with significantly less functional myocardial tissue. Extensive necrosis, despite late reperfusion, leads to significant ventricular remodeling characterized by dilation of the left ventricular cavity, thinning of the infarcted tissue, and electrical remodeling, which dramatically increases the risk of sudden cardiac death *(11,12)*. These patients also go on to have

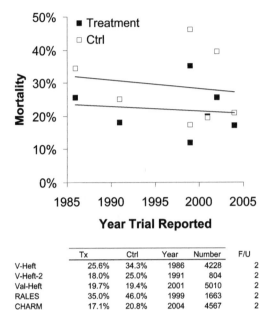

	Tx	Ctrl	Year	Number	F/U
V-Heft	25.6%	34.3%	1986	4228	2
V-Heft-2	18.0%	25.0%	1991	804	2
Val-Heft	19.7%	19.4%	2001	5010	2
RALES	35.0%	46.0%	1999	1663	2
CHARM	17.1%	20.8%	2004	4567	2
COPERNICUS	25.6%	39.4%	2002	2289	2
CIBIS-II	11.8%	17.3%	1999	2647	1.3

Fig. 3. Graph (top) and listing (bottom) of reported 2-year mortality in representative trials studying medical treatment strategies in patients with chronic heart failure. Tx; treatment arm; Ctrl; control arm. *Note:* Not all trials were placebo-controlled. Year, year the trial results were reported; F/U was the average time for follow-up in the study; Number represents the total number of patients in the trial.

additional MIs. Studies on the genetics of MI have clearly demonstrated that MI and atherosclerosis are distinct processes *(13–15)*. Thus, a patient who has had an MI is at higher risk of having another MI than is a patient with stable coronary disease without a history of MI *(16)*.

One strategy to prevent the development of CHF aggressively pursued over the past decade is to optimize the left ventricular remodeling process. We know that the higher the white blood cell count or other markers of inflammation at the time of MI, the higher the likelihood that the patient will develop CHF and have a worse outcome *(17,18)*. We have learned that the inflammatory response following MI has a significant role in the thinning and dilation of the injured myocardial tissue *(19,20)*. However, beyond restoration of myocardial blood flow, none of the strategies put forth have proven effective in clinical trials *(21,22)*.

At the end of the day, we have an increasing number of patients surviving acute ischemic events who are living to have further ischemic events, further decreasing the amount of viable myocardial tissue and increasing the prevalence of CHF. This, combined with the impressive decrease in mortality associated with the implantation of implantable cardiac defibrillators *(12)* and/or cardiac resynchronization *(23)*, indicates that we have reached a point of truly diminishing returns.

Optimal medical therapy with angiotensin-converting enzyme inhibitors, β-blockers, and aldactone clearly decreases symptoms and improves outcomes. The data in Fig. 3 show the 2-year mortality in a series of heart failure trials that have studied the combination of hydralazine and nitrates, angiotensin-converting enzyme inhibitors, β-blockers, and aldactone. Although the data in Fig. 3 would suggest no significant decline in mortality in patients with CHF over the past two decades, it should be noted that over this period of time the severity of heart failure studied has significantly increased.

Cardiac transplantation is an effective therapy but will never be available to all the patients at need given the fixed number of donors available. It is in this setting that we hailed the results of the Randomized Evaluation of Mechanical Assistance Therapy as an Alternative in Congestive Heart Failure (REMATCH) trial, which showed "improved outcomes" with destination left ventricular assist device placement *(24)*. Although an important, even heroic trial, the improvement in medial survival was only 258 days. This is not the level of success that we have come to expect from major cardiovascular trials. Although it is likely that destination mechanical pump therapy will have a significant role in the treatment of severe CHF, it is years from mainstream use and is likely not to repair, but rather replace heart function. Of note, all the patients in the control arm of the REMATCH trial were dead at 26 months, demonstrating that the mortality associated with patients with severe heart failure rivals that of virtually any neoplasm.

It is in this setting of desperation to treat a growing patient population with or at risk for CHF that the cardiovascular medicine and surgery community, and to a great extent our patients, have grabbed hold of the potential of stem cell therapy. Although clinical trials have commenced in the arena of stem cell therapy, investigation needs to focus on patient populations that are not already well treated by contemporary therapy. Given the past successes, the challenges for successful stem cell-based therapies are great.

REFERENCES

1. Robbins MA, O'Connell JB. Economic impact of heart failure. In: Rose EA, Stevenson Lw, eds. Management of End-Stage Heart Disease. Lippincott-Raven, Philadelphia, 1998, pp. 3–13.
2. Randomized factorial trial of high-dose intravenous streptokinase, of oral aspirin and of intravenous heparin in acute myocardial infarction. ISIS (International Studies of Infarct Survival) pilot study. Eur Heart J 1987;8:634–642.
3. Stone GW, Grines CL, Cox D, et al. Comparison of angioplasty with stenting, with or without abciximab, in acute myocardial infarction. N Engl J Med 2002;346:957–966.
4. The PURSUIT Trial Investigators. Inhibition of platelet glycoprotein IIb/IIIa with eptifibatide in patients with acute coronary syndromes. Platelet glycoprotein IIb/IIIa in unstable angina: receptor suppression using integrilin therapy. N Engl J Med 1998;339:436–443.
5. Platelet Receptor Inhibition in Ischemic Syndrome Management in Patients Limited by Unstable Signs and Symptoms (PRISM-PLUS) Study Investigators. Inhibition of the platelet glycoprotein IIb/IIIa receptor with tirofiban in unstable angina and non-Q-wave myocardial infarction. N Engl J Med 1998;338:1488–1497.
6. Cannon CP, Weintraub WS, Demopoulos LA, et al. Comparison of early invasive and conservative strategies in patients with unstable coronary syndromes treated with the glycoprotein IIb/IIIa inhibitor tirofiban. N Engl J Med 2001;344:1879–1887.
7. Steinhubl SR, Berger PB, Mann JT, III, et al. Early and sustained dual oral antiplatelet therapy following percutaneous coronary intervention: a randomized controlled trial. JAMA 2002;288: 2411–2420.
8. Versaci F, Gaspardone A, Tomai F, Crea F, Chiariello L, Gioffre PA. A comparison of coronary-artery stenting with angioplasty for isolated stenosis of the proximal left anterior descending coronary artery. N Engl J Med 1997;336:817–822.
9. Randomised trial of cholesterol lowering in 4444 patients with coronary heart disease: the Scandinavian Simvastatin Survival Study (4S). Lancet 1994;344:1383–1389.
10. Nissen SE, Tuzcu EM, Libby P, et al. Effect of antihypertensive agents on cardiovascular events in patients with coronary disease and normal blood pressure: the CAMELOT study: a randomized controlled trial. JAMA 2004;292:2217–2225.
11. Kadish A, Dyer A, Daubert JP, et al. Prophylactic defibrillator implantation in patients with nonischemic dilated cardiomyopathy. N Engl J Med 2004;350:2151–2158.

12. Bardy GH, Lee KL, Mark DB, et al. Amiodarone or an implantable cardioverter-defibrillator for congestive heart failure. N Engl J Med 2005;352:225–237.
13. McCarthy JJ, Parker A, Salem R, et al. Large scale association analysis for identification of genes underlying premature coronary heart disease: cumulative perspective from analysis of 111 candidate genes. J Med Genet 2004;41:334–341.
14. Wang L, Fan C, Topol SE, Topol EJ, Wang Q. Mutation of MEF2A in an inherited disorder with features of coronary artery disease. Science 2003;302:1578–1581.
15. Wang Q, Rao S, Shen GQ, et al. Premature myocardial infarction novel susceptibility locus on chromosome 1P34-36 identified by genomewide linkage analysis. Am J Hum Genet 2004;74:262–271.
16. Haffner SM, Lehto S, Ronnemaa T, Pyorala K, Laakso M. Mortality from coronary heart disease in subjects with type 2 diabetes and in nondiabetic subjects with and without prior myocardial infarction. N Engl J Med 1998;339:229–234.
17. Bhatt DL, Chew DP, Lincoff AM, et al. Effect of revascularization on mortality associated with an elevated white blood cell count in acute coronary syndromes. Am J Cardiol 2003;92:136–140.
18. Barron HV, Cannon CP, Murphy SA, Braunwald E, Gibson CM. Association between white blood cell count, epicardial blood flow, myocardial perfusion, and clinical outcomes in the setting of acute myocardial infarction: a thrombolysis in myocardial infarction 10 substudy. Circulation 2000;102: 2329–2334.
19. Vasilyev N, Williams T, Brennan ML, et al. Myeloperoxidase-generated oxidants modulate left ventricular remodeling but not infarct size after myocardial infarction. Circulation 2005;112:2812–2820.
20. Askari A, Brennan ML, Zhou X, et al. Myeloperoxidase and plasminogen activator inhibitor-1 play a central role in ventricular remodeling after myocardial infarction. J Exp Med 2003;197:615–624.
21. Baran KW, Nguyen M, McKendall GR, et al. Double-blind, randomized trial of an anti-CD18 antibody in conjunction with recombinant tissue plasminogen activator for acute myocardial infarction: limitation of myocardial infarction following thrombolysis in acute myocardial infarction (LIMIT AMI) study. Circulation 2001;104:2778–2783.
22. Ross AM, Gibbons RJ, Stone GW, Kloner RA, Alexander RW. A randomized, double-blinded, placebo-controlled multicenter trial of adenosine as an adjunct to reperfusion in the treatment of acute myocardial infarction (AMISTAD-II). J Am Coll Cardiol 2005;45:1775–1780.
23. Cleland JG, Daubert JC, Erdmann E, et al. The effect of cardiac resynchronization on morbidity and mortality in heart failure. N Engl J Med 2005;352:1539–1549.
24. Rose EA, Gelijns AC, Moskowitz AJ, et al. Long-term mechanical left ventricular assistance for end-stage heart failure. N Engl J Med 2001;345:1435–1443.

I

CELLS OF INTEREST FOR MYOCARDIAL REGENERATION

2

Hematopoietic Stem Cells for Myocardial Regeneration

Donald Orlic, PhD
and Richard O. Cannon III, MD

SUMMARY

Adult bone marrow consists of several populations of stem cells that are the focus of investigations into their potential to regenerate nonhematopoietic tissues. According to this hypothesis, bone marrow stem cells display a plasticity not previously recognized. Although data supporting bone marrow stem cell plasticity is extensive, many researchers dispute this concept. One of the most controversial aspects of stem cell plasticity relates to regeneration of heart muscle following acute myocardial infarction (MI). When experimentally induced MIs in rodents were analyzed for regeneration of the heart tissues, it was reported that cardiomyocyte renewal was achieved as a result of bone marrow stem cell infiltration of the damaged tissue. Evidence continues to accumulate in support of and against the potential for myocardial regeneration, indicating the need for a better scientific basis for the possible involvement of bone marrow-derived stem cells in myocardial regeneration.

In order to achieve a higher level of acceptance for myocardial regeneration, researchers must develop more exacting methodologies to monitor repair over time at the cellular level. A major effort must be undertaken to identify the signals required for stem cell mobilization and trafficking to infarcted cardiac tissue and to define the genetic mechanisms involved in stem cell plasticity. To answer these questions it will be necessary to establish the exact identity of the stem cell population involved. Controversies regarding myocardial regeneration in rodent models will require additional experiments using large animal models, with an emphasis on tracking of labeled donor cells. These preclinical experiments will also enable testing cell-delivery devices and noninvasive modalities for detecting improvement in regional and global myocardial function. If key questions relating to transdifferentiation potential, cell survival, and function can be resolved, we may one day be able to fully exploit the potential of stem cells for myocardial repair.

Key Words: Myocardial regeneration; stem cell plasticity; ischemia; myocardial infarction.

STEM CELLS FOR TISSUE REGENERATION

Investigators in the nascent field of stem cell therapy propose the lofty goal that one day it may be within our capacity to regulate the regeneration of tissues and organs. There is a biological basis for some of the enthusiasm for regenerative medicine: in

From: *Contemporary Cardiology: Stem Cells and Myocardial Regeneration*
Edited by: M. S. Penn © Humana Press Inc., Totowa, NJ

normal growth and especially following injury, tissues undergo regeneration, and in many instances the stem cells involved in regeneration have been identified.

The most thoroughly investigated developmental pathway from a stem cell to a mature functional cell is the renewal of blood cells through hematopoiesis. From early fetal life and throughout adult life, the bone marrow consists of hematopoietic stem cells (HSCs) that give rise to multiple populations of descendants referred to as progenitor cells. The progeny of these progenitor cells acquire specific molecular patterns that characterize unique blood cell lineages. Each blast cell transits through several levels of cell maturation accompanied by a series of cell divisions, leading to the formation of a cluster of 8–32 erythrocytes or leukocytes.

HSCs in adult bone marrow are a rare population of cells. The best estimates of their frequency, obtained largely from mouse studies, suggest that they occur at a ratio of approx 1:10,000 or 1:100,000 cells. Their enrichment, utilizing lineage-specific markers and several HSC-specific markers, by flow cytometry has enabled basic researchers and clinicians to better define the molecular and cellular events that occur in bone marrow and achieve a degree of control over hematopoietic tissue regeneration. Advances such as these, over many years, have provided insight into normally occurring processes in tissue regeneration.

Currently, several stem cell populations, most prominently HSCs and neural stem cells (NSCs), are being investigated for a newly proposed attribute referred to as stem cell plasticity or transdifferentiation. According to this hypothesis, stem cells from one specific tissue may differentiate into cells of a different tissue, even one whose origin is from another embryonic germ layer. The concept of stem cell plasticity has provoked enormous interest from biologists and clinicians. The excitement in some quarters, however, is matched by skepticism in others. In this chapter we will attempt to define what has been achieved thus far and what future studies may be needed to establish bone marrow stem cell plasticity as a basic component of today's science as well as its potential in treating human diseases.

STEM CELLS IN ADULT BONE MARROW

Initially, hematopoietic stem cells arise in the yolk sac (1) and aorta–gonad–mesonephros (2,3) region of the developing embryo. During fetal development, these stem cells are believed to colonize the liver, spleen, and, at mid-gestation, the bone marrow. After birth, hematopoietic activity in bone marrow is under the control of resident HSCs. However, in addition to HSCs, the cells that infiltrate the cavities of fetal bone marrow also give rise to mesenchymal stem cells (MSCs), which survive the lifetime of the individual, and perhaps a third class of stem cells referred to as multipotent adult progenitor cells (MAPCs). With this hierarchy in mind, it is clear that HSCs and bone marrow stem cells (BMSCs) are not synonymous. Thus, HSCs are one of several stem cell populations in adult bone marrow (Fig. 1). Unfortunately, the literature is replete with examples in which authors use the term HSCs to describe transdifferentiation events when working with a combination of BMSCs.

Hemangioblasts are believed to represent a population of bone marrow cells more primitive than HSCs. They are present initially in yolk sac blood islands, where they appear to give rise to the primitive red blood cells of the embryo and the endothelial cells that form channels, the vitelline veins, through which newly formed red cells circulate to the embryo proper. This developmental pattern may simply be an attribute of a cell population with dual differentiation pathways. Alternatively, because endothelial cells and red blood cells do not share a common morphology or function, hemangioblast activity may represent an example of stem cell plasticity in adult bone marrow. Although their phenotype is not well characterized, hemangioblasts appear to co-purify with HSCs. A recent investigation showed that a single donor lineage-negative (Lin[-]) Sca-1[+] CD45[+] green fluorescent protein-positive (GFP[+]) bone marrow-derived stem cell reconstituted ablated recipient bone marrow within 30 days of transplantation. Subsequently, following laser beam-induced damage to the retinal vasculature, the progeny of this single GFP[+] bone marrow reconstituting cell trafficked to the site of retinal ischemia and engaged in neovasculogenesis (4). From this observation and many others (5–12), there is growing support for the concept of a rare population of adult bone marrow cells that is endowed with hematopoietic and vasculogenic potential.

HSCs are capable of unlimited cell proliferation in bone marrow. They have a relatively well-defined surface phenotype (Fig. 1) by which they can be enriched using fluorescence-activated flow cytometry. Mouse HSCs are classified as Lin[-] Sca-1[+] (13) and c-kit[+] (14,15). However, they cannot be purified because their phenotype is shared in part with their immediate progeny, the committed progenitor cells that give rise to the myeloid and lymphoid lineages, and also, to a more limited extent, with MSCs, MAPCs, and the bone marrow-derived endothelial progenitor cells (EPCs), which have the potential to generate endothelium. By comparison, based on difficulties involved in following HSC activity in human bone marrow, the phenotype of human HSCs is less well defined. There is general agreement, however, that human HSCs are Lin[-] CD34[+] CD38[-] cells, but several cell types share the Lin[-] CD34[+] phenotype, and CD38 is not a well-defined marker. Finally, HSCs, the ultimate ancestor of the blood cell hierarchy, share with all developing and mature blood cells the CD45 common leukocyte marker.

Are HSCs the bone marrow component that some believe exhibit plasticity, and, if so, should they be considered prime candidates for initiatives in cellular therapy? This concept is fraught with difficulties. For decades scientists and hematologists have struggled with the difficulty that HSCs cannot be purified based on phenotypical characteristics and, perhaps more importantly, cannot be expanded and cloned ex vivo. Recent evidence has emerged suggesting that HSCs can be expanded ex vivo (16) and that this occurs by forced expression of the Polycomb group gene *Bmi-1 (17)*, but there is still no evidence to support the idea of clonality. For these reasons HSCs are not ideally suited for in vitro experiments designed to test plasticity. In this regard HSCs differ dramatically from MSCs in bone marrow and NSCs in the central nervous system, both of which can be clonally derived and tested for multiple differentiation pathways. Some of the best evidence to date regarding HSC plasticity is from mouse experiments that involved the injection of a single bone marrow-derived stem cell that initially reconstitutes the bone marrow and subsequently gives rise to cells with a capacity to form endothelium (4) and epithelium in multiple organs (18).

Although HSCs reside primarily in bone marrow, small numbers can be isolated from the circulation. However, the relatively few HSCs in blood under normal conditions can be greatly enhanced in response to a series of daily injections of granulocyte–colony-stimulating factor (G-CSF) and stem cell factor (SCF) (19,20). The cytokine G-CSF induces neutrophils in bone marrow to release their granular content of proteolytic enzymes, including matrix metalloproteinase-9 and elastase (21–24). This change in the bone marrow microenvironment alters the steady-state conditions, and following proteolytic cleavage of stromal-derived factor-1 (SDF-1) from its receptor

Multipotent Adult Progenitor Cells

	Mouse	Human
fibronectin adherent:	yes	yes
expandable ex vivo:	yes	yes
cell doublings:	120	180
phenotype:	CD34-	CD34-
	CD45-	CD45-
	CD44-	CD44-
	c-kit-	c-kit- (CD117)
	class I HLA-	class I HLA-
plasticity:	yes	yes

Endothelial Progenitor Cells

	Mouse	Human
fibronectin adherent:	yes	yes
expandable ex vivo:	yes	yes
phenotype:	CD133+	CD133+
	KDR+	KDR+
	CD31-	CD31-
	???	VEGFR2+
plasticity:	yes (?)	yes (?)

Bone Marrow Stem Cells

Hematopoietic Stem Cells

	Mouse	Human
plastic adherent:	no	no
expandable ex vivo:	no	no
phenotype:	lineage-	lineage-
	c-kit+	c-kit+ (CD117)
	Sca-1+	Sca-1-
	CD34 (?)	CD34+
	CD45+	CD45+
plasticity:	yes	yes

Mesenchymal Stem Cells

	Mouse	Human
plastic adherent:	yes	yes
expandable ex vivo:	yes	yes
cell doublings:	14-21 days	14-21 days
phenotype:	CD34-	CD34+
	CD45-	CD45-
	CD31-	CD31-
	Sca-1+	CD90+
	Class II HLA-	CD106+
plasticity:	yes	yes

CXCR4, the previously tethered HSCs are released into the circulation. HSCs obtained from bone marrow and blood can reconstitute bone marrow, but there is evidence that some physiological features of HSCs residing in bone marrow differ from those within the circulation. Gene expression analysis, using cDNA microarray technology, has identified nine genes associated with cell cycling expressed at two- to fivefold higher levels in CD34$^+$ cells residing in bone marrow compared with circulating CD34$^+$ cells (25). This raises the question: Is one or the other population more suited to respond to chemokine signals that emanate from injured myocardium by homing to the zone of infarction? This and many other questions remain unanswered; however, cytokine mobilization of stem cells retains its appealing and innovative promise for the initiation of clinical trials involving cell therapy in patients with cardiac disease.

Mesenchymal or stromal cells are a second population of stem cells in bone marrow (Fig. 1). They are a Lin$^-$ CD34 low/- c-kit$^+$ Sca-1$^+$ CD45$^-$ nonhematopoietic cell population in bone marrow (26,27) and are generally considered to be a structural component of bone marrow with little or no ability to enter the circulation. Recent experiments demonstrate their capacity to produce soluble factors important for establishing the bone marrow microenvironment (28) needed for HSC homing and tethering during steady-state conditions (29–31). It is also becoming clear that mesenchymal/stromal stem cells are capable of multilineage differentiation (32). This finding has generated excitement because MSCs appear to avoid detection by the immune system of recipients following transplantation (33). Thus, they are prime candidates for regenerative cell therapy.

MAPCs isolated from mouse bone marrow are a less well-defined bone marrow stem cell subpopulation (34) (Fig. 1). They co-purify with MSCs in the bone marrow mononuclear cell fraction, are CD45$^-$, are TER119$^-$, and display adherence to the surface of culture dishes. When injected into the tail vein of nonirradiated nonobese diabetic/severe combined immunodeficient (NOD/SCID) mice, MAPCs colonized several but not all rapidly renewing epithelial structures. Importantly, they were not detected in the heart and brain. These reported regenerative findings have yet to be confirmed in parallel studies, but it is hoped that the study of MAPCs will contribute substantially to the study of stem cell plasticity.

Endothelial progenitor cells, or angioblasts, derived from bone marrow enter the blood in small numbers and are the immediate precursors for endothelial cells during neovasculogenesis (for review, see ref. 35) (Fig. 1). Their phenotype includes the markers CD34, CD133, and one of the receptors for vascular endothelial growth factor (VEGFR-2) (36,37). Within a few days to a week in culture, EPCs differentiate into

---

Fig. 1. *(Opposite page)* Adult bone marrow is the source of several populations of stem cells. These are rare cells. Estimates indicate that hematopoietic stem cell incidence ranges from 1:10,000 to 1:100,000 and mesenchymal stem cells may be as rare as 1:200,000 bone marrow mononuclear cells. The number of hematopoietic stem cells remains relatively constant in vivo, with little or no capacity to proliferate ex vivo. In contrast, mesenchymal stem cells, multipotent adult progenitor cells, and endothelial progenitor cells proliferate extensively ex vivo. Some of the similarities and differences between mouse and human stem cells within each stem cell population are indicated. Each stem cell population is characterized by its specific surface phenotype and its ability to differentiate into multiple cell types. We thank the publishers for permission to reproduce the photographs of mesenchymal stem cells from Cardiovasc Res 2005;65:334–344 and of multipotent adult progenitor cells from J Clin Invest 2005;25(5):535–537.

mature CD31$^+$ CD144$^+$ endothelial cells that bind acetylated low-density lipoprotein and synthesize nitric oxide. The level of circulating EPCs measured by colony formation in vitro proved to be a strong indicator of endothelial function and, by extension, potential cardiovascular risk among men of average age 50 years *(38)*. Mouse *(39)* and human *(40)* bone marrow-derived EPCs are capable of restoring vasculogenesis in aging and immunodeficient murine recipients, respectively. In addition to the evidence for EPC origin of endothelial cells, several reports suggest that cells positive for the monocytic surface marker CD14 show outgrowth of endothelial cells from clusters grown on fibronectin-coated dishes *(41,42)*.

In summary, HSCs, MSCs, MAPCs, and EPCs are distinct stem/progenitor cell populations in bone marrow. These cell types differ in size, surface markers, and ability to proliferate and differentiate. For these reasons the term "bone marrow stem cell" may be more suitable when referring to findings based on transplants consisting of a mononuclear fraction of bone marrow cells. Reference to HSCs, which may be uniquely committed to hematopoiesis, rather than BMSCs has created considerable confusion among researchers in the nascent field of cellular plasticity.

THE CONTROVERSY: STEM CELL PLASTICITY OR CELL FUSION?

Many studies that report BMSC generation of multiple cell types (Fig. 2), including skeletal myocytes *(43–46)*, hepatocytes *(18)*, epithelium *(47,48)*, neurons *(49,50)*, and cardiomyocytes *(55,56)*, have been criticized recently. Some of the criticism derives from utilizing the Y chromosome as the primary indicator of transdifferentiation. More exacting studies, based on karyotyping and DNA content, have provided in vitro evidence of fusion of male bone marrow mononuclear cells with female-derived embryonic stem cells *(57)*. Individual cells within the clones produced by these fused cells displayed tetraploidy—three X chromosomes and one Y chromosome—and contained a 4 N nuclear content of DNA. Additional studies have demonstrated in vivo cell–cell fusion following transplantation of *Cre* recombinase engineered bone marrow cells into transgenic R26R, β-galactosidase-positive (β-gal$^+$) recipients *(58)*. Cell–cell fusion was observed following *Cre* recombinase excision of the *loxP*-flanked stop cassette in recipient nuclei resulting in expression of the *LacZ* reporter.

Fusion occurred in hepatocytes, neurons, and cardiomyocytes at a frequency of approx 1:1000 cells.

HSCs cannot be cloned, unlike mouse NSCs (mNSCs), and thus cannot be analyzed in vitro for plasticity. When enhanced GFP$^+$ (EGFP$^+$) mNSCs were co-cultured with fresh or paraformaldehyde-fixed human endothelial cells (hECs), the mNSCs were coaxed into adopting a mEC phenotype *(59)*. Cell surface contact was proposed as the mechanism driving transdifferentiation. These findings challenge the theory that no cellular crossover of the embryonic germ layer boundaries occurs in adult tissues and establish the experimental standard needed to achieve acceptance for BMSC plasticity.

DO STEM CELL NICHES EXIST IN MYOCARDIUM?

The existence of cellular niches in the microenvironment of tissues has been extensively studied in bone marrow. Although without compelling evidence, local niches are nevertheless considered the basis for HSC homing to specific sites within bone marrow following their exit from the circulation *(60–63)*. These presumed but poorly

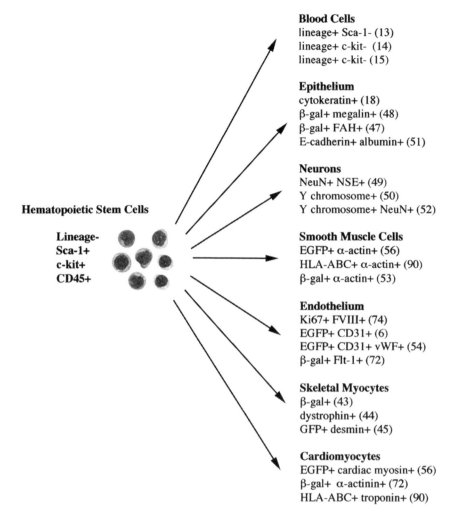

Blood Cells
lineage+ Sca-1- (13)
lineage+ c-kit- (14)
lineage+ c-kit- (15)

Epithelium
cytokeratin+ (18)
β-gal+ megalin+ (48)
β-gal+ FAH+ (47)
E-cadherin+ albumin+ (51)

Neurons
NeuN+ NSE+ (49)
Y chromosome+ (50)
Y chromosome+ NeuN+ (52)

Hematopoietic Stem Cells

Lineage-
Sca-1+
c-kit+
CD45+

Smooth Muscle Cells
EGFP+ α-actin+ (56)
HLA-ABC+ α-actin+ (90)
β-gal+ α-actin+ (53)

Endothelium
Ki67+ FVIII+ (74)
EGFP+ CD31+ (6)
EGFP+ CD31+ vWF+ (54)
β-gal+ Flt-1+ (72)

Skeletal Myocytes
β-gal+ (43)
dystrophin+ (44)
GFP+ desmin+ (45)

Cardiomyocytes
EGFP+ cardiac myosin+ (56)
β-gal+ α-actinin+ (72)
HLA-ABC+ troponin+ (90)

Fig. 2. The most widely studied stem cells in bone marrow are the hematopoietic stem cells. Their role in blood cell formation is well characterized. Of great interest is the recent flurry of papers describing their possible role in the generation of cells outside the hematopoietic system. The claims of hematopoietic stem cell plasticity are based largely on molecular features that the cells acquire during their transdifferentiation into cells of nonmesodermal origin. However, many of the molecular findings that support the concept of hematopoietic stem cell plasticity are being called into question. EGFP, enhanced green fluorescent protein; HLA, human leukocyte antigen; GFP, green fluorescent protein.

defined niches in bone marrow may be the product of secretions from osteoblasts and/or the endosteal cells that form the boundary between bone and bone marrow *(62,63)*. The molecular components of bone marrow niches are believed to provide the appropriate signals needed to anchor stem cells in a milieu conducive for self-renewal and differentiation.

Recent attempts to define microenvironmental niches have been spurred by studies suggesting that BMSCs home to ischemic tissue when they engage in tissue regeneration. Although niches are not well defined within infarcted myocardium, infiltrating or local inflammatory cells, as well as damaged fibroblasts, endothelial cells, mast cells, and even cardiomyocytes may help to establish the myocardial niche by secreting cytokines, chemokines, and angiogenic factors. This hypothesis suggests that neovasculogenesis and myogenesis may occur in the ischemic zone of infarcted myocardium when BMSCs respond to locally secreted β-fibroblast growth factor, VEGF, angiopoietin 1 and 2, interleukin (IL)-1β and -6, and SDF-1 (64–69). One example of early changes in the myocardial microenvironment involves the accumulation of SDF-1 within the zone of infarction induced by ligation of the left anterior descending coronary artery in a rat model. The level of SDF-1 increased within hours and remained high for a week before dropping to preinfarction levels (70). Expression of SDF-1 in ischemic myocardium was found to induce circulating CXCR4+ c-kit+ stem cells to home to the infarction, resulting in improved cardiac function (70). A major difficulty in proposing that vascular endothelial cells, fibroblasts, and especially cardiomyoctes within the zone of infarction participate in niche formation derives from indications that apoptosis is initiated within 30 minutes of the onset of ischemia (71). Exploration of the manner by which constituents of the microenvironment are generated is at a rudimentary stage, but it is likely that real progress in cardiovascular repair will be achieved only when our understanding of the molecular signaling pathways is more complete.

Regardless of our inability to define the composition of stem cell niches in mouse myocardium, it was reported that nonmobilized EGFP+ bone marrow stem cells traffic to the zone of infarction, albeit in small numbers, where they infiltrate the tissue (72). Their numbers increased substantially following daily cytokine therapy with G-CSF and SCF (73), resulting in improved cardiac function. In a nonhuman primate model, cytokine mobilized stem cells homed to the site of myocardial infarctions and provided evidence of neovascularization accompanied by a 26% increase in blood flow in the zone of infarction (74). It is unclear whether the cytokine therapy utilized in these experiments also induced mobilization of stem cells in other organs. G-CSF and/or SCF therapy may trigger mobilization of endogenous cardiac stem cells residing in atrial and/or ventricular myocardium (75) or bone marrow-derived stem cells present in skeletal muscle (76–78).

DOES MYOCARDIUM REGENERATE?

The dogma that defines myocardium as a tissue incapable of self-renewal may no longer be tenable. Several reports now suggest that cardiomyocytes are produced throughout the lifetime of the adult (79,80), but at a low frequency compared with rapidly renewing tissues such as epithelium and bone marrow. However, even a low rate of cardiomyocyte proliferation coupled with an extended cellular half-life may account for a significant level of myocardial renewal during the lifetime of an individual. Although medication is effective in prolonging life in patients with heart disease, there is a strong interest among basic researchers and clinicians to develop a means for repair of injured myocardium. This research is focused on attempts to identify a population of stem cells that would expand the naturally occurring low level of regenerative potential that exists in myocardium. As indicated previously, many believe that myocardial renewing cells can be derived from bone marrow. In addition, skeletal muscle (81) and cardiac tissue (82–87) appear to contain stem cells with a capacity for myocardial regeneration. To date, none of these three sources has emerged as the leading candidate for repair, but BMSCs have been most frequently studied (Table 1).

Table 1
Animal Studies of Myocardial Cell Therapy Using Bone Marrow-Derived Stem Cells[a]

Reference	Cell source	Donor species	Cardiac injury	Follow-up	Outcome
Jackson et al., 2001 (72)	Nonmobilized BM cells	Mouse	LAD ligation	2 and 4 weeks	Cardiomyocyte and endothelial cell regeneration
Orlic et al., 2001 (56)	Lin- c-kit+ BM cells	Mouse	LAD ligation	11 days	Myocardial regeneration, improved LVEDP and LVDP
Orlic et al., 2001 (73)	G-CSF/SCF mobilized BM cells	Mouse	LAD ligation	28 days	Myocardial regeneration, improved LVEF
Kamihata et al., 2001 (88)	BM-derived mononuclear cells	Rat	LAD ligation	3 weeks	Neovascularization, cytokine secretion
Kocher et al., 2001 (89)	Mobilized CD34+ BM cells	Human	LAD ligation	2 and 15 weeks	Vasculogenesis, improved systolic function
Yeh et al., 2003 (90)	Nonmobilized PB CD34+ cells	Human	LAD ligation	2 months	Myocardial regeneration
Norol et al., 2003 (74)	G-CSF/SCF mobilized BM cells	Baboon	CCA ligation	2 months	Angiogenesis, no improvement in LV systolic function
Balsum et al., 2004 (91)	Lin- c-kit+ BM cells	Mouse	LAD ligation	2 and 6 weeks	No myocardial regeneration, improved LVEDD, LVESD, FS
Murry et al., 2004 (92)	Lin- c-kit+ BM cells	Mouse	LAD ligation	2–10 weeks	No myocardial regeneration
Henning et al., 2004 (93)	CB-derived mononuclear cells	Human	LAD ligation	1–4 months	Reduced infarct size, improved LVEF and LV dP/dt
Soukiasian et al., 2004 (94)	B2-microglobulin-BM cells	Rat	Cryoinjury	6 and 8 weeks	Cardiomyocyte regeneration
Zhang et al., 2004 (95)	Nonmobilized PB CD34+ cells	Human	LAD ligation	60 days	Cardiomyocyte and endothelial cell regeneration

(Continued)

Table 1 (*Continued*)

Reference	Cell source	Donor species	Cardiac injury	Follow-up	Outcome
Thompson et al., 2005 (*96*)	Mixed BM-derived Progenitor cells	Rabbit	Cryoinjury	4 weeks	Cardiomyocyte regeneration, improved LVEDP and LV dP/dt
Fukuhara et al., 2005 (*97*)	G-CSF mobilized BM cells	Mice	LAD ligation	4 weeks	Myocytes derived mostly from non-BM sources
Yoshioka et al., 2005 (*98*)	BM CD34+ cells	Monkeys	LAD ligation	2 weeks	No cardiomyocyte regeneration, donor cell secretion of VEGF
Deten et al., 2005 (*99*)	G-CSF/SCF mobilized and iv injected BM cells	Mice	LAD ligation	6 weeks	No cardiac regeneration, LVSP decreased, LVEDP increased
Yoon et al., 2005 (*100*)	Multipotent BM-derived stem cells	Human	LAD ligation	4 weeks	Myocardial regeneration, improved LVEDD, LVESD, FS

[a]Mesenchymal/stromal stem cells, multipotent adult progenitor cells and endothelial progenitor cells are present in adult bone marrow but are not included in this table. BM, bone marrow; LAD, left anterior descending (coronary artery); LVEDP, left ventricle end diastolic pressure; LVDP, left ventricle-developed pressure; G-CSF, granulocyte-colony stimulating factor; SCF, stem cell factor; LVEF, left ventricle ejection fraction; PB, peripheral blood; CCA, circumflex coronary artery; LVEDD, left ventricle end diastolic diameter; LVESD, left ventricle end systolic diameter; FC, fractional shortening; CB, cord blood; LV dP/dt, left ventricle rate of pressure change; VEGF, vascular endothelial growth factor; LVSP, left ventricle systolic pressure.

CAN TRANSPLANTED STEM CELLS REGENERATE MYOCARDIUM?

At 600 beats per minute, the anterior wall of the left ventricle in adult mice is a difficult target for cell transplantation, especially if aiming for the border zone of an infarction. In our experience, of 30 mice injected with a 2.5-μL bolus of EGFP$^+$ Lin$^-$ c-kit$^+$ BMSCs, only 12 displayed tissue regeneration *(56)*. Upon examination by confocal microscopy and immunochemistry, the regenerating EGFP$^+$ cardiomyocytes resembled fetal cardiomyocytes. They expressed Nkx2.5, MEF-2, and GATA-4, transcriptional factors associated with early cardiomyocyte maturation. EGFP$^+$ endothelial cells expressed Ki67, suggesting proliferation and a role in neovascularization. Following stem cell therapy, left ventricular function was improved. In contrast, when the stem cell-depleted Lin$^-$ c-kit$^-$ fraction of bone marrow *(15)* was injected, there was no improvement in cardiac function. Because cardiomyocytes undergo apoptosis soon after exposure to ischemia, and because developing EGFP$^+$ cardiomyocytes averaged 500–2500 μm^3, whereas mature mouse cardiomyocytes average 25,000 μm^3, our findings are consistent with the concept of cardiomyocyte renewal rather than cell fusion.

In subsequent investigations, human CD34$^+$ cells isolated from peripheral blood *(69,90)* or cord blood *(11)* were injected into ischemic myocardium of NOD/SCID mice or nude rats. These studies and those involving a swine model of myocardial infarction *(68)* demonstrated an increase in the number of capillaries lined with human CD34$^+$ endothelial cells and improved regional blood flow. In contrast, several studies failed to achieve cardiomyogenesis or neovasculogenesis in infarcted mouse hearts *(91,92,101)*. In addition, they reported either no evidence of donor cell–cardiomyocyte fusion or cardiomyocyte–donor cell fusion in less than 1:1000 cardiomyocytes counted *(101)*. Of interest, in one experiment *(91)*, although microscopic analysis did not reveal any myocardial regeneration at an early time interval, mice examined at 6 weeks postinfarction demonstrated significantly improved cardiac function. Unfortunately, the basis for the partial recovery was not determined. Since scar tissue is expected to be well formed at 6 weeks post infarction, it is unfortunate that the contractile basis for this improvement was not established.

The controversy arising from these contrasting animal findings may serve to motivate researchers in this field to be more rigorous in experimental design and data reporting. It is clear that to advance research on BMSCs in regenerative medicine, it is incumbent on us to resolve these many issues. This lack of agreement regarding myocardial regeneration, however, has not halted ongoing clinical trials that continue to provide a modest degree of encouragement. Indeed, early data suggested that intracardiac injection of host-derived bone marrow mononuclear cells may provide benefit for patients with heart disease.

CLINICAL TRIALS IN ISCHEMIC HEART DISEASE

Heart disease is a leading cause of death worldwide, with nearly 50% of deaths resulting from ischemic heart disease. Nearly 1.1 million myocardial infarctions occur in the United States alone each year. Myocardial infarction is an irreversible injury that severely affects both men and women. When a coronary artery is occluded, regional systolic function and metabolism decrease suddenly and the affected cardiomyocytes undergo changes, leading to apoptosis within 30 minutes of the onset of ischemia *(71)*. Angioplasty and thrombolytic agents can significantly limit the extent of the infarction by reducing the duration and severity of the perfusion defect and thus improve the prognosis of patients suffering an infarction, but there is no treatment to replace a myocardial scar with healthy contractile tissue. Thus, there is a need to investigate possible regenerative therapies.

Several clinical trials are currently underway in Europe, the Far East, Brazil, and the United States to test the regenerative capacity of autologous bone marrow-derived cells following an acute myocardial infarction. With one exception in which CD133+ cells were injected *(102)*, most trials to date have utilized density gradient separated bone marrow mononuclear cells *(103–113)* consisting of a mixture of primitive hematopoietic, endothelial, and mesenchymal stem cell populations as well as mature monocytes and lymphocytes. The cells were delivered percutaneously to the zone of infarction by a series of transendocardial injections or were infused in a series of pulses into the infarct-related coronary artery using a balloon catheter. These trials were based on results from animal experiments that were not designed to determine the appropriate cell type for transplantation or the optimum number of cells needed to achieve a positive outcome. Likewise, the most efficacious route for cell delivery is still an open question. Several reports indicated a modest degree of short-term (2–4 month) efficacy in regard to reperfusion of the infarcted zone with improved survival of cardiomyocytes distal to the occluded artery. However, critics point to major short-comings of these trials, including the small number of patients enrolled and the fact that the studies, with a single exception thus far, were not randomized or double-blinded. Even stronger criticism is directed at the concept of initiating clinical proto-cols prior to establishing positive outcomes in nonhuman primate studies. However, clinicians conducting trials argue, with considerable justification, that patients with severely damaged heart muscle are in need of novel attempts to improve symptoms and prognosis. They also argue that no adverse effects have been observed to date among the more than 200 patients treated with stem cell therapy.

One clinical trial *(108)* that received considerable attention was designed to sat-isfy some of the objections raised against the earlier trials. Sixty patients were enrolled, with 30 randomly assigned to the control group and 30 to the cell therapy group. All patients received percutaneous coronary intervention with stent implanta-tion prior to entry in the trial and were maintained on medication. Magnetic reso-nance imaging of global left ventricular ejection fraction was designated the primary end point. Autologous bone marrow cells were obtained from the posterior iliac crest within 4–8 days after percutaneous coronary intervention but prior to the onset of fibrous tissue formation. A total of approx 2.5–3.0×10^9 mononuclear cells, including 1.0–1.2×10^7 CD34+ cells, were infused during four or five occlusions of the infarct-related coronary artery via an over-the-wire inflated balloon catheter to prevent retrograde cell migration. Each occlusion lasted 2.5–4 minutes, after which the balloon was deflated and the tissue reperfused for several minutes to prevent mini-infarctions. Six months after treatment, all patients were assayed by scintilla-tion angiography using fluorodeoxyglucose–positron emission tomography. The cell therapy group demonstrated enhanced global and regional contraction and a modest but significant 6% increase in left ventricular ejection fraction from a baseline value of 51 to 57% ($p = 0.0026$). The 30 patients enrolled as control subjects showed a nonsignificant 0.7% increase in left ventricle ejection fraction. No attempt was made to uncover the molecular or cellular mechanisms responsible for this improvement, but it has been suggested that the transplanted cells may have secreted cytokines or chemokines that favored cardiomyocyte recovery from the ischemic episode. Of concern, the heart sizes in diastole were greater in cell therapy-treated patients compared with untreated patients, which is contrary to expectation of a favorable effect on healing of the infarct.

In a follow-up to the early 6-month report on the BOOST trial in which 60 patients were randomized to receive placebo or BM transfer, cardiac MRI was repeated at 18 months after treatment. The significant improvement in mean global LV ejection fraction seen early in the study was no longer apparent at 18 months (3.1% increase in controls vs 5.7% in BM recipients, $p = 0.27$). The authors concluded that a single dose of BM cells infused via the infarct-related coronary artery did not provide long-term improvement in LV systolic function (109). This observation differed substantially from the data obtained in the TOPCARE-AMI trial that demonstrated a continuous rise in LV ejection fraction in a cohort of similarly treated patients assessed at 4, 12, and 24 months after BM cell transfer. Global LV ejection fraction in the BM treated group increased progressively from 47 + 10% to 63 + 10% for a mean increase of 15.8% at 24-month follow-up (110).

A randomized, double blind, placebo-controlled study was recently reported that included 67 patients with ST-elevation acute myocardial infarction (111). Patients received autologous BM cells or placebo by intracoronary transfer within 24 hours following reperfusion therapy. Global LV ejection fraction assessed by MRI at 4 months did not show improvement following BM cell transfer. The increase from 48.5 to 51.8% was comparable to the increase from 46.9 to 49.1% observed in control patients ($p = 0.36$). In contrast, infarct size decreased significantly from 21 to 10 g in recipients of BM cells compared with a reduction from 22 to 15 g in the placebo controls. This 28% treatment effect ($p = 0.036$) may represent a favorable effect on myocardial remodeling. Similarly, findings were obtained when intracoronary transplantation was performed on a small cohort of 18 patients with chronic coronary artery disease (112). Infarct size was reduced by 30% at 3 months following transplantation along with a 15% improvement in global LV ejection fraction and a 57% increase in infarction wall movement velocity.

The infarct-related coronary artery is the most common route for infusing BM cells acutely following an infarction. However, in treating patients with chronic ischemic heart failure an attempt has been made to utilize the transendocardial route for cell delivery (113). This clinical trial followed a study in adult pigs (114), in which transendocardial injections of autologous BM cells resulted in enhanced collateral perfusion. In the clinical study, a cohort of 18 nonrandomized patients received transendocardial transplantation of autologous BM cells using a NOGA catheter. At 4 months, the authors reported an improvement in LV ejection fraction from 20 to 27% ($p = 0.003$) and a significant reduction in end systolic volume ($p = 0.03$).

In addition to clinical trials involving coronary artery or transendocardial infusion of BM stem cells, several papers report the use of subcutaneous injections of G-CSF in order to mobilize BM stem cells. Regardless of whether cytokine treatment was initiated on day 1 or day 5 after acute myocardial infarction there was no detectable influence on LV ejection fraction between the G-CSF group and the placebo group (0.5 vs 2.0%, $p = 0.14$) (115), no reduction in infarct size (6.2 vs 4.9%, $p = 0.56$) (115) and no systolic wall thickening in the infarct area (17 vs 17%, $p = 1.0$) (116) at 4–6 months compared with randomized, double-blind, placebo-controlled patients. It was concluded that G-CSF treatment is safe but fails to produce positive effects in acute myocardial infarction patients. The 4- to 5-day delay in achieving large numbers of mobilized BM CD34+ cells following the onset of G-CSF therapy may in part be responsible for the lack of a positive outcome.

SUMMARY

Since the mid-1990s when reports began to appear suggesting the possibility of regenerating damaged myocardial tissue following coronary artery occlusion or cryoinjury, numerous studies have explored the potential regenerative capacity of embryonic stem cells, fetal stem cells, cardiac stem cells, and adult BMSCs. These early experiments in rodents, dogs, pigs, and nonhuman primates have provided some insight into myocardial regeneration, but much remains obscure. Perhaps the highest priority at this time is the need to precisely identify the cells with the best prospect for tissue regeneration. This has not been accomplished in any of the animal models to date, but once identified it will be possible to study the genetic and cellular regulatory mechanisms involved. There is an urgent need to expand the use of large animal models in regenerative studies. This will enable researchers to determine the optimum time and route of stem cell delivery and establish the number of stem cells required to regenerate a unit volume of infarcted myocardium.

Reports indicating some success in regenerating myocardium in small animal studies have stimulated a desire among clinicians to initiate trials in patients with acute myocardial infarction and ischemic heart failure. Most of these clinical efforts have utilized a mixture of adult bone marrow cells that included several populations of stem cells. These trials have provided modest but encouraging achievements, and, not withstanding all the controversy, it is clear that we are entering an exciting period in cardiovascular medicine. We eagerly await the outcome from long-term randomized trials conducted at multiple clinical centers. If stem cell therapy for regenerative medicine can be widely validated, perhaps one day it will become standard therapy.

ACKNOWLEDGMENT

This research was supported by the Intramural Research Program of the National Heart Lung and Blood Institute, NIH, Bethesda, MD.

REFERENCES

1. Yoder MC, Papaioannou VE, Breitfield PP, et al. Murine yolk sac endoderm- and mesoderm-derived cell lines support in vitro growth and differentiation of hematopoietic cells. Blood 1994;83: 2436–2343.
2. Xu MJ, Tsuji K Ueda T, et al. Stimulation of mouse and human primitive hematopoiesis by murine embryonic aorta-gonad-mesonephros-derived stromal cell lines. Blood 1998;92:2032–2040.
3. Oostendorp RA, Harvet KN, Kusadasi N, et al. Stromal cell lines from mouse aorta-gonad-mesonephros subregions are potent supporters of hematopoietic stem cell activity. Blood 2002;99:1183–1189.
4. Grant MB, May WS, Caballero S, et al. Adult hematopoietic stem cells provide functional hemangioblast activity during retinal neovascularization. Nat Med 2002;8:607–612.
5. Lacaud G, Robertson S, Palis J, et al. Regulation of hemangioblast development. Ann NY Acad Sci 2001;938:96–108.
6. Otani A, Kinder K, Ewalt K, et al. Bone marrow-derived stem cells target retinal astrocytes and can promote or inhibit retinal angiogenesis. Nat Med 2002;8:1004–1010.
7. Ema M, Faloon P, Zhang WJ, et al. Combinatorial effects of Flk1 and Tal1 on vascular and hematopoietic development in the mouse. Genes Dev 2003;17:380–393.
8. Liu YJ, Lu SH, Xu B, et al. Hemangiopoietin, a novel human growth factor for the primitive cells of both hematopoietic and endothelial cell lineages. Blood 2004;103:4449–4456.
9. Cogle CR, Wainman D., Jorgensen ML, et al. Adult human hematopoietic cells provide functional hemangioblast activity. Blood 2004;103:133–135.
10. Wang LS, Li L, Shojaei F, et al. Endothelial and hematopoietic cell fate of human embryonic stem cells originates from primitive endothelium with hemangioblastic properties. Immunity 2004;21:31–41.

11. Botta R, Gao E, Stassi G, et al. Heart infarct in NOD/SCID mice: therapeutic vasculogenesis by transplantation of human CD34(+) cells and low dose CD34(+) KDR(+) cells. FASEB J 2004;18:1392–1394.

12. Bailey AS, Jiang S, Afentoulis M, et al. Transplanted adult hematopoietic stem cells differentiate into endothelial cells. Blood 2004;103:13–19.

13. Spangrude GJ, Heimfeld S, Weissman IL. Purification and characterization of mouse hematopoietic stem cells. Science 1988;241:58–62.

14. Okada S, Nakauchi H, Nagayoshi K, et al. Enrichment and characterization of murine hematopoietic stem cells that express c-kit molecule. Blood 1991;78:1706–1712.

15. Orlic D, Fischer R, Nishikawa S, et al. Purification and characterization of heterogeneous pluripotent hematopoietic stem cell populations expressing high levels of c-kit receptor. Blood 1993;82: 762–770.

16. Zhang CC, Lodish HF. Murine hematopoietic stem cells change their surface phenotype during ex vivo expansion. Blood 2005;105:4314–4320.

17. Iwama A, Oguro H, Negishi M, et al. Enhanced self-renewal of hematopoietic stem cells mediated by the polycomb gene product Bmi-1. Immunity 2004;21:843–851.

18. Krause DS, Theise ND, Collector MI, et al. Multi-organ, multi-lineage engraftment by a single bone marrow-derived stem cell. Cell 2001;105:369–377.

19. Bodine DM, Seidel NE, Gale MS, et al. Efficient retrovirus transduction of mouse pluripotent hematopoietic stem cells mobilized into the peripheral blood by treatment with granulocyte colony-stimulating factor and stem cell factor. Blood 1994;84:1482–1491.

20. Andrews RG, Briddell R., Knitter GH, et al. In vivo synergy between recombinant human stem cell factor and recombinant human granulocyte colony-stimulating factor in baboons enhanced circulation of progenitor cells. Blood 1994;84:800–810.

21. Pettit I, Szyper-Kravitz M, Nagler A, et al. G-CSF induces stem cell mobilization by decreasing bone marrow SDF-1 and up-regulating CXCR4. Nat Immunol 2002;3:687–694.

22. Levesque JP, Hendy J, Takamatsu Y, et al. Disruption of the CXCR4/CXCL12 chemotactic interaction during hematopoietic stem cell mobilization induced by GCSF or cyclophosphamide. J Clin Invest 2003;111:187–196.

23. Carstanjen D, Ulbricht N, Iacone A, et al. Matrix metalloproteinase-9 (gelatinase B) is elevated during mobilization of peripheral blood progenitor cells by G-CSF. Transfusion 2002;42:588–596.

24. Heissig B, Hattori K, Dias S, et al. Recruitment of stem and progenitor cells from the bone marrow niche requires mmp-9 mediated release of kit-ligand. Cell 2002;109:625–637.

25. Steidl U, Kronenwett R, Rohr U-P, et al. Gene expression profiling identifies significant differences between the molecular phenotypes of bone marrow-derived and circulating human CD34+ hematopoietic stem cells. Blood 2002;99:2037–2044.

26. Pittenger MF, Martin BJ. Mesenchymal stem cells and their potential as cardiac therapeutics [a review]. Circ Res 2004;95:9–20.

27. Gojo S, Gojo N, Takeda Y, et al. In vivo cardiovasculogenesis by direct injection of isolated adult mesenchymal stem cells. Exp Cell Res 2003;288:51–59.

28. Kinnaird T, Stabile E, Burnett MS, et al. Local delivery of marrow-derived stromal cells augments collateral perfusion through paracrine mechanisms. Circulation 2004;109:1543–1549.

29. Peled A, Grabovsky V, Habler L, et al. The chemokine SDF-1 stimulates integrin-mediated arrest of CD34(+) cells on vascular endothelium under shear flow. J Clin Invest 1999;104:1199–1211.

30. Mohle R, Bautz F, Rafii S, et al. The chemokine receptor CXCR-4 is expressed on CD34+ hematopoietic progenitors and leukemic cells and mediates transendothelial migration induced by stromal cell-derived factor-1. Blood 1998;91:4523–4530.

31. Kollet O, Spiegel A, Peled A, et al. Rapid and efficient homing of human CD34(+)CD38(-/low)CXCR4(+) stem and progenitor cells to the bone marrow and spleen of NOD/SCID and NOD/SCID/B2m(null) mice. Blood 2001;97:3283–3291.

32. Prockop DJ. Marrow stromal cells as stem cells for nonhematopoietic tissues. Science 1997;276:71–74.

33. Mahmud N, Pang W, Cobbs C, et al. Studies of the route of administration and role of conditioning with radiation on unrelated allogeneic mismatched mesenchymal stem cell engraftment in a nonhuman primate model. Exp Hematol 2004;32:494–501.

34. Jiang Y, Jahagirdar BN, Reinhardt RL, et al. Pluripotency of mesenchymal stem cells derived from adult marrow. Nature 2002;418:41–49.

35. Cannon RO. Cardiovascular potential of BM-derived stem and progenitor cells. Cytotherapy 2004;602–607.

36. Asahara T, Murohara T, Sullivan A, et al. Isolation of putative progenitor endothelial cells for angiogenesis. Science 1997;275:964–967.

37. Peichev M, Naiyer AJ, Pereira D, et al. Expression of VEGFR-2 and AC133 by circulating CD34+ cells identifies a population of functional endothelial precursors. Blood 2000;95:952–958.
38. Hill JM, Zalos G, Halcox JP, et al. Circulating endothelial progenitor cells, vascular function, and cardiovascular risk. N Engl J Med 2003;348:593–600.
39. Edelberg JM, Tang L, Hattori K, et al. Young adult bone marrow-derived endothelial precursor cells restore aging-impaired cardiac angiogenic function. Circ Res 2002;90:E89–93.
40. Kocher AA, Schuster MD, Szabolcs MJ, et al. Neovascularization of ischemic myocardium by human bone-marrow-derived angioblasts prevents cardiomyocyte apoptosis, reduces remodeling and improves cardiac function. Nat Med 2001;7:430–436.
41. Rehman J, Li J, Orschell CM, March KL. Peripheral blood endothelial progenitor cells are derived from monocyte/macrophages and secrete angiogenic growth factors. Circulation 2003;107: h1164–1169.
42. Urbich C, Heeschen C Aicher A, et al. Relevance of monocytic features for neovascularization capacity of circulating endothelial progenitor cells. Circulation 2003;108:2511–2516.
43. Ferrari G, Cusella-DeAngelis G, Colletta M, et al. Muscle regeneration by bone marrow-derived myogenic progenitors. Science 1998;279:1528–1530.
44. Gussoni E, Soneoka Y, Strickland CD, et al. Dystrophin expression in the mdx mouse restored by stem cell transplantation. Nature 1999;401:390–394.
45. LaBarge MA, Blau HM. Biological progression from adult bone marrow to mononucleate muscle stem cell to multinucleate muscle fiber in response to injury. Cell 2002;111:589–601.
46. Doyonnas R, LaBarge MA, Sacco A, et al. Hematopoietic contribution to skeletal muscle regeneration by myelomonocytic precursors. Proc Natl Acad Sci USA 2004;101:13,507–13,512.
47. Lagasse E, Connors H, Al Dhalimy M, et al. Purified hematopoietic stem cells can differentiate into hepatocytes in vivo. Nat Med 2000;6:1229–1234.
48. Kale S, Karihaloo A, Clark PR, et al. Bone marrow stem cells contribute to repair of the ischemically injured renal tubule. J Clin Invest 2003;112:42–49.
49. Mezey E, Chandross KJ, Harta G, et al. Turning blood into brain: cells bearing neuronal antigens generated in vivo from bone marrow. Science 2000;290:1779–1782.
50. Weimann JM, Charlton CA, Brazelton TR, et al. Contribution of transplanted bone marrow cells to Purkinje neurons in human adult brains. Proc Natl Acad Sci USA 2003;100:2088–2093.
51. Jang Y-Y, Collector MI, Baylin SB, et al. Hematopoietic stem cells convert into liver cells within days without fusion. Nat Cell Biol 2004;6:532–539.
52. Mezey E, Key S, Vogelsang G, et al. Transplanted bone marrow generates new neurons in human brains. Proc Natl Acad Sci 2003;100:1364–1369.
53. Sata M, Saiura A, Kunisato A, et al. Hematopoietic stem cells differentiate into vascular cells that participate in the pathogenesis of atherosclerosis. Nat Med 2002;8:403–409.
54. Bailey AS, Jiang S, Afentoulis, et al. Transplanted adult hematopoietic stem cells differentiate into functional endothelial cells. Blood 2004;103:13–19.
55. Tomita S, Li R-K, Weisel RD, et al. Autologous transplantation of bone marrow cells improves damaged heart function. Circulation 1999;100(suppl II);247–256.
56. Orlic D, Kajstura J, Chimenti S, et al. Bone marrow cells regenerate infarcted myocardium. Nature 2001;410:701–705.
57. Terada N, Hamazaki T, Oka M, et al. Bone marrow cells adopt the phenotype of other cells by spontaneous cell fusion. Nature 2002;416:542–545.
58. Alvares-Dolado M, Pardal R, Garcia-Verdugo JM, et al. Fusion of bone marrow-derived cells with Purkinje neurons, cardiomyocytes and hepatocytes. Nature 2003;425:968–973.
59. Wurmser AE, Nakashima K, Summers RG, et al. Cell fusion-independent differentiation of neural stem cells to the endothelial lineage. Nature 2004;430:350–356.
60. Papayannopoulou T, Craddock C, Nakamoto B, et al. The VLA4/VCAM-1 adhesion pathway defines contrasting mechanisms of lodgement of transplanted murine hemopoietic progenitors between bone marrow and spleen. Proc Natl Acad Sci USA 1995;92:9647–9651.
61. Simmons PJ, Masinovsky B, Longenecker BM, et al. Vascular cell adhesion molecule-1 expressed by bone marrow stromal cells mediates the binding of hematopoietic progenitor cells. Blood 1992;80:388–595.
62. Zhang J, Niu C, Ye L, et al. Identification of the haematopoietic stem cell niche and control of the niche size. Nature 2003;423:302–305.
63. Calvi LM, Adams GB, Weilbrecht KW, et al. Osteoblastic cells regulate the haematopoietic stem cell niche. Nature 2003;425:841–846.

64. Hiasa K, Ishibashi M, Ohtani K, et al. Gene transfer of stromal cell-derived factor-1alpha enhances ischemic vasculogenesis and angiogenesis via vascular endothelial growth factor/endothelial nitric oxide synthase-related pathway: next-generation chemokine therapy for therapeutic neovascularization. Circulation 2004;109:2454–2461.

65. Deten A, Volz HC, Briest W, Zimmer. Cardiac cytokine expression is upregulated in the acute phase after myocardial infarction. Experimental study in rats. Cardiovasc Res 2002;55:329–340.

66. Matsunaga T, Warltier DC, Tessmer J, et al. Expression of VEGF, angiopoietins-1 and -2 during ischemia-induced coronary angiogenesis. Am J Physiol Heart Circ Physiol 2003;285:H352–358.

67. Matsumura G, Miyagawa-Tomita S, Shin'oka T, et al. First evidence that bone marrow cells contribute to the construction of tissue-engineered vascular autografts in vivo. Circulation 2003;108:1729–1734.

68. Kamihata H, Matsubara H, Nishiue T, et al. Implantation of bone marrow mononuclear cells into ischemic myocardium enhances collateral perfusion and regional function via side supply of angioblasts, angiogenic ligands, and cytokines. Circulation 2001;104(9):1046–1052.

69. Kawamoto A, Tkebuchava T, Yamaguchi J-I, et al. Intramyocardial transplantation of autologous endothelial progenitor cells for therapeutic neovascularization of myocardial ischemia. Circulation 2003;107:461–470.

70. Askari AT, Unzek S, Popovic ZB, et al. Effect of stromal-cell-derived factor 1 on stem-cell homing and tissue regeneration in ischaemic cardiomyopathy. Lancet 2003;362:697–703.

71. Heyndrickx GR, Baig H, Nellens P, et al. Depression of regional blood flow and wall thickening after brief coronary occlusions. Am J Physiol 1978;234:H653–659.

72. Jackson KA, Majka SM, Wang H, et al. Regeneration of ischemic cardiac muscle and vascular endothelium by adult stem cells. J Clin Invest 2001;107:1395–1402.

73. Orlic D, Kajstura J, Chimenti S, et al. Mobilized bone marrow cells repair the infarcted heart, improving function and survival. Proc Natl Acad Sci USA 2001;98:10,344–10,349.

74. Norol F, Merlet P, Isnard R, et al. Influence of mobilized stem cells on myocardial infarct repair in a nonhuman primate model. Blood 2003;102:4361–4368.

75. Beltrami AP, Barlucchi L, Torella D, et al. Adult cardiac stem cells are multipotent and support myocardial regeneration. Cell 2003;114:763–776.

76. Kawada H, Ogawa M. Bone marrow origin of hematopoietic progenitors and stem cells in murine muscle. Blood 2001;98:2008–2013.

77. Issarachai S, Priestley GV, Nakamoto B, Papayannopoulou T. Cells with hemopoietic potential residing in muscle are itinerant bone marrow-derived cells. Exp Hematol 2002;30:366–373.

78. McKinney-Freeman SL, Jackson KA, et al. Muscle-derived hematopoietic stem cells are hematopoietic in origin. Proc Natl Acad Sci USA 2002;99:1341–1346.

79. Kajstura J, Leri A, Finato N, et al. Myocyte proliferation in end-stage cardiac failure in humans. Proc Natl Acad Sci USA 1998;95:8801–8805.

80. Beltrami AP, Urbanek K, Kajstura J, et al. Evidence that human cardiac myocytes divide after myocardial infarction. N Engl J Med 2001;344:1750–1757.

81. Winitsky SO, Gopal TV, Hassanzadeh S, et al. Adult murine skeletal muscle contains cells that can differentiate into beating cardiomyocytes in vitro. PLoS 2005;3:e87.

82. Hierlihy AM, Seale P, Lobe CG, et al. The post-natal heart contains a myocardial stem cell population. FEBS Letters 2002;530:239–243.

83. Urbanek K, Quaini F, Tasca G, et al. Intense myocyte formation from cardiac stem cells in human cardiac hypertrophy. Proc Natl Acad Sci 2003;100:10,440–10,445.

84. Oh H, Bradfute SB, Gallardo TD, et al. Cardiac progenitor cells from adult myocardium: homing, differentiation, and fusion after infarction. Proc Natl Acad Sci USA 2003;100:12,313–12,318.

85. Matsuura K, Nagai T, Nishigaki N, et al. Adult cardiac Sca-1 positive cells differentiate into beating cardiomyocytes. J Biol Chem 2004;79:11,384–11,391.

86. Torella D, Rota M, Nurzynska D, et al. Cardiac stem cell and myocyte aging, heart failure, and insulin-like growth factor-1 overexpression. Circ Res 2004;94:514–524.

87. Messina E, De Angelis L, Frati G, et al. Isolation and expansion of adult cardiac stem cells from human and murine heart. Circ Res 2004;95:911–921.

88. Kamihata H, Matsubara H, Nishiue T, et al. Implantation of bone marrow mononuclear cells into ischemic myocardium enhances collateral perfusion and regional function via side supply of angioblasts, angiogenic ligands, and cytokines. Circulation 2001;104(9):1046–1052.

89. Kocher AA, Schuster MD, Szabolcs MJ, et al. Neovascularization of ischemic myocardium by human bone-marrow-derived angioblasts prevents cardiomyocyte apoptosis, reduces remodeling and improves cardiac function. Nat Med 2001;7:430–436.

90. Yeh ET, Zhang S, Wu HD, Korbling M, et al. Transdifferentiation of human peripheral blood CD34+-enriched cell population into cardiomyocytes, endothelial cells, and smooth muscle cells in vivo. Circulation 2003;108:2070–2073.

91. Balsam LB, Wagers AJ, Christensen JL, et al. Haematopoietic stem cells adopt mature haematopoietic fates in ischaemic myocardium. Nature 2004;428:668–673.

92. Murry CE, Soonpaa MH, Reinecke H, et al. Haematopoietic stem cells do not transdifferentiate into cardiac myocytes in myocardial infarcts. Nature 2004;428:664–668.

93. Henning RJ, Abu-Ali H, Balis JU, et al. Human umbilical cord blood mononuclear cells for the treatment of acute myocardial infarction. Cell Transplant 2004;13:729–739.

94. Soukiasian HJ, Czer LSC, Avital I, et al. A novel sub-population of bone marrow-derived myocardial stem cells: Potential autologous cell therapy in myocardial infarction. J Heart Lung Transplant 2004;23:873–880.

95. Zhang S, Wang D, Estrov Z, et al. Both cell fusion and transdifferentiation account for the transformation of human peripheral blood CD34-positive cells into cardiomyocytes in vivo. Circulation 2004;110:3803–3807.

96. Thompson RB, van den Bos EJ, Davis BH, et al. Intracardiac transplantation of a mixed population of bone marrow cells improves both regional systolic contractility and diastolic relaxation. J Heart Lung Transplant 2005;24:205–214.

97. Fukuhara S, Tomita S, Nakatani T, et al. Endogenous bone marrow-derived stem cells contribute only a small proportion of regenerated myocardium in the acute infarction model. J Heart Lung Transplant 2005;24:67–72.

98. Yoshioka T, Ageyama N, Shibata H, et al. Repair of infarcted myocardium mediated by transplanted bone marrow-derived CD34+ stem cells in a nonhuman primate model. Stem Cells 2005;23:355–364.

99. Deten A, Volz HC, Clamors S, et al. Hematopoietic stem cells do not repair the infarcted mouse heart. Cardiovasc Res 2005;65:52–63.

100. Yoon Y-S, Wecker A, Heyd L, et al. Clonally expanded novel multipotent stem cells from human bone marrow regenerate myocardium after myocardial infarction. J Clin Invest 2005;115:326–338.

101. Nygren JM, Jovinge S, Breitbach M, et al. Bone marrow-derived hematopoietic cells generate cardiomyocytes at a low frequency through cell fusion, but not transdifferentiation. Nat Med 2004;10:494–501.

102. Stamm C, Westphal B, Kleine HD, et al. Autologous bone-marrow stem-cell transplantation for myocardial regeneration. Lancet 2003;361:45, 46.

103. Strauer BE, Brehm M, Zeus T, et al. Repair of infarcted myocardium by autologous intracoronary mononuclear bone marrow cell transplantation in humans. Circulation 2002;106:1913–1918.

104. Assmus B, Schachinger V, Teupe C, et al. Transplantation of progenitor cells and regeneration enhancement in acute myocardial infarction (TOPCARE-AMI). Circulation 2002;106:3009–3017.

105. Tse HF, Kwong YL, Chan JK, Lo G, et al. Angiogenesis in ischaemic myocardium by intramyocardial autologous bone marrow mononuclear cell implantation. Lancet 2003;361:47–49.

106. Perin EC, Dohmann HF, Borojevic R, et al. Transendocardial, autologous bone marrow cell transplantation for severe, chronic ischemic heart failure. Circulation 2003;107:2294–2302.

107. Fernandez-Aviles F, Roman JAS, Garcia-Frade J, et al. Experimental and clinical regenerative capability of human bone marow cells after myocardial infarction. Circ Res 2004;95:742–748.

108. Wollert KC, Meyer GP, Lotz J, et al. Intracoronary autologous bone-marrow cell transfer after myocardial infarction: the BOOST randomised controlled clinical trial. Lancet 2004;364:141–148.

109. Meyer GP, Wollert KC, Lotz J, et al. Intracoronary bone marrow cell transfer after myocardial infarction. Circulation 2006;113:1287–1294.

110. Britten MB, Assmus B, Abolmaali ND, et al. Preserved functional improvement and evidence for reverse ventricular remodeling 2 years after intracoronary progenitor cell therapy in patients with acute myocardial infarction. Circulation 2005;112(17):Supplement II-632.

111. Janssens S, Dubois C, Bogaert J, et al. Autologous bone marrow-derived stem cell transfer in patients with ST-segment elevation myocardial infarction:double-blind, randomized controlled trial. Lancet 2006;367:113–121.

112. Strauer BE, Brehm M, Zeus T, et al. Regeneration of human infarcted heart muscle by intracoronary autologous bone marrow cell transplantation in chronic coronary artery disease. J Am Coll Cardiol 2005;46:1651–1658.

113. Perin EC, Dohmann HFR, Borojevic R, et al. Transendocardial, autologous bone marrow cell transplantation for severe, chronic ischemic heart failure. Circulation 2003;107:2294–2302.

114. Fuchs S, Baffour R, Zhou YF, et al. Transendocardial delivery of autologous bone marrow enhances collateral perfusion and regional function in pigs with chronic experimental ischemia. J Am Coll Cardiol 2001;37:1726–1732.
115. Zohlnhofer D, Ott I, Mehilli J, et al. Stem cell mobilization by granulocyte colony-stimulating factor in patients with acute myocardial infarction. JAMA 2006;295:1003–1010.
116. Ripa RS, Jorgensen E, Wang Y, et al. Stem cell mobilization induced by subcutaneous granulocyte colony-stimulating factor to improve cardiac regeneration after acute ST-elevation myocardial infarction. Circulation 2006;113:1983–1992.

3

Mesenchymal Stem Cells for Cardiac Therapy

Mark F. Pittenger, PhD

SUMMARY

Mesenchymal stem cells (MSCs) are multipotential cells that can be isolated from a number of tissues but are readily isolated from bone marrow. These cells grow in culture as attached fibroblastic cells that expand readily in culture but maintain their contact inhibition as they reach confluence. Flow cytometry analysis of surface markers on MSCs shows that the cultured cells are very homogeneous, and differentiation assays indicate their potential to differentiate into a variety of cell types. Numerous experiments have demonstrated that these multipotential cells are not rejected by the immune system and therefore it may be possible to use the MSCs from one donor in multiple recipients. Additionally, these remarkable cells, found in all individuals, have the natural ability to migrate to sites of injury in the body, a finding the meaning of which is only beginning to be understood. Cardiac injury results in the loss of cardiomyocytes and reduced heart function. Cardiomyoplasty with MSCs is seen as a way to augment the myocardium with multipotential cells that may aid in repairing the heart and improving function. Animal studies have supported this approach, and human clinical trials have now begun.

Key Words: Cardiomyoplasty; cardiac myocytes; cell differentiation; immune rejection.

INTRODUCTION

The mammalian heart develops early in embryogenesis and is easily discernable by its rhythmic contractions, which become more rhythmic and stronger over time as new cells are added. The stem or progenitor cells that form the heart are derived from the primary mesenchyme, but it is an ongoing question as to how many cells may also migrate to the nascent heart from the secondary or head mesenchyme during early development and undergo differentiation in response to signals in the cardiogenic field. Similarly, the degree to which cellular apoptosis and morphogenesis modify the original population of heart forming cells remains to be further understood. Like all of early development, heart embryogenesis is a balance of the expansion of stem and progenitor cells and cell death.

It was thought by most scientists that after birth the heart only grew by hypertrophy—that there was no new genesis of cardiomyocytes and that, subsequently, repair processes are very limited in the heart. This may be largely correct because the heart, once damaged, does not repair very well and heart disease remains the number one

From: *Contemporary Cardiology: Stem Cells and Myocardial Regeneration*
Edited by: M. S. Penn © Humana Press Inc., Totowa, NJ

cause of death in the Western world. However, new findings about the nature of cells derived from heart tissue continue to add to our collective understanding of the heart and the potential repair processes in the body (e.g., *see* Chapter 7). Because of the recognized need for new cells that would form new tissue and repair the heart, cardiomyoplasty is envisioned as a potential therapeutic process to add necessary cells to the damaged heart *(1,2)*. With that premise, a major question becomes determining which cells can be isolated in sufficient numbers and engrafted in the damaged heart to provide a lasting physiological benefit. Recently, a number of laboratories have identified evidence that several types of progenitor cells or stem cells engrafting in the damaged heart may undergo varying degrees of differentiation and can modify the remodeling that occurs in the injured heart. Among these are the mesenchymal stem cells (MSCs) discussed in this chapter, the skeletal myoblasts *(3,4)*, side population cells *(5,6)*, endothelial progenitor cells *(7–9)*, c-kit$^+$ progenitor cells *(10,11)*, Sca-1$^+$ progenitor cells *(12)*, and perhaps one or two others. The relationships between these different stem and progenitor cells are not yet clear because no unique surface markers for the cells are under investigation. This is true for many stem cells; they express small amounts of many different surface markers, whereas differentiated cell types tend to make larger amounts of more specific surface molecules. Studies with skeletal myoblasts have been begun, and this approach has progressed to the phase II clinical testing stage (*see* Chapter 18). Endothelial progenitors are similarly undergoing testing (*see* Chapter 17). MSCs have been characterized and their biology studied for many years, and they are the focus of this chapter. MSCs have many characteristics that make them ideal for developing cellular therapeutics. They are undergoing clinical testing in the cancer transplantation field and entered phase I testing in patients with acute myocardial infarction (MI) in Spring 2005.

MESENCHYMAL STEM CELLS

MSCs were examined in a number of fields before they were introduced into cardiac research. Understanding some of this background will give the reader an appreciation for the cross-discipline nature of current stem cell research. MSCs have been isolated and characterized in a number of laboratories, the original work focusing on the osteochondral differentiation of these cells and their potential to repair bone and cartilage.

Certain early studies will not be examined here because of space considerations. These include studies of bone marrow transfer to ectopic sites, where subsequent histological analysis revealed unexpected tissue formation; starting in the mid-1960s, the first studies to isolate and culture bone marrow-derived osteoprogenitor cells were the work of Alexander Friedenstein of the Gamaleya Institute in Moscow. Bone marrow was taken from guinea pigs and later rabbits and placed in culture dishes in nutrient medium. The cells that attached to the substrate and grew in culture were then reimplanted into ectopic sites. Histology later revealed the presence of bone and cartilage at these sites *(13)*. That the cultured cells were participating in the new tissue formation rather than inducing endogenous cells to differentiate became apparent through further studies. Study of these connective tissue stem cells continued in the 1980s and 1990s by Owens and several other groups *(14–16*; *see* reviews in refs. *17,18,22–24)*, but was perhaps overshadowed by the rapid developments in studies of hematopoietic stem cells (HSCs) and their life-saving therapeutic use. Interestingly, HSCs were difficult to culture ex vivo and required a "stromal cell feeder layer" that contained MSCs as well as other cell types. Hence, many researchers continue to refer to MSCs as marrow stromal cells, although the culture, characterization, and understanding of MSCs have been significantly refined. Human MSCs (hMSCs) were first isolated by Arnold Caplan and colleagues at Case Western Reserve University from small bone marrow samples drawn through the skin under local anesthetic (19,20). A key step was using a tour de force approach for selecting optimal lots of fetal bovine serum (FBS) that included placing the cultured cells on ceramic carriers and implanting the cells/carriers in athymic mice for several weeks to allow in vivo differentiation (21). The histological examination of the retrieved carriers for the presence of differentiated cell types (bone, cartilage, etc.) indicated the optimal lots of FBS that allowed cell expansion and also preserved the multipotential nature of the hMSCs during in vitro culture. The selection of optimal lots of FBS still offers advantages, although now that the growth and cell characteristics of MSCs are better understood, the serum-selection process is not always performed by the MSC investigator. Space does not allow for a detailed review of the contributions to the field of MSC research from many groups, but the above-mentioned reviews are informative.

STEM VS PROGENITOR CELLS

The ability of multipotential cells to differentiate to several cell types under the appropriate conditions raises the question of whether they should be termed progenitor cells or can be properly called stem cells. With the fertilized egg as the ultimate stem cell, followed by the embryonic stem cell and the embryonic germ cell, how many different stem and progenitor cells persist in the adult remains under investigation. In the adult there are a number of tissues that certainly harbor stem cells, most notably the HSCs found in bone marrow, the epithelial stem cells of the intestinal crypts, and dermal stem cells of skin; others include the neural stem cells of the subventricular zone. The HSC is certainly the best described among these stem cells. In the bone marrow, about 1 in 1000 nucleated cells is a HSC, capable of producing all the myeloid and lymphoid cell lineages. HSCs can be isolated but grow poorly in the laboratory. For clinical use, they are usually mobilized in situ by the administration of a growth factor, granulocyte–colony-stimulating factor (G-CSF), and then collected from the peripheral blood. As to the number of MSCs in bone marrow, they are less common than HSCs. Plating studies that examine colony formation from single cells suggest the MSCs are present at a rate of 1 in 10,000–100,000, diminishing as one ages. Although rare, once placed in culture and given room to expand, MSCs expand readily manyfold, with a single cell giving rise to 1 million in about 3 weeks (25). The MSCs remain "contact inhibited," and as they approach confluence the cells slow and stop dividing, remaining quiescent for long periods; perhaps this is why the MSCs are not abundant in vivo. Their controlled expansion capacity is one of the positive attributes of MSCs for developing cellular therapy methods because, after many years of experience, they do not appear to grow in vivo to cause tumors. The expanded MSCs can be tested for homogeneity, sterility, and cellular potency, and in vitro assays are available to show progression to several different lineages. The in vitro differentiation assays are particularly good for osteogenic, adipogenic, and chondrogenic differentiation (see Fig.1), producing full differentiation with mature tissue-like attributes (25). Implantation studies or other assays produce MSCs with characteristics of muscle cells, and even characteristics of nonmesenchymal lineages, as differentiation to lung epithelium or neural gene expression can be demonstrated (26–28). It is this multilineage potential of these

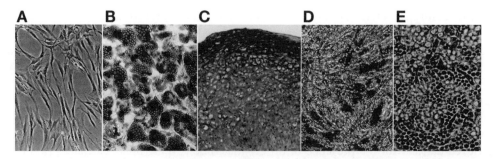

Fig. 1. Mesenchymal stem cells (MSCs) growing in culture **(A)** can be induced to differentiate to the adipogenic lineage **(B)** with the accumulation of lipid vacuoles stained with oil red O. **(C)** Chondrogenic lineage with the expression of collagen type II stained brown. **(D)** Osteogenic lineage with the expression of alkaline phosphatase (stained red) and the accumulation of supracellular calcium nodules (stained black with silver). **(E)** MSCs can form a feeder layer underneath the hematopoietic stem cells that show a characteristic cobblestone appearance. (*See* color insert following p. 114.)

cultured cells that led to their being called mesenchymal stem cells. Some scientists suggest "mesenchymal progenitor cell" is more accurate than stem cell, reserving stem cell for only the very few cells that can be proven to grow indefinitely and differentiate to all appropriate lineages. However, in order to understand the biology and signaling of cellular ontogeny and to increase the potential avenues for the development of cellular therapies for the repair of damaged tissues, the stem cell and cellular therapy fields embrace the terms progenitor and stem cell alike.

MSCs PRODUCE GROWTH FACTORS AND CYTOKINES

MSCs are also studied for their ability to supply a stromal function and support hematopoietic stem cells. Indeed, the MSCs produce an important array of growth factors and cytokines, including macrophage–, granulocyte–, and granulocyte macrophage–colony-stimulating factors (M-, G-, and GM-CSF), stem cell factor-1, leukemia inhibitory factor, stromal cell-derived factor-1, Flt-3 ligand, and interleukins (IL)-1, 6, 7, 8, 11, 14, and 15 *(29,30)*. MSCs have been shown to produce a useful feeder layer for the ex vivo expansion of HSCs *(31)*. Recently, human MSCs were also shown to support human embryonic stem (ES) cells, thereby providing for an all-human culture system allowing for the production of ES cells for therapeutic use without the concerns of xenobiotic transfer of viruses that prohibit the use of human ES cells grown on mouse feeder layers, such as is the case for the original ES cell lines approved for study *(32)*.

Because of their ability to support HSCs, the first clinical testing of MSCs involved their ability to aid engraftment in oncology patients receiving bone marrow transplantation. The phase I study results were recently published *(33)*, but the follow-up phase II study of MSCs in bone marrow transplantation (BMT) was modified to reflect new research and clinical results suggesting that the greater value to the BMT recipient may be that the MSCs can modulate the immune response in the allogeneic recipients. Therefore, the phase II trial will evaluate MSC treatment of graft-vs-host (GVH) disease, a life-threatening complication associated with many allogeneic BMT procedures.

MSCs MODULATE THE ALLOGENEIC IMMUNE RESPONSE

In vitro studies examined the interaction of MSCs with allogeneic T-cells in experiments that were designed to test the ability of MSCs to present antigen to T-cells

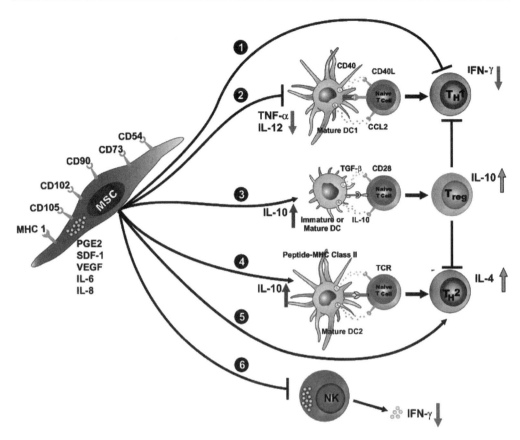

Fig. 2. Mesenchymal stem cells (MSCs) mediate their immuno-modulatory effects by interacting with cells from both the innate (dendritic cells [DCs], pathways 2–4; natural killer [NK] cells, pathway 6) and adaptive immunity systems (T-cell pathways 1 and 5). MSC inhibition of tumor necrosis factor (TNF)-α secretion and promotion of interleukin (IL)-10 secretion may affect DC maturation state and functional properties, resulting in skewing the immune response toward in an anti-inflammatory/tolerant phenotype. Alternatively, when MSCs are present in an inflammatory microenvironment, they inhibit interferon (IFN)-γ secretion from T-helper (T_H)1 and NK cells and increase IL-4 secretion from T_H2 cells, thereby promoting a T_H1→T_H2 shift. It is likely that MSCs also mediate their immuno-modulatory actions by direct cell–cell contact by secreted factors. Several MSC cell surface molecules and secreted molecules are depicted. (From ref. *39*.)

(34). It became apparent that allogeneic immune cells (T-cells) were not stimulated and would not proliferate when MSCs were present in the standard mixed lymphocyte reaction, yet also that MSCs at low numbers could produce cytokines to maintain support of T-cells *(34–39)*. The nonresponding T-cells were not apoptotic or impaired, because they could be isolated and responded to other stimuli. These studies also attempted to define the mechanism associated with the lack of T-cell response to allogeneic MSCs. Our recent studies *(39)* continued that quest and tested the response of human MSCs to isolated subpopulations of immune cells (isolated populations of T helper-1 [T_H1], T_H2, T-regulatory, matured dendritic cells [DC]-1 and -2, and natural killer [NK] cells). The results indicate that MSCs interact with each of these types of immune cells to alter their cytokine production such that pro-inflammatory DC-1 decrease secretion of tumor necrosis factor (TNF)-α and anti-inflammatory DC-2 increase IL-10 secretion; MSCs caused pro-inflammatory T_H1 cells to decrease secretion

of interferon (IFN)-γ and caused anti-inflammatory T_H2 cells to increase secretion of IL-4; MSCs caused an increase of T_{Reg} cells and the associated secretion of IL-10. Finally, MSCs caused decreased expression of inflammatory IFN-γ from NK cells (40). Overall, the results indicate that MSCs, if present in the appropriate amounts, can modify the immune response to decrease the inflammatory response and create a more "tolerogenic" environment (see Fig. 2). Such a response may serve to limit rejection or GVH disease in the transplant setting and may have useful effects in autoimmune diseases. A recent review offers greater insight into the properties and uses of allogeneic MSCs (40).

OTHER MSC-LIKE CELLS

In recent years, several populations of stem and progenitor cells have been isolated and characterized from bone marrow and other tissue sources that are similar to MSCs, but some of these may have additional properties, so scientists continue to evaluate which cell type may be better for regeneration studies in different tissues. To date, most of these other MSC-like cells are not as far along and not as much data is available as for MSCs. These include the mesenchymal adult progenitor cells (MAPCs) (41–43), the rapidly cycling stromal cells (RS-1) (44), and the adipose-derived adipose progenitor cells (APCs) (45,46) and pluripotent liposuction aspirate-derived cells (PLAs) (47,48). The MAPCs have generated much interest because published work indicates that these cells can differentiate to endodermal-derived and ectodermal-derived tissues as well as mesodermal tissues. Hence, the MAPCs may have a differentiation potential that rivals the ES cells if the process can be understood and consistently reproduced. The relationship of MAPCs, RS-1, APCs, and PLAs to MSCs is not clear, but the cell populations have many overlapping characteristics (see Table 1). Attempts to directly compare these cell populations in one laboratory, assuring the same methods are applied to each population, gave very similar results, suggesting few differences (49).

It is likely that similar reparative cells in different tissues in the body exhibit distinctive characteristics, depending on the tissues in which they are found, but share similar differentiation potential. Also, although certain reparative cells may reside in the tissues of the organ that is damaged, additional reparative cells may migrate to the injury from other tissues. For example, there is growing evidence that MSCs derived from bone marrow share many properties with the microvascular pericytes or mural cells found surrounding small blood vessels throughout the body. This is interesting because the pericytes may represent the peripheral version of MSCs found in bone marrow, and the pericytes would form a line of "first responders" to tissue injury. The potential presence of multiple stem cells in tissues has led to the suggestion that it is the specialized niche that preserves and determines the type of stem cell that may be present.

For developing cellular therapeutics, our approach working with MSCs has been to study the progenitor cell that has the best attributes for development of cellular therapeutics. That is, ease of isolation, extensive ex vivo expansion capacity, produces important growth factors and cytokines, stability of phenotype, contact inhibited, ability to differentiate to multiple cell types, and suitable immunological properties. Whether another stem cell will prove superior to the MSC for regeneration therapy of a particular tissue, such as the damaged heart, remains to be determined.

Table 1

Surface antigen	MSCs ref. 14	MAPCs ref. 31	RS-1 ref. 32	PLAs ref. 35	APCs ref. 34
CD9					+
CD10		−	−		+
CD11[a,b]	−		−		−
CD13	+	+		+	+
CD14	−		−	−	−
CD18 Integrin β_2	−				−
CD29	+			+	+
CD31 PECAM	−	−	±	−	
CD34	−	−	−	−	+
CD44	+		+	+	+
CD45	−[a]	−	−	−	−
CD49b Integrin α_2	+	+			
CD49d Integrin α_4	−			+	+
CD49e Integrin α_5	+		+		+
CD50 ICAM3	−	−			−
CD54 ICAM1	+				+
CD56 NCAM				−	−
CD62E E-Selectin	−	−		−	−
CD71 Transferrin Rec	+		+	+	
CD73 SH-3	+			+	
CD90 Thy-1	+	+	±	+	
CD105 Endoglin, SH-2	+			+	+
CD106 VCAM	+	−		−	+
CD117	−	−			
CD133	−	(+)	−	−	
CD166 ALCAM	+				+
Other markers					
β_2-Microglobulin	+	+			
Nestin	+			+	
p75	+			+	
HLA ABC	+	−	±		+
HLA DR	− induc	−	−		−
SSEA-4	+	+			
TRK (ABC)	+		+		
Differentiation in vitro					
Osteo	+	+	+	+	+
Adipo	+	+	+	+	+
Chondro	+	+	+	+	
Neural	(+)			(+)	
Stromal	+	+			
Myoblast Sk	(+)	+			+
Endothelial	(+)	+			

+, positive; −, negative; (+), detection varied.

MSC, mesemchymal stem cell; MAPC, mesenchymal adult progenitor cell; RS, rapidly cycling stromal cell; PLA, pluripotent liposuction aspirate-derived cell; APC, adult progenitor cell; induc, inducible with interferon-γ.

[a]Positive upon isolation, lost in culture.

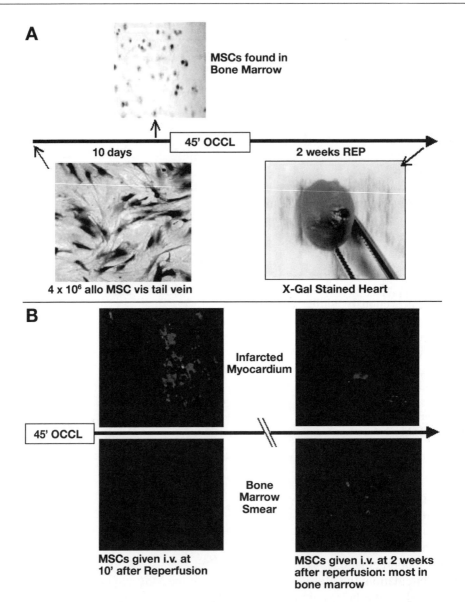

Fig. 3. (A) Mesenchymal stem cells (MSCs) were transduced in vitro with the β-galactosidase (β-gal) reporter gene to follow their distribution following intravenous delivery. (Left panel) Nearly 100% of the transduced MSCs stained positive for β-gal activity prior to injection. 3.9×10^6 MSCs were injected into the tail vein of healthy Fisher rats. β-gal-positive cells were only detected in the bone marrow 10 days post-MSC delivery. When these animals were then subjected to 45' of ischemia and 2 weeks of reperfusion, labeled MSCs migrated to the site of infarction. Labeled cells were not detected in noncardiac tissues at 2 weeks postinfarction. **(B)** To determine if MSCs could home to sites of infarction when administered systemically at reperfusion, 2×10^6 DiI-labeled rMSCs were delivered intravenously either 10 minutes (left panels) or 14 days (right panels) postreperfusion. In both groups the animals were sacrificed 14 days post-cell injection and the hearts (top panels) and bone marrow (bottom panels) examined for the presence of DiI-positive MSCs. Qualitative assessment suggests that MSC delivery at 10 days postreperfusion results in a greater degree of MSC engraftment in the infarcted myocardium than delivery at 14 days. Conversely, MSC engraftment in the bone marrow is increased with delayed administration. (*See* color insert following p. 114.) (From ref. *52*.)

MIGRATION OF MSCs TO SITES OF TISSUE INJURY

An unexpected finding was that MSCs migrate to sites of tissue injury. This is exciting because it indicates that stem cells can play an active role in tissue repair, even if the cells are initially present at a site distant from the injury, perhaps obviating the need for local administration. Bittner et al. reported that mouse models of muscular dystrophy showed engraftment of genetically marked cells in not only skeletal muscle, but also cardiac tissue, sites of tissue damage in the *mdx* mouse *(50)*. Chiu and colleagues at McGill University, working with an experimental rat model of cardiac infarction, showed that cultured MSC-like cells, when injected into the tail vein, would migrate to the damaged cardiac tissue *(51)*. We have repeated and confirmed this finding; an example is shown in Fig. 3 *(52)*. Furthermore, it is apparent that MSC migration to the cardiac injury is enhanced when the MSCs are administered soon after the infarction, and the strength of the homing effect diminishes with time (Fig. 3B). Similar homing-to-injury results obtained in the acutely infracted porcine model *(53)* and in a rat model of chronic rejection *(54)* suggest that MSC migration to injury may have a positive impact on either acute or chronic injuries. We recently reported in vivo monitoring and visualization of intravenously administered MSCs that were dual labeled with [111]indium and ferumoxides, followed by single-photon emission computed tomography (SPECT/CT) with x-ray CT and magnetic resonance imaging (MRI) techniques, respectively, in the canine infarct model *(55)*. Further careful analysis of large animal models should establish safety, dose, and efficacy parameters before human studies are undertaken.

It appears that MSCs migrate towards factors that are present as a part of the tissue injury/inflammation cascade, although the active component is not yet known (perhaps TNF-α, IFN-γ, other?). What role the homing of MSCs to injury and the apparent diminishing level of MSCs available as one ages plays in age-related tissue degeneration remains to be explored.

CARDIAC IMPLANTATION STUDIES WITH MSCs

The availability of well-characterized human MSCs prompted our studies implanting human MSCs into the heart. We first studied the delivery of *lac* Z-labeled human MSCs into SCID/*beige* immunodeficient mice by injection into the ventricle chamber through a diaphragmatic approach *(55)*. About 5% of the heart output goes through the coronary circulation; therefore, only this portion of the MSCs likely reaches the cardiac capillary beds, with the remaining 95% moving out through the aorta to the rest of the body. Many MSCs were found in the lungs, liver, and spleen at the early time points, but these redistributed with time, and a portion of the human MSCs appeared to persist in the bone marrow. Of the human MSCs found to persist in the heart, the cells were monodisperse and surrounded by cardiomyocytes. Counting the number of MSCs found in sections of the recipients' cardiac tissue, only 5–10% of the 5% that entered the coronary circulation persisted at 2 weeks, and later cell counts decreased somewhat. For the animals sacrificed during the first 14 days, histology and immunostaining did not reveal differentiation of the MSCs to a cardiac phenotype, but all cells found at 30–60 days appeared to be differentiated and expressed cardiac isoforms of the sarcomeric proteins myosin heavy chain, troponin I, α-actinin. There was also new expression of the cardiac calcium-handling protein phospholamban and the muscle intermediate filament protein desmin, all at levels that were indistinguishable from the surrounding cardiomyocytes. When the plane of sectioning was optimal, sarcomeric organization was evident in the engrafted MSCs *(55)*. Because every identified MSC beyond 30 days was found to express cardiac proteins, which is much higher than the very low expected percentage that might occur if spontaneous cell fusion was occurring, we believe the results indicate that MSCs can differentiate to cardiomyocytes under the right conditions.

Recognizing that MSC cellular therapy for cardiac infarction may provide benefits to the damaged heart by (1) production of important growth factors and cytokines, (2) modifying the tissue damage/inflammation cascade, (3) providing cells that survive in infracted tissue, and (4) potentially differentiating to maturing cardiomyocytes, we began experiments in porcine models of MI with Dr. W. Baumgartner and colleagues in the Division of Cardiac Surgery at Johns Hopkins University School of Medicine *(56,57)*. The initial studies used an open chest surgical procedure with a 45-minute occlusion of the left anterior descending artery. The artery was then reopened to simulate catheter or surgical reperfusion. MSCs were injected into a limited region of the infarct bounded by implanted sonocrystals to provide for accurate wall thickness and contractility measurements over time. Approximately 20 million MSCs were delivered to the sonocrystal field area of the infracted heart. Results indicated a 30% improvement in ventricular wall thickness in the area of MSC injection.

In further studies, in order to test a therapeutic scenario, the number of MSCs injected was increased 10-fold to 200 million, and the cells were injected at 20 sites to broadly cover the infarction. Additionally, the recognition of the lack of rejection of MSCs allowed for the testing of allogeneic porcine MSCs without the use of immunosuppression. Overall, there was a approx 30% improvement in ventricular wall thickness and 50% reduction in left ventricular end-diastolic pressure in animals that received MSCs, suggesting less deleterious remodeling with improved dynamics compared to control animals *(58)*. However, there was not a measurable improvement in the systolic pressure. Histology and immunostaining indicated the expression of low levels of cardiac proteins but no sarcomeric organization or gap junctions, perhaps explaining the lack of improvement in systolic contractility.

To date, areas of damaged myocardium that receive MSCs do not become as "good as new," but the outcomes appear favorable compared to the hearts that do not receive them. The hearts that do not receive MSCs continue to undergo deleterious remodeling as the heart attempts to compensate for decreased cardiomyocytes, reduced perfusion, and the associated altered electrical patterns. Those that receive cells appear to maintain a thicker ventricle wall, show increased ejection fraction, and have reduced pressure at rest (diastole).

Taylor and colleagues have recently begun the important work of evaluating progenitor cell implantation in a side-by-side manner *(4)*. These researchers isolated skeletal myoblasts and cultured MSC-like bone marrow cells and evaluated their performance following injection into cardiac cryo-injuries, a reproducible model of infarction. They reported similar improvements in regional systolic heart function for both populations of implanted cells.

IMAGING STUDIES FOR MSC THERAPY

We and others have used a variety of methods to label and track MSCs and other cells types in order to follow their biodistribution in the recipients. These methods include (1) dye labeling of membranes or surface proteins such as Di I, (2) labeling of

DNA with intercalating fluors such as DAPI, (3) gene tagging of cells by transfection such as the gene for lac Z or green fluorescent protein, (4) *in situ* hybridization for the Y chromosome in female recipients of male cells, (5) polymerase chain reaction for a transgene or Y chromosome, (6) radiolabeling with [111]indium for γ imaging, (7) iron particle labeling with agents such as Feridex for detection by MRI *(55,59–61)*, and (8) iridium labeling of MSCs and detection by neutron activation analysis. Each has its uses and its limitations. In all cases, increasing the amount of label on the MSCs improves detection, but too much can interfere with some properties of the cells. This was the case for MSC labeling with the MRI contrast agent Feridex, where interference with chondrogenic differentiation was evident at the higher labeling levels *(60)*.

Because each cell-labeling method has its limitations, it may be that the most useful imaging information will come from combining labeling/detection methods. Most recently, working with our colleagues at Johns Hopkins, MSCs that have been dual labeled with MRI tracers and radiolabels and delivered by intravenous administration have been tracked in vivo in the canine model of infarction *(55)*. Towards this end, MSCs were surface labeled with the radio-tracer [111]indium-oxime and internally labeled with the ferumoxide MRI agent Feridex, providing two signals that can be independently imaged and electronically registered, providing superior spatial resolution. With this system it is possible to obtain the MRI image of the MSCs in the body and use radiolabel imaging to obtain semi-quantitative information about the relative number of stem cells in the tissue. The MSCs are seen to first deposit in the lungs for 24 hours, after which a portion of the MSCs migrated to the infracted heart, and these persisted for at least 1 week. Using this type of imaging, we are gaining a better understanding of the biodistribution of the MSCs and their homing to infarcted heart tissue after systemic delivery. Such questions are particularly important in developing clinical protocols where optimization of dosage may be necessary for therapeutic success.

CLINICAL TRIALS

Clinical trials with autologous skeletal myoblasts were begun a few years ago. Some of the patients encountered arrhythmias as a result of the electrogenic nature of the myoblasts, which were not faithfully coupled to the endogenous cardiac tissue. The solution to this was to assure that patients receiving skeletal myoblast injections also receive an implantable cardiac defibrillator to protect against any future arrhythmia.

Several recent clinical trials have utilized whole bone marrow delivered to patients with MIs, and these studies have begun the important work of bringing new therapies to cardiac patients. Strauer and Wernet and colleagues at the Division of Cardiology of Heinrich-Heine University in Düsseldorf treated 10 patients who had received standard of care with autologous mononuclear bone marrow cells delivered by percutaneous transluminal coronary angioplasty (balloon catheter dilation). The reported 3-month follow-up results indicated decreased infarct region and increased wall motion in the cell-treated patients compared to control patients. Further analysis of the cell-treated patients indicated improved myocardial perfusion, contractility, and stroke volume index *(62)*. Gustav Steinhoff and his team at the University of Rostock initiated a phase I study of patients with MI longer than 10 d with previous autologous stem cell transplant utilizing AC133 (CD133) immunoselected bone marrow cells without culture expansion of the cells. The first 12 patients showed no new arrhythmia and improved left ventricular end diastolic volume as well as left ventricular ejection fraction *(63)*.

Although this is a small patient sampling, the results are encouraging and the study will be extended to additional patients.

Perin, Willerson, and colleagues at the Texas Heart Institute in Houston and the Federal University in Rio de Janiero have treated and reported on 20 patients with end-stage cardiomyopathy who received autologous bone marrow mononuclear cells (all cell types without selection), delivered by transendocardial catheter with the aid of electromechanical mapping *(64)*. The results were reported for 6 and 12 months on the 11 treated patients vs the 9 controls and demonstrated improved perfusion and improved capacity for exercise in the 6-minute walk test in the cell-treated patients.

Perhaps the most advance clinical trial to date is the so-called TOPCARE trial for acute MI wherein 30 patients were given circulating progenitor cells and 29 were given bone marrow-derived progenitor cells via intracoronary circulation *(65,66)*. The study report following 1 year of data collection reported improvement in left ventricular ejection fraction, reduced infarct size, and improved end-systolic volume. The results were similar for both types of injected cells.

Bone marrow contains a variety of stem and progenitor cells, and it is possible that the combination of cell types present in marrow can provide for repair and rejuvenation of the damaged heart. However, it will be important to identify the cell types and/or factors in bone marrow that provide the greatest benefit so that these can be optimized.

Given all of the in vitro and in vivo animal data on allogeneic MSCs and their ability to home to the sites of injury, including cardiac infarcts, and the human exposure data from hematological malignancy patients suggesting that MSCs can be safely administered to patients, Osiris Therapeutics Inc., of Baltimore, Maryland initiated a placebo-controlled dose escalation phase I clinical trial of allogeneic MSCs administered intravenously 1–10 days after infarction in Spring 2005. The results of this 60-patient study should be available at the end of 2006. We all look forward to the outcome report.

CONCLUSIONS

MSCs represent well-characterized progenitor cells with attributes that lend themselves to the development for cellular therapeutics for several important tissues. Their ability to produce important growth factors and cytokines that support other cell types has been demonstrated, and their capacity to differentiate to multiple important lineages favors their use in tissue-regeneration studies. The promising potential for MSCs to be used as a treatment for hearts damaged by ischemia, disease, injury, or genetic abnormalities is undergoing careful evaluation. The lack of immune rejection may allow the use of allogeneic MSCs in several areas of tissue regeneration. MSCs are currently undergoing clinical evaluation for treatment of cardiac and cancer patients. Many studies remain, yet MSC-based therapy is potentially one of the most promising cellular therapies under evaluation for adoption into clinical practice.

REFERENCES

1. Kao RL, Chiu RC. Cellular Cardiomyoplasty: Myocardial Repair with Cell Implantation. Landes Bioscience, Austin, TX, 1997.
2. Kessler PD, Byrne BJ. Myoblast cell grafting into heart muscle: cellular biology and potential applications. Annu Rev Physiol 1999;61:219–242.
3. Menasche P, Hagege AA, Vilquin JT, et al. Autologous skeletal myoblast transplantation for severe postinfarction left ventricular dysfunction. J Am Coll Cardiol 2003;41:1078–1083.

4. Thompson RB, Emani SM, Davis BH, et al. Comparison of intradcardiac cell transplantation: Autologous skeletal myoblasts versus bone marrow cells. Circulation 2003;108(suppl II):264–271.
5. Jackson KA, Tiejuan M, Goodell MA. Hematopoietic potential of stem cells isolated from murine skeletal muscle. Proc Natl Acad Sci 1999;96:14482–14486.
6. Pfister O, Mouquet F, Jain M, et al. CD31- but not CD31+ cardiac side population cells exhibit functional cardiomyogenic differentiation. Circ Res 2005;97:52–61.
7. Ii M, Nishimura H, Iwakura A, et al. Endothelial progenitor cells are rapidly recruited to myocardium and mediate protective effect of ischemic preconditioning via "imported" nitric oxide synthase activity. Circulation 2005;111:114–1120.
8. Asahara T, Masuda H, Takahashi T, et al. Bone marrow origin of endothelial progenitor cells responsible for postnatal vasculogenesis in physiologic and pathological neovascularization. Circ Res 1999;85:221–228.
9. Vasa M, Fichtlscherer S, Aicher A, et al. Number and migratory activity of circulating endothelial progenitor cells inversely correlate with risk factors for coronary artery disease. Circ Res 2001;89:E1–E7.
10. Orlic D, Kajstura J, Chimenti S, et al. Mobilized bone marrow cells repair the infarcted heart, improving function and survival. Proc Natl Acad Sci USA 2001;98:10,344–10,349.
11. Messina E, DeAngelis L, Frati G, et al. Isolation and expansion of adult cardiac stem cells from human and murine heart. Circ Res 2004;95:911–921.
12. Oh H, Bradfute SB, Gallardo TD, et al. Cardiac progenitor cells from adult myocardium: homing, differentiation, and fusion after infarction. Proc Natl Acad Sci USA 2003;100:12,313–12,318.
13. Friedenstein AJ, Petrakova KV, Kurolesova AI, Frolova GP. Heterotopic of bone marrow. Analysis of precursor cells for osteogenic and hematopoietic tissues. Transplantation 1968;6:230–247.
14. Friedenstein AJ, Chailakhyan RK, Gerasimov UV. Bone marrow osteogenic stem cells: in vitro cultivation and transplantation in diffusion chambers. Cell Tissue Kinet 1987;20:263–272.
15. Ashton BA, Allen TD, Howlett CR, Eaglesom CC, Hattori A, Owen M. Formation of bone and cartilage by marrow stromal cells in diffusion chambers in vivo. Clin Orthop 1980;115:294–307.
16. Owen M, Friedenstein AJ. Stromal stem cells: marrow-derived osteogenic precursors. Ciba Found Symp 1988;136:42–60.
17. Pittenger MF, Marshak DR. Regenerative mesenchymal stem cells from adult bone marrow. In: Gardner R, Gottlieb D, Marshak D, eds. Stem Cells. Cold Spring Harbor Press, Cold Spring Harbor, NY, 2001, pp. 349–373.
18. Bianco P, Riminucci M, Gronthos S, Robey PG. Bone marrow stromal stem cells: nature, biology and potential applications. Stem Cells 2001;19:180–192.
19. Caplan AI. Mesenchymal stem cells. J Orthop Res 1991;9:641–650.
20. Haynesworth SE, Goshima J, Goldberg VM, Caplan AI. Characterization of cells with osteogenic potential from human bone marrow. Bone 1992;13:81–88.
21. Lennon DP, Haynesworth SE, Bruder SP, Jaiswal N, Caplan AI. Development of a serum screen for mesenchymal progenitor cells from bone marrow. In Vitro Animal Cell Dev Biol 1996;32:602–611.
22. Pittenger MF, Mackay AM. Multipotential human mesenchymal stem cells. Graft 2000;3:288–294.
23. Deans RJ, Moseley AB. Mesenchymal stem cells: biology and potential clinical uses. Exp Hematol 2000;28:875–884.
24. Pittenger MF, AM Flake, Deans RJ. Human mesenchymal stem cells from adult bone marrow for tissue engineering. In: Atala A, Lanza R, eds. Methods in Tissue Engineering. Academic Press, Inc., San Diego, 2002, pp. 1461–1470.
25. Pittenger MF, Mackay AM, Beck SC, et al. Multilineage potential of adult human mesenchymal stem cells. Science 1999;284:143–147.
26. Pereira RF, Halford KW, O'Hara MD, et al. Cultured adherent cells from marrow can serve as long lasting precursor cells for bone, cartilage, and lung in irradiated mice. Proc Natl Acad Sci 1995;92:4857–4861.
27. Kopen GC, Prockop DJ, Phinney DG. Marrow stromal cells migrate throughout forebrain and cerebellum, and they differentiate into astrocytes after injection into neonatal mouse brains. Proc Natl Acad Sci USA 1999;96:10,711–10,716.
28. Hofstetter CP, Schwarz EJ, Hess D, et al. Marrow stromal cells form guiding strands in the injured spinal cord and promote recovery. Proc Natl Acad Sci USA 2002;99:2199–2204.
29. Haynesworth SE, Baber MA, Caplan AI. Cytokine expression by human marrow-derived mesenchymal progenitor cells in vitro: effects of dex and IL-1α. J Cell Physiol 1996;66:585–592.
30. Majumdar MK, Thiede MA, Mosca JD, Moorman M, Gerson SL. Phenotypic and functional comparison of marrow-derived mesenchymal stem cells and stromal cells. J Cell Physiol 1998;176:57–66.

31. Reese JS, Koc ON, Gerson SL. Human mesenchymal stem cells provide stromal support for efficient CD34+ transduction. J Hematother Stem Cell Res 1999;8:515–523.
32. Cheng L, Hammond H, Ye Z, Zhan X, Dravid G. Human adult marrow cells support prolonged expansion of human embryonic stem cells in culture. Stem Cells 2003;21:131–142.
33. Lazarus HM, Koc ON, Devine SM, et al. Cotransplantation of HLA-identical sibling culture expanded mesenchymal stem cells and hematopoietic stem cells in hematologic malignancy patients. Biol Blood Marrow Transplant 2005;11:389–398.
34. Klyushnenkova E, Mosca JD, Zernetkina V, et al. T cell responses to allogeneic human mesenchymal stem cells: immunogenicity, tolerance and suppression. J Biomed Sci 2005;12:47–57.
35. Di Nicola M, Carlo-Stella C, Magni M, et al. Human bone marrow stromal cells suppress T-lymphocyte proliferation induced by cellular or nonspecific mitogenic stimuli. Blood 2002;99:3838–3843.
36. Tse WT, Pendleton JD, Beyer WM, Egalka MC, Guinan EC. Suppression of allogeneic T-cell proliferation by human marrow stromal cells: implications in transplantation. Transplantation 2003;75: 389–397.
37. Le Blanc K, Tammik C, Rosendahl K, Zetterberg E, Ringden O. HLA expression and immunologic properties of differentiated and undifferentiated mesenchymal stem cells. Exp Hematol 2003;31:890–896.
38. Le Blanc K, Tammik L, Sundberg B, Haynesworth SE, Ringden O. Mesenchymal stem cells inhibit and stimulate mixed lymphocyte cultures and mitogenic responses independently of the major histocompatibility complex. Scand J Immunol 2003;57:11–20.
39. Aggarwal S, MF Pittenger. Human mesenchymal stem cells modulate immune cell responses. Blood 2005;105:1815–1822.
40. Le Blanc K, Pittenger MF. Mesenchymal stem cells: progress toward promise. Cytotherapy 2005;7:36–45.
41. Jiang Y, Jahagirdar BN, Reinhardt RL, et al. Pluripotency of mesenchymal stem cells derived from adult marrow. Nature 2002;418:41–49.
42. Reyes M, Dudek A, Jahagirdar B, Koodie L, Marker PH, Verfaillie CM. Origin of endothelial progenitors in human postnatal bone marrow. J Clin Invest 2002;109:337–346.
43. Reyes M, Lund T, Lenvik T, Aguiar D, Koodie L, Verfaillie CM. Purification and ex vivo expansion of postnatal human marrow mesodermal progenitor cells. Blood 2001;98:2615–2625.
44. Colter DC, Class R, DiGirolamo CM, Prockop DJ. Rapid expansion of recycling stem cells in cultures of plastic-adherent cells from human bone marrow. Proc Natl Acad Sci USA 2000;97: 3213–3218.
45. Halvorsen YC, Wilkison WO, Gimble JM. Adipose-derived stromal cells—their utility and potential in bone formation. Int J Obes Relat Metab Disord. 2000;24:S41–S44.
46. Gronthos S, Franklin DM, Leddy HA, Robey PG, Storms RW, Gimble JM. Surface protein characterization of human adipose tissue-derived stromal cells. J Cell Physiol 2001;189:54–63.
47. Zuk PA, Zhu M, Ashjian P, et al. Human adipose tissue is a source of multipotent stem cells. Mol Biol Cell 2002;13:4279–4295.
48. Zuk PA, Zhu M, Mizuno H, et al. Multilineage cells from human adipose tissue: implications for cell-based therapies. Tissue Eng 2001;7:211–228.
49. Lodie TA, Blickarz CE, Devarakonda TJ, et al. Systematic analysis of reportedly distinct populations of multipotent bone marrow-derived stem cells reveals a lack of distinction. Tissue Eng 2002;8:739–751.
50. Bittner RE, Schofer C, Weioltshammer K, et al. Recruitment of bone-marrow-derived cells by skeletal and cardiac muscle in adult dystrophic mdx mice. Anat Embryol (Berlin) 1999;5:391–396.
51. Saito T, Kuang JQ, Bittira B, Al-Khaldi A, Chiu RC. Xenotransplant cardiac chimera: immune tolerance of adult stem cells. Ann Thorac Surg 2002;74:19–24.
52. Pittenger MF, Martin BJ. Mesenchymal stem cells and their potential as cardiac therapeutics. Circ Res 2004;95:9–20.
53. Price MJ, Frantzen M, Kar S, et al. Intravenous allogeneic mesenchymal stem cells home to myocardial injury and reduce left ventricular remodeling in a porcine balloon occlusion-reperfusion model of myocardial infarction. J Am Coll Card 2003;41:269A.
54. Wu GD, Nolta JA, Jin YS. Migration of mesenchymal stem cells to heart allografts during chronic rejection. Transplantation 2003;75:679–685.
55. Kraitchman DL, Tatsumi M, Gilson WD, et al. Dynamic imaging of allogeneic stem cells homing to myocardial infarction. Circulation 2005;112:1451–1461.

56. Toma C, Pittenger MF, Cahill KS, Byrne BJ, Kessler PD. Human mesenchymal stem cells differentiate to a cardiomyocyte phenotype in the adult murine heart. Circulation 2002;105:93–98.

57. Shake JG, Gruber PJ, Baumgartner WA, et al. Mesenchymal stem cell implantation in a swine myocardial infarct model: engraftment and functional effects. Ann Thorac Surg 2002;73:1919–1926.

58. Caparrelli DJ, Cattaneo SM, Shake JG, et al. Cellular myoplasty with mesenchymal stem cells results in improved cardiac performance in a swine model of myocardial infarction. Circulation 2001;104:II-599.

59. Kraitchman DL, Heldman AW, Atalar E, et al. In vivo magnetic resonance imaging of mesenchymal stem cells in myocardial infarction. Circulation 2003;107:2290–2293.

60. Hill JM, Dick AJ, Raman VK, et al. Serial cardiac magnetic resonance imaging of injected mesenchymal stem cells. Circulation 2003;108(8):1009–1014.

61. Kostura L, Kraitchman DL, Mackay AM, Pittenger MF, Bulte JW. Feridex labeling of mesenchymal stem cells inhibits chondrogenesis but not adipogenesis or osteogenesis. Nuclear Magnetic Resonance Biomed 2004;17(7):513–517.

62. Strauer BE, Brehm M, Zeus T, et al. Repair of infarcted myocardium by autologous intracoronary mononuclear bone marrow cell transplantation in humans. Circulation 2002;106:1913–1918.

63. Stamm C, Westphal B, Kleine HD, et al. Autologous bone-marrow stem-cell transplantation for myocardial regeneration. Lancet 2003;361:45–46.

64. Perin EC, Dohmann HF, Borojevic R, et al. Transendocardial, autologous bone marrow cell transplantation for severe, chronic ischemic heart failure. Circulation 2003;107:2294–3018.

65. Schachinger V, Assmus B, Britten MB, et al. Transplantation of progenitor cells and regeneration enhancement in acute myocardial infarction. Final one-year results of the TOPCARE-AMI trial. J Am Coll Cardiol 2004;44:1690–1699.

66. Schachinger V, Assmus B, Honold J, et al. Normalization of coronary blood flow in the infarct-related artery after intracoronary progenitor cell therapy: intracoronary Doppler substudy of the TOPCARE-AMI trial. Clin Res Cardiol 2006;95(1):13–22.

4

Multipotent Adult Progenitor Cells

*Wouter van't Hof, PhD, Niladri Mal, MD,
Amy Raber, Ming Zhang, MD, PhD,
Anthony Ting, PhD, Marc S. Penn, MD, PhD,
and Robert Deans, PhD*

SUMMARY

In 2001 the laboratory of Catherine Verfaillie at the University of Minnesota described the multipotent adult progenitor cell (MAPC) as a novel progenitor cell present in adult marrow that is biologically and antigenically distinct from the mesenchymal stem cell (MSC). MAPCs represent a more primitive progenitor cell population than MSCs and demonstrate remarkable differentiation capability along the epithelial, endothelial, neuronal, myogenic, hematopoeitic, osteogenic, hepatic, chondrogenic, and adipogenic lineages. MAPCs thus embody a unique class of adult stem cells that emulate the broad biological plasticity characteristic of embryonic stem (ES) cells, while maintaining the characteristics that make adult stem cells more amenable to therapeutic application. MAPCs have been reported to be capable of prolonged culture without loss of differentiation potential, and of showing efficient, long-term engraftment and differentiation along multiple developmental lineages in nonobese diabetic (NOD)–severe combined immunodeficient (SCID) mice without evidence of teratoma formation. Based on these findings, there is great interest in evaluating the therapeutic value of MAPCs for a variety of human genetic and degenerative ailments, including cardiovascular disease.

This chapter will focus on reviewing MAPCs and other adult stem cells displaying broad, pluripotent differentiation potential as cellular therapeutics with application for myocardial repair in heart disease. For clarity, the MAPC acronym will be used specifically to represent the cell population originally described by or acquired from the laboratory of Catherine Verfaillie and collaborators. Pluripotent adult stem cell cultures reported by other researchers will be referred to in accordance with designations used in the original publications.

Key Words: Multipotent adult progenitor cell; mesenchymal stem cell; adult stem cell; pluripotency; myocardial infarct; heart failure; stem cell therapy; regenerative medicine.

STEM CELL THERAPY FOR HEART DISEASE

Chronic heart failure (CHF) is a clinical condition in which a primary or secondary circulatory system disease causes abnormal cardiac pressure or performance characteristics that lead to pulmonary congestion *(1)*. CHF is most often caused by myocardial

From: *Contemporary Cardiology: Stem Cells and Myocardial Regeneration*
Edited by: M. S. Penn © Humana Press Inc., Totowa, NJ

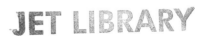

infarction (MI), but other causes include hypertension, anemia, and cardiomyopathy *(2)*. When cardiac dysfunction instigates insufficient perfusion of peripheral tissues, compensatory mechanisms are stimulated that can cause many of the clinical signs and symptoms of CHF. Currently, the main treatment strategy for CHF includes the use of small molecule therapeutics that target disruption of the compensatory systems. For example, various clinical trials with angiotensin-converting enzyme inhibitors, β-blockers, and aldosterone-receptor antagonists have shown that it is possible to block the production of factors that are upregulated in CHF, thereby increasing survival. However, none of these pharmacological intervention approaches improve the underlying pathophysiology of CHF. Surgical intervention to treat CHF is limited, and cardiac transplantation options, the mainstay of treatment for patients with end-stage cardiomyopathies such as CHF, are curtailed by the scarcity of donor organs and complications such as graft rejection and allograft coronary vasculopathy *(3)*.

Stem cell therapy holds great promise in regenerative medicine, with potential application in both acute tissue repair as well as healing of chronic degenerative disease. It offers the hope of treating MI and CHF with a pharmacological agent that would be capable not only of limiting inflammatory tissue damage or enhancing reperfusion through angiogenic stimulation, but also directly replacing the affected tissue, thereby treating the underlying cause of disease. Stem cells that possess the ability to replicate extensively and give rise to the variety of the body's cells and organs can be obtained from both embryonic and adult sources *(4–8)*. The most important feature attributed to embryonic stem (ES) cells is pluripotency—the ability to differentiate into virtually any cell type in the body. Adult stem cells are dispersed throughout the body and can be isolated from a number of tissue sources, including organs, bone marrow, and blood. The adult stem cells are free from many of the ethical and safety issues associated with ES cells *(9)* and have not been linked to the growth of ectopic tissue or teratomas or tumors, as are found at high frequency in ES cell transplantation studies. Still, adult stem cells have shown limitations in their potential for therapeutic application in that their differentiation potential generally appears to be restricted to narrowly defined cell lineages or tissues, typically reflecting the tissue or organ from which the cells were isolated *(4–6)*, and their expansion capacity in vitro is limited by replicative senescence.

POTENTIAL MECHANISMS FOR ADULT STEM CELL
BENEFIT IN CARDIAC REPAIR

Cardiac Repair

Following an MI, healthy tissue may be replaced by fibrotic scar tissue in conjunction with significant remodeling of the left ventricular wall. The magnitude of this progression is in part determined by neovascularization, especially in the border zone of the infarct. The deleterious effects of remodeling and recovery of function correlate with the limited regenerative capacity of native cardiomyocytes and circulating stem cells. The surviving cardiomyocytes bordering the infarct zone become hypertrophied following MI as a part of an adaptive mechanism to compensate for the loss of myocardium. Late perfusion of vascular beds in the area of infarct in human and animal models improves ventricular remodeling and survival. However, after MI, normal angiogenesis is usually insufficient to meet the greater demands for oxygen and nutrients and to prevent apoptosis of hypertrophied cardiomyocytes and continued loss

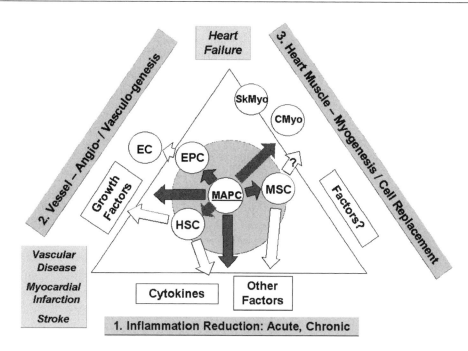

Fig. 1. Concept for mechanisms of stem cell benefit. Each side of the triangle represents one of three different primary pathways for stem cell-mediated improvement in ischemic heart injury, consisting of (1) trophic influences, (2) neo-angiogenesis, and (3) regeneration of new heart muscle tissue. Trophic influences could logically be seen with transplants of hematopoietic stem cells (HSCs), multi-potent adult progenitor cells (MAPC), or mesenchymal stem cells (MSCs). In addition to the production of vascular endothelial growth factor (VEGF) or other factors, delivered stem or progenitor cells contributing to the generation of endothelial and smooth muscle compartments in neoangiogenesis might achieve improved reperfusion of damaged tissue. Endothelial cells (ECs) or endothelial progenitor cells (EPCs) may be present in bone marrow treatments or, similar to purified HSCs, delivered as an enriched cell population. Replacement of fibrotic tissue with new muscle might be achieved by engraftment of skeletal myoblasts (SkMyo), endogeneous cardiac stem cells (CMyo), or cells derived from MSC preparations. Among these stem cell populations, MAPCs are unique as a reservoir for all stem and progenitor cell types and hence have unique therapeutic potential.

of contractile function. Therefore, increasing perfusion to infarcted myocardium to enhance oxygen and nutrient delivery through the formation of new blood vessels has the potential to improve cardiac function.

Concept for Stem Cell Benefit in Repair of Tissue Damage

Preclinical studies of acute MI in small and large animal models have determined that protection from progressive fibrosis by injection of cells into ischemic tissue or the border zone surrounding ischemic damage can confer functional improvement. As highlighted in other chapters, many cell types, including skeletal myoblasts, mesenchymal stem cells (MSCs), and fractionated or nonfractionated bone marrow cells, have shown benefit and supported early clinical trials in both the acute and chronic states. However, the long-term cell fate of injected cells and physiological mechanisms for benefit remain unclear and likely vary reflective of differences in therapeutic cell types. Short-term trophic influences mediating inflammatory damage, vascular permeability, cell survival, or homing of repair cells to sites of damage may be common to many cell types tested, whereas angiogenic benefit may be limited to endothelial progenitors or stem cells with endothelial plasticity. In chronic ischemia, modulation of the inflammatory response by trophic factors is unlikely to play a key role, and vasculogenesis and regeneration of healthy myocardium become the therapeutic pathways. This concept for different modes of benefit depending on the cell type used in cellular therapy is illustrated in Fig. 1.

PROPERTIES OF ADULT STEM CELLS
USED FOR CARDIOVASCULAR THERAPY

The three major classes of adult stem cells studied to date in cardiovascular disease include hematopoietic stem cells (HSCs), MSCs, and multipotent adult progenitor cells (MAPCs). These different stem cell types can be distinguished by a number of properties in addition to biological lineage capacity (5,6,10). This chapter focuses on describing the potential and preliminary experiences in studying the utilization of MAPCs for cardiac repair. Additional descriptions of HSCs and MSCs and their application in cellular therapy for heart disease can be found in other chapters of this book.

Hematopoietic Stem Cells

HSCs have been utilized therapeutically for several decades in immune reconstitution settings. These cells have been available clinically through the identification of unique cell surface receptors allowing their direct isolation from bone marrow, peripheral blood, or cord blood. This was enabled initially using antibodies recognizing the CD34 receptor (11) and later with antibiotics with specificity for the CD133 receptor (12). Although a minor population in blood tissue, their relative abundance has allowed direct isolation and redelivery without the need for ex vivo expansion. These cell-separation procedures do not provide a pure biological population, but rather contain progenitor and mature cell populations as well. Interestingly, in the context of bone marrow treatment of acute or chronic MI, it is conceivable that endothelial cell progenitors are co-delivered with HSCs based on CD34 antigen expression, and it is therefore an intriguing possibility that this may be the effector cell providing benefit by stimulating angiogenic pathways. It is clear that HSC populations are not suitable for allogeneic cell therapy because they can be contaminated with immune stimulatory cells and T-cells, causing graft rejection or graft-vs-host disease (GVHD). In addition, the HSC does not contribute to significant myocardial tissue regeneration, as evidenced in two recent and thorough studies examining marked HSCs in several models (13,14).

MSCs

Another bone marrow-derived stem cell, the MSC, is derived from the adherent stromal cell compartment of adult bone marrow and other tissues, including adipose. These cells are capable of differentiating along osteogenic, chondrogenic, and adipogenic lineages while retaining their self-renewal properties over limited cell doublings (15). Preclinical data reported in both rat and pig models have demonstrated significant protective benefit from progressive heart failure in acute MI settings, although cell fate in these reports has been inconsistent and apparently restricted to smooth muscle and endothelial fates (16,17). A recent study showed evidence of severe calcification after transplantation of bone marrow cells in a rat MI model (18). This implies that the MSC or MSCs committed to differentiation into bone cell progenitors may cause unwanted side effects after transplantation into the heart.

MAPCs

Dr. Catherine Verfaillie at the Stem Cell Institute of the University of Minnesota identified a progenitor cell that is biologically and antigenically distinct from MSCs (19). This cell, the MAPC, represents a more primitive progenitor cell population than the MSC (19,20). MAPC cultures have demonstrated differentiation capability encompassing the epithelial, endothelial, neural, myogenic, hematopoeitic, osteogenic, hepatogenic, chondrogenic, and adipogenic lineages (5,19–22). These cells thus represent a unique class of adult stem cell that exhibit the broad biological plasticity characteristic of ES cells, while maintaining safety characteristics that make adult stem cells appealing. For example, MAPCs are capable of extensive culture without loss of differentiation potential and show efficient, long-term engraftment and differentiation along multiple developmental lineages in nonobese diabetic (NOD)–severe combined immunodeficient (SCID) mice without evidence of teratoma formation (23). In an elegant demonstration of the clonal potency of some cells within a MAPC culture, single genetically marked MAPCs were injected into mouse blastocysts. These blastocysts were successfully implanted and the resulting embryos developed to term (22). Postnatal analysis in highly chimeric animals showed reconstitution of all tissues and organs, and, interestingly, no abnormalities or organ dysfunction were observed in any of these animals. Importantly, dual staining experiments also demonstrated that gene-marked MAPCs contributed to a significant percentage of apparently functional cardiomyocytes in these chimeric animals (22). These animals did not show any heart abnormalities or irregularities in either the embryological or the adult state, suggesting that the MAPCs are capable of differentiating into healthy heart cells with normal functionality.

DEVELOPMENT OF MAPCs FOR CLINICAL USE

The clinical use of MAPCs requires development of a consistent ex vivo expansion process, yielding cell numbers in the range of 50–500 million cells per dose, with characterization of phenotype and lineage potency. We have established routine protocols for human, rat, and pig stem cell expansion enabling preclinical model testing for benefit in ischemic injury (24). The ideal cell product for therapeutic use will have broad potential for allogeneic usage, exerting functional benefit without stimulating a strong allogeneic tissue response.

Expansion Capacity

The extensive replicative capacity of MAPCs (6,7,19,22), a property not found in other adult stem cell types (15,25), is a key component in cell expansion strategies to use these cells for clinical or research use. This stem cell population was initially isolated from bone marrow but subsequently established from other tissues, including brain, muscle (19), umbilical cord blood and umbilical cord matrix tissue (data not shown). Adherent cells from bone tissue are enriched in a media containing low serum (2%), dexamethasone, endothelial growth factor, platelet-derived growth factor, and other additives and grown at relatively low cell density under conditions of low oxygen tension (26). At early culture points, more heterogeneity is detected in the population, but many adherent stromal cells undergo replicative senescence around cell doubling 20, and a

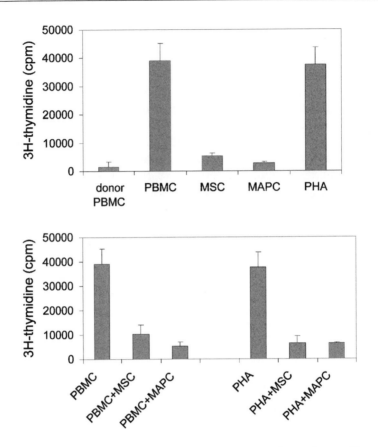

Fig. 2. Low in vitro immunogenicity of human pluripotent progenitor cultures. (Top panel) Mixed lymphocyte reactions using allogeneic peripheral blood mononuclear cells (PBMCs), mesenchymal stem cells (MSCs), or multipotent adult progenitor cells (MAPCs). Donor PBMCs were incubated with irradiated stimulator cells, including donor PBMCs, allogeneic PBMCs, MSCs, or MAPCs. As a positive control, donor PBMCs were stimulated with 2 ng/mL (PHA). (Bottom panel) Immunosuppressive effects of MSCs and MAPCs on allogeneic MLR. Donor PBMCs were incubated with allogeneic PBMCs in the presence or absence of MSCs or MAPCs. Donor PBMCs were also stimulated with 2 ng/mL PHA in the presence or absence of MSCs or MAPCs.

more morphologically homogeneous population of cells continues to expand, associated with telomerase expression and absence of telomere shortening. A key parameter in expansion is the maintenance of cells at low density (500–5000 cells/cm^2). Higher cell density results in maturation of cells along primarily mesenchymal pathways with reduced replicative potential.

Low Immunogenicity

MAPCs have immunological properties similar to those of MSCs. MAPCs do not express class II human leukocyte antigen and do not express T-cell co-stimulatory molecules (A. Raber et al., unpublished data). MSCs have demonstrated low in vitro immunogenicity and the ability to engraft across in allogeneic recipients (27–29). A recent report suggests that production of prostaglandins by activated mesenchymal stem cells results in activation of a dendritic cell population DH2, which acts to immunosuppress inflammatory T-cells, whereas others have pointed to an upregulation of interleukin-10 as an immunosuppressive cytokine (27,29). These processes are likely not exclusive, and a recruited MAPC or MSC at the site of injury may thus play a downmodulating role in the inflammatory response and signal the initiation of repair. Recently, a report by LeBlanc in *Lancet* documented the remarkable recovery from steroid-resistant grade IV GVHD by delivery of haploidentical MSCs from mother to patient (30). This is the strongest evidence to date that cells with the immune phenotype of MSCs might be used clinically to dampen and resist allogeneic reactivity.

We have performed preliminary experiments that show that our human pluripotent progenitor cultures exhibit low in vitro immunogenicity and, analogous to MSC, are immunosuppressive when added to otherwise potent T-cell mixed lymphocyte reactions (MLRs) (Fig. 2). Responder and stimulator cells were prepared, and MLRs were performed according to described procedures (28). The observations are consistent across various sets of donor and responder pairs tested. These findings prompted evaluation of allogeneic MAPCs in animal models of ischemic heart injury.

BENEFIT OF ADULT PLURIPOTENT STEM CELLS IN CARDIOVASCULAR DISEASE MODELS

MAPCs have previously been shown to differentiate into cardiomyocyte-like cells and engraft in cardiac tissue in animal studies (22). Consequently, they likely hold potential to repair damage in the heart caused by MI, CHF, and vascular disorders.

MAPCs and Acute Ischemic Injury

We have performed initial proof of concept studies in collaboration with Dr. Marc Penn of the Cleveland Clinic. MAPC benefit was evaluated in a Lewis rat model for myocardial infarction in which permanent ischemia was induced by direct surgical ligation of the left anterior descending artery (LAD). The stem cells used in these experiments were isolated from the bone marrow of Sprague-Dawley rats and stably labeled by using a lentiviral construct encoding green fluorescent protein (GFP). In vitro differentiation of the GFP-labeled MAPCs into the endothelial (mesodermal), hepatic (endodermal), and neuronal (ectodermal) lineages and subsequent analysis of lineage-specific marker expression by quantitative polymerase chain reaction (qPCR) confirmed that the GFP-labeled MAPCs had retained tri-lineage differentiation potential (Fig. 3). These stem cells were at population doubling numbers greater than 200 and displayed normal karyotypes and telomere lengths comparable to early bone marrow cultures (data not shown).

To test the hypothesis that delivery of MAPCs to the myocardium in the peri-infarct region can help to improve cardiac function, Lewis rats received allogeneic MAPCs immediately after LAD ligation by direct injection into the infarct border zone (five injections of 400,000 cells per injection). This experiment was designed to provide proof of concept for allogeneic cell use with secondary endpoints of benefit. When echocardiography was performed at 2 weeks post-MI, we observed a significant increase in shortening fraction in those animals that received direct injection of MAPCs compared to the phosphate-buffered saline vehicle control group ($13.9 \pm 2.2\%$ [$n = 4$] vs $24.0 \pm 6.6\%$ [$n = 7$]; $p < 0.5$) (*see* Fig. 4). Shortening fraction is calculated as a percentage of end-diastoloic minus end-systolic two-dimensional dimension divided by end-diastolic length.

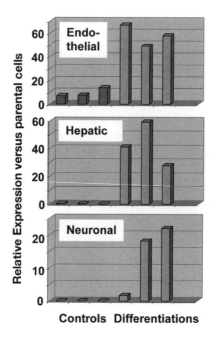

Fig. 3. Tri-lineage differentiation of rat multipotent adult progenitor cells (MAPCs). For endothelial differentiation, MAPCs were cultured on fibronectin-coated plates in the presence of vascular endothelial growth factor-B. For hepatocyte differentiation, MAPCs were grown on matrigel-coated plates and treated with fibroblast growth factor (FGF)-4 and hepatocyte growth factor. Neuronal differentiation was induced by sequential treatment with basic-FGF (bFGF), with both FGF-8 and Sonic Hedgehog, and with brain-derived neurotrophic factor. After 2 wk mRNA was extracted from cells and applied to qPCR analysis using primers specific for detection of various lineages markers. In all assays, cells cultured in the absence of lineage-inducing cytokines served as controls. The expression levels of lineage markers were first normalized to an internal control (GAPDH), and differentiation success was then assessed by calculation of the relative expression in the differentiated or the control cells compared to the levels in the parental MAPC line, using an increase of more than fivefold in the relative expression as a cutoff for successful differentiation. Differentiated rat MAPCs displayed significant expression of the endothelial markers, von Willebrand factor (top panel), and PECAM-1, the hepatic markers albumin (middle panel), cytokeratin-18, and HNF-1α, and the neuronal/astrocyte markers GFAP (bottom panel), nestin, and NF-200.

Subsequent histological analysis of the hearts confirmed that all of the animals that displayed increased shortening fractions after stem cell injection had received prior successful LAD ligation, as evidenced by the presence of extended zones of infarcted tissue in the left ventricular wall areas of the heart (Fig. 5A). In addition, in all animals that received the MAPCs by direct myocardial injection, GFP-positive cells were identified in infarcted heart tissue and in the infarct border zones after immunofluorescence analysis (Fig. 5B,C). Interestingly, an absence of inflammatory lymphocytes in H&E sections of heart that were positive for donor cells, either in the fibrotic ischemia zone or in healthy myocardium, was observed. In addition, no allogeneic antibody (Ab) response could be detected using serial dilutions of plasma against either donor stem cells or Sprague-Dawley splenocytes. Detection was performed using anti-rat κ Ab, and controls against peripheral blood and isotype Ab showed the ability to detect all classes of rat immunoglobulin (data not shown). Mixed lymphocyte reactions were performed using blood cells collected at time of sacrifice tested against irradiated stem

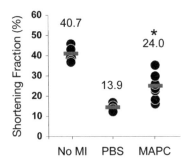

Fig. 4. Assessment of the shortening fraction two weeks after myocardial infarct (MI) induction and multipotent adult progenitor cell (MAPC) injection. Lewis rats received either no MI surgery (no MI) or LAD artery ligation followed by myocardial administration of phosphate-buffered saline (PBS) or 2 million MAPCs in five separate injections of 400,000 cells in the infarct border zone. After 2 wk animals were subjected to M-mode echocardiography for measurement of the shortening fraction. For each animal the left ventricular end-diastolic dimension (LVEDD) and the left ventricular end-systolic dimension (LVESD) were measured five separate times, and the mean values were used to calculate the shortening fraction (SF) according to the following formula: SF = (LVEDD – LVESD)/LVEDD × 100. The asterisk in the figure indicates a significant difference between the MAPC and the PBS control group (Dunn's test, nonparametric multiple comparisons).

cells or Sprague-Dawley splenocytes. No shift in peak MLR kinetics was seen in treated vs control animals, consistent with a lack of immune sensitization at this time point (data not shown). More extensive analysis of allogeneic reactivity in long-term studies, inclusive of additional strain combinations, is currently underway.

These first observations support the hypothesis that administering MAPCs to the injured heart can aid in improvement of heart function. Subsequent experiments are in progress to evaluate dose–response characteristics and to assess functional benefit at longer time scales.

Bone-Derived Adult Pluripotent Stem Cells

A recent report from the laboratory of Dr. Losordo provides independent corroboration that pluripotent stem cells derived from bone marrow (bone marrow stem cells [BMSCs]) show physiological benefit in rodent acute ischemia models (31). Although culture conditions vary compared to MAPC protocols (22), primarily in the context of serum concentration in media formulation, this stem cell population reiterates the retention for primitive germ layer regenerative capacity with extended replication capacity as reported for MAPCs. In these studies, nude rats were used in an experimental model of acute left ventricular ischemia to evaluate the benefit and cell fate of human pluripotent stem cell cultures. A total of 800,000 human BMSC were injected into the peri-infarct zone of animals undergoing a permanent LAD ligation shortly after treatment. Echocardiography was used to determine heart wall function expressed as fractional shortening and regional wall motion scores at 3 days and 4 weeks posttreatment. Pluripotent stem cell-treated animals showed statistically significant improvements compared with vehicle controls and animals treated with total bone marrow cells (31).

The tracking of donor cells marked with a viable fluorescent dye was performed for cell fate analysis. By these criteria, fluorescent cells could be found at 4 weeks in both the infarct zone and, encouragingly, in healthy heart tissue, with the labeled cells

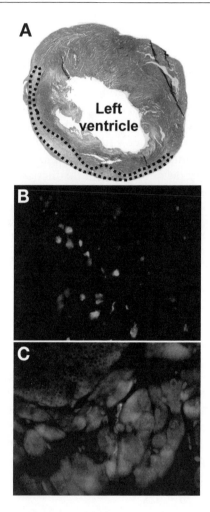

Fig. 5. Analysis of myocardial infarct (MI) induction and multipotent adult progenitor cell (MAPC) engraftment. Two weeks after MI surgery and MAPC injection, animals were sacrificed and the hearts were harvested for histological analysis. **(A)** Semi-thin cross-sections of paraffin-embedded tissue were stained with hematoxylin/eosin for gross morphological evaluation. The infarcted region in the left ventricular wall is highlighted by the dotted line. **(B,C)** Sections were labeled with primary goat anti-green fluorescent protein (GFP) antibody, followed by secondary Alexa-fluor conjugated anti-goat IgG antibody and DAPI staining. Nuclei are blue and GFP-positive cells are green. Autofluorescent signals in the tissue are caused by lipofuscins (pink) and myofbrils (yellow). The orange signal is caused by erythrocytes in blood vessels. In panel **C**, note the presence of an extended GFP-positive cell intercalated within an area of cardiac myofibrils. (*See* color insert following p. 114)

displaying characteristics of cardiomyocytes *(31)*. Because the animals were immune deficient in this xenogeneic model, no comments can be made regarding potential allogeneic cell utility.

CONCLUSIONS AND FUTURE DIRECTIONS

The studies described above illustrate the potential of pluripotent stem cells to restore cardiac function in acute ischemic injury, likely through trophic benefit at early times postinjury (Fig. 3). Yoon et al. suggest that this potency may be greater than that of total bone marrow cells *(31)*. Preliminary observations from our own studies support previous findings reported in the MSC literature that adherent BMSCs may be immune privileged and therefore have therapeutic value in an allogeneic setting as an off-the-shelf product. These data, however, are still preliminary, and parameters such as dose regimen, route of delivery, cell fate, and adjunct therapy require further analysis to validate allogeneic clinical strategies.

It will also be important that further progress is made in standardizing the definitions and descriptions of pluripotent stem cell properties and the experimental models in which they are tested. For example, many of the phenotypic markers used in the early descriptions of MSC biology do not provide a distinction between adherent marrow stromal cell cultures that display noticeable variations in tissue regenerative capacity. It will be essential to classify stem cells based on markers of lineage potency, such as transcription factors like Oct4, and to more precisely determine what effects cell culture conditions, including oxygen tension, cell density, serum levels, and substratum modifications, have on both stem cell marker expression and stem cell lineage differentiation potential.

ACKNOWLEDGMENTS

We thank Jim Kovach for the design of Fig. 1 and Mark Frey for the qPCR analysis described in Fig. 3.

REFERENCES

1. Zhang J, Narula J. Molecular biology of myocardial recovery. Surg Clin North Am 2004;84(1):223–242.
2. Lee MS, Lill M, Makkar RR. Stem cell transplantation in myocardial infarction. Rev Cardiovasc Med 2004;5(2):82–98.
3. Fedak PW, Weisel RD, Verma S, Mickle DA, Li RK. Restoration and regeneration of failing myocardium with cell transplantation and tissue engineering. Semin Thorac Cardiovasc Surg 2003;15(3):277–286.
4. Raff M. Adult stem cell plasticity: fact or artifact? Annu Rev Cell Dev Biol 2003;19:1–22.
5. Verfaillie CM. Adult stem cells: assessing the case for pluripotency. Trends Cell Biol 2002;12(11): 502–508.
6. Verfaillie CM, Pera MF, Lansdorp PM. Stem cells: hype and reality. Hematology (Am Soc Hematol Educ Program) 2002:369–391.
7. Verfaillie CM, Schwartz R, Reyes M, Jiang Y. Unexpected potential of adult stem cells. Ann N Y Acad Sci 2003;996:231–234.
8. Wagers AJ, Weissman IL. Plasticity of adult stem cells. Cell 2004;116(5):639–648.
9. Cai J, Rao MS. Stem cell and precursor cell therapy. Neuromolecular Med 2002;2(3):233–249.
10. Verfaillie CM. Hematopoietic stem cells for transplantation. Nat Immunol 2002;3(4):314–317.
11. Palaganas J, Civin CI. Two steps forward: keeping the momentum in stem cell research. Stem Cells 2004;22(3):240–241.
12. Ivanovic Z, Hermitte F, de la Grange PB, et al. Simultaneous maintenance of human cord blood SCID-repopulating cells and expansion of committed progenitors at low O2 concentration (3%). Stem Cells 2004;22(5):716–724.
13. Murry CE, Soonpaa MH, Reinecke H, et al. Haematopoietic stem cells do not transdifferentiate into cardiac myocytes in myocardial infarcts. Nature 2004;428(6983):664–668.
14. Balsam LB, Wagers AJ, Christensen JL, Kofidis T, Weissman IL, Robbins RC. Haematopoietic stem cells adopt mature haematopoietic fates in ischaemic myocardium. Nature 2004;428(6983):668–673.
15. Pittenger MF, Mackay AM, Beck SC, et al. Multilineage potential of adult human mesenchymal stem cells. Science 1999;284(5411):143–147.
16. Pittenger MF, Martin BJ. Mesenchymal stem cells and their potential as cardiac therapeutics. Circ Res 2004;95(1):9–20.
17. Shake JG, Gruber PJ, Baumgartner WA, et al. Mesenchymal stem cell implantation in a swine myocardial infarct model: engraftment and functional effects. Ann Thorac Surg 2002;73(6):1919–1926.

18. Yoon YS, Park JS, Tkebuchava T, Luedeman C, Losordo DW. Unexpected severe calcification after transplantation of bone marrow cells in acute myocardial infarction. Circulation 2004;109(25): 3154–3157.
19. Jiang Y, Vaessen B, Lenvik T, Blackstad M, Reyes M, Verfaillie CM. Multipotent progenitor cells can be isolated from postnatal murine bone marrow, muscle, and brain. Exp Hematol 2002;30(8): 896–904.
20. Reyes M, Verfaillie CM. Characterization of multipotent adult progenitor cells, a subpopulation of mesenchymal stem cells. Ann NY Acad Sci 2001;938:231–235.
21. Anjos-Afonzo F, Bonnet D. SSEA-1 defines the most primitive cell-type in adult murine mesenchymal stem cell (MUMSCS) compartment with multipotential activity in vitro and in vivo including hematopoietic reconstitution capacity. In: Third Annual Meeting of the International Society for Stem Cell Research, 2005, San Francisco, CA, 2005, p. 35.
22. Jiang Y, Jahagirdar BN, Reinhardt RL, et al. Pluripotency of mesenchymal stem cells derived from adult marrow. Nature 2002;418(6893):41–49.
23. Jahagirdar BN, Miller JS, Shet A, Verfaillie CM. Novel therapies for chronic myelogenous leukemia. Exp Hematol 2001;29(5):543–556.
24. Yasuhara T, Matsukawa N, Yu G, et al. Transplantation of cryopreserved human bone marrow-derived multipotent adult progenitor cells for neonatal hypoxic-ischemic injury: targeting the hippocampus. Rev Neurosci 2006;17(1,2):215–225.
25. Pittenger MF, Mosca JD, McIntosh KR. Human mesenchymal stem cells: progenitor cells for cartilage, bone, fat and stroma. Curr Top Microbiol Immunol 2000;251:3–11.
26. Jiang Y, Breyer A, Lien L, Blackstad M, Verfaillie C. Culture of multipotent adult progenitor cells (MAPCs). ASH Annual Meeting Abstracts 2004;104(11):23–29.
27. Di Nicola M, Carlo-Stella C, Magni M, et al. Human bone marrow stromal cells suppress T-lymphocyte proliferation induced by cellular or nonspecific mitogenic stimuli. Blood 2002;99(10): 3838–3843.
28. Tse WT, Pendleton JD, Beyer WM, Egalka MC, Guinan EC. Suppression of allogeneic T-cell proliferation by human marrow stromal cells: implications in transplantation. Transplantation 2003;75(3): 389–397.
29. Barry FP, Murphy JM, English K, Mahon BP. Immunogenicity of adult mesenchymal stem cells: lessons from the fetal allograft. Stem Cells Dev 2005;14(3):252–265.
30. Le Blanc K, Rasmusson I, Sundberg B, et al. Treatment of severe acute graft-versus-host disease with third party haploidentical mesenchymal stem cells. Lancet 2004;363(9419):1439–1441.
31. Yoon YS, Wecker A, Heyd L, et al. Clonally expanded novel multipotent stem cells from human bone marrow regenerate myocardium after myocardial infarction. J Clin Invest 2005;115(2):326–338.

5

Mesenchymal Progenitor Cells for Vascular Network Formation and Cardiac Muscle Regeneration

Silviu Itescu, MD, Fiona See, PhD, and Timothy Martens, MD

SUMMARY

Mammalian bone marrow contains mesenchymal lineage progenitors that have high proliferative capacity, are clonogenic in vitro, and demonstrate the ability to differentiate to multiple mesenchymal lineage tissue types, including bone, cartilage, fat, smooth muscle, and cardiac muscle. Isolation of these cells on the basis of their physical properties results in clonal outgrowth with functional in vitro heterogeneity. Prospective immunoselection of mesenchymal lineage precursor cells enhances reproducible functional outgrowth, and the phenotype STRO-1brightVCAM-1$^+$ characterizes a multipotent mesenchymal precursor cell in vivo, which gives rise to a 50% frequency of multipotential clonal outgrowth in vitro. These cells are anatomically located in perivascular niches in the bone marrow and throughout the body and demonstrate phenotypic and genetic identity to vascular pericytes. Consistent with the pivotal role played by pericytes in formation of vascular structures during embryogenesis, cumulative data show that mesenchymal precursors regulate adult vasculature formation. In addition, under appropriate differentiation conditions, mesenchymal precursors give rise to new cardiomyocytes. Because vascular network formation is a prerequisite for long-term survival of cardiomyocyte precursors implanted into ischemic myocardium, mesenchymal lineage precursors appear to be ideal candidates for enhancing both cardiac neovascularization and myogenesis. Clinical protocols using these cells will require optimization of serum-free culture methodologies and biological scaffolds/matrices for enhancing survival of implanted cells. Finally, recent data indicating that mesenchymal lineage precursors evade immune recognition raise the exciting prospect that allogeneic use of these cells may be feasible.

Key Words: Cardiomyocyte; progenitor cells; clonal expansion; pericytes.

INTRODUCTION

The mammalian bone marrow comprises two distinct stem cell populations that cooperate and are functionally interdependent: the hematopoietic and mesenchymal lineage progenitors. Traditionally, mesenchymal lineage progenitors within the bone marrow stroma have been viewed largely in terms of their well-documented role in supporting the proliferation, differentiation, and maturation of hematopoietic stem

From: *Contemporary Cardiology: Stem Cells and Myocardial Regeneration*
Edited by: M. S. Penn © Humana Press Inc., Totowa, NJ

cells. However, although hematopoietic lineage stem cells appear to be relatively restricted in their range of tissue differentiation to cells of hematopoietic and endothelial lineage, mesenchymal lineage progenitors have more recently been shown to contain multipotent stem cells with the capacity to give rise to a variety of differentiated cell lineages, including bone, cartilage, adipose, smooth muscle, and even cardiac muscle tissue.

The increasing recognition of the multipotential properties of mesenchymal lineage progenitor cells, together with their apparent ease of culture manipulation, has generated great interest in using these cells for diverse clinical applications. More intriguing recent data have focused on the ability of these cells to evade recognition by the immune cells of unrelated recipients, raising the possibility that they may potentially constitute a source of allogeneic cellular therapeutic products. This chapter will give an overview of the identity, nature, developmental origin, and functional characteristics of mesenchymal lineage progenitor cells, their amenability to ex vivo culture manipulation, and existing data in support of their therapeutic potential, particularly for patients with cardiovascular disease.

MESENCHYMAL LINEAGE PROGENITORS IN MAMMALIAN MARROW

Friedenstein and colleagues (1) were the first to establish a reproducible biological assay to identify the presence of cells in mammalian bone marrow capable of giving rise to multiple tissues of mesenchymal lineage, including bone, cartilage, and fat. Using gentle mechanical disruption of bone marrow tissue, they were able to readily dissociate stromal and hematopoietic cells into a single-cell suspension. The bone marrow stromal cells rapidly adhere, can be easily separated from the nonadherent hematopoietic cells by repeated washing, and, under appropriate culture conditions, give rise to distinct colonies. The clonogenic stromal progenitor cells responsible for colony growth under these conditions were termed fibroblast colony-forming cells (CFU-F) and described as rapidly adherent, nonphagocytic clonogenic cells capable of extended proliferation in vitro (1).

The degree of CFU-F proliferative activity in vitro is greatly dependent on the mitogenic factors present in the culture media. The most important of these include platelet-derived growth factor (PDGF), epidermal growth factor (EGF), basic fibroblast growth factor, transforming growth factor-β, and insulin-like growth factor-1 (2,3). Under optimal conditions, cultured cells combined from multiple CFU-F colonies can undergo more than 50 cell doublings, or more than 25 culture passages, demonstrating extensive self-replicative capacity.

FUNCTIONAL IN VITRO HETEROGENEITY OF MARROW MESENCHYMAL LINEAGE PROGENITORS

Neither CFU-F outgrowth nor expression of osteogenic, chondrogenic, or adipogenic phenotypic markers in culture (detected by either mRNA expression or histochemical techniques) necessarily constitutes multipotency of a given clone (4). Typically, CFU-F outgrowth is heterogeneous and is characterized by a broad range of colony sizes and different cell morphologies, representing varying growth rates of different cell types ranging from spindle-shaped cells to large flat cells. Moreover, different clones may spontaneously differentiate to different tissues under inductive conditions in vitro or following transplantation in vivo (5,6).

Interestingly, the bone marrow stromal population from which mesenchymal lineage stem cells are derived shares properties with cells of fibroblast, myofibroblast, and endothelial cell lineage, expressing matrix proteins, α-smooth muscle actin (α-SMA), as well as endoglin (CD105) and MUC-18 (CD146). Despite attempts to use only those clones that have been distinctively characterized phenotypically following ex vivo culture and passage of cells initially isolated from bone marrow stroma by simple density gradient separation and plastic adherence, the resulting clones continue to display varying degrees of multipotentiality *(7)*. To date, no surface marker expressed by in vitro cultured mesenchymal lineage cells has consistently shown predictability of the biological behavior of any given clone either in vitro or in vivo.

PROSPECTIVE IMMUNOSELECTION OF MESENCHYMAL LINEAGE PRECURSOR CELLS AND REPRODUCIBLE FUNCTIONAL OUTGROWTH

To generate mesenchymal lineage stem cells with sufficient functional reproducibility to enable clinical use, investigators have sought to develop more precise methods to identify and isolate the subset of marrow mesenchymal lineage precursors with the most extensive replication and differentiation potential. This requires prospective linkage between surface phenotype, genotype, and multipotency displayed in transplantation assays. By immunizing mice with human mesenchymal lineage precursors, several laboratories have developed monoclonal antibodies reactive with and suitable for isolation of highly purified mesenchymal precursor cell populations *(8–11)*. Use of a monoclonal antibody reactive with an antigen termed STRO-1 enables identification of a population of marrow stromal cells that are clonogenic (STRO-1+bright) *(12)* and results in a 10- to 20-fold enrichment of CFU-F relative to their incidence in unseparated bone marrow *(13)*. Freshly isolated STRO-1+bright cells containing multipotent stromal/mesenchymal lineage stem cells have been extensively characterized for a long list of markers expressed by fibroblasts, myofibroblasts, endothelial cells, and hematopoietic cells in several different laboratories *(14–17)*. In these studies, combined use of monoclonal antibodies against STRO-1 and vascular cell adhesion molecule-1 (VCAM-1/CD106) results in up to 1000-fold enrichment of CFU-F relative to their incidence in unseparated bone marrow, with a CFU-F incidence of approximately one per two cells plated *(17)*. At a clonal level, STRO-1bright/VCAM-1+ cells are devoid of hematopoietic, fibroblast, or endothelial lineage cells and demonstrate multipotential capability, differentiating to bone, cartilage, and adipose tissue. Thus, in order to maximize functional reproducibility, all efforts should be made to initiate mesenchymal lineage stem cell culture expansion with as pure and homogeneous a population of STRO-1bright/VCAM+ cells as possible.

ANATOMICAL LOCATION OF MESENCHYMAL LINEAGE PRECURSOR CELLS SUGGESTS SHARED IDENTITY WITH VASCULAR PERICYTES

There are now cumulative data from a number of investigators that convincingly point toward the identity of clonogenic stromal/mesenchymal lineage stem cell precursors as being cells intimately associated with blood vessel walls, generally referred to as vascular smooth muscle cells (vSMCs) or pericytes. By immunohistochemistry, STRO-1+ cells in human bone marrow as well as at other sites, including abdominal fat, dental pulp, skin, and liver, are predominantly localized anatomically to perivascular and sinusoidal sites *(18)*. Here they are found to co-express markers typically associated with both vascular smooth muscle, such as α-SMA, and with endothelium, such as MUC-18/CD146.

Observations from cultured bone marrow-derived stromal cells support the interpretation that mesenchymal precursor cells are vascular pericytes in vivo. Cultured stromal cells/mesenchymal lineage stem cells co-express α-SMA as well as other markers of pericytes/smooth muscle cells such as caldesmon, metavinculin, calponin, and smooth muscle myosin heavy chains *(19)*. Moreover, cultured pericytes and marrow stromal cells synthesize very similar extracellular matrix proteins, which include a variety of basal lamina and interstitial collagens *(20,21)*. In addition, marrow stromal cells respond exuberantly to culture with PDGF-BB *(22)*, a cytokine whose interaction with its cognate receptor is involved in pericyte recruitment and viability *(23)*. Finally, vascular pericytes isolated from blood vessels or the retina fulfill the criteria for being multipotential mesenchymal precursors, demonstrating capability for differentiation into a variety of cell types, including osteoblasts, adipocytes, chondrocytes, and fibroblasts *(24–29)*.

FORMATION OF VASCULAR STRUCTURES DURING EMBRYOGENESIS: INTERRELATIONSHIP BETWEEN PERICYTES AND ENDOTHELIAL PRECURSORS

In order to develop successful methods for inducing neovascularization of the adult heart, one needs to understand the process of definitive vascular network formation during embryogenesis. In the prenatal period, hemangioblasts derived from the human ventral aorta give rise to cellular elements involved in both vasculogenesis, or formation of the primitive capillary network, and hematopoiesis *(30,31)*. Under the regulatory influence of various transcriptional and differentiation factors, embryonic hemangioblasts mature, migrate, and differentiate to become endothelial lining cells and create the primitive vasculogenic network. Subsequent to capillary tube formation, the newly created vasculogenic vessels undergo sprouting, tapering, remodeling, and regression under the direction of vascular endothelial growth factor (VEGF), angiopoietins, and other factors, a process termed angiogenesis. The final component required for definitive vascular network formation to sustain embryonic organogenesis is influx of mesenchymal lineage cells to form the vascular supporting mural cells such as vSMCs and pericytes.

The embryological origins of pericytes and vSMCs include mesenchymal cells surrounding the dorsal aorta *(32,33)*, neural crest cells in the forebrain and cardiac outflow tract *(34)*, and epicardial cells in heart coronary vessels *(35)*. In the mature vascular system, the endothelium is supported by mural cells, with the smallest capillaries partially covered by solitary pericytes and arteries and veins surrounded by single or multiple layers of vSMC. It has been suggested that pericytes and vSMCs represent a continuum of a common mural cell lineage and that pericytes may give rise to vSMCs during vessel enlargement or remodeling (arteriogenesis) *(36)*. The vSMCs provide structural support to large vessels and are important regulators of arteriolar blood flow because of contractile characteristics. Whereas pericytes com in direct contact with endothelial cells via N-cadherin- and β-catenin-based adherens junctions *(37)*, vSMCs are separated from the endothelium by a basement membrane and in larger arteries by the intima.

Pericytes form intimate connections with endothelial cells, with alterations in these interactions having significant consequences on microvasculature morphology and physiology. Injecting N-cadherin-neutralizing antibodies into the developing chick brain has profound effects on vascular integrity *(38)*, whereas injecting neutralizing PDGFR-β antibodies into newborn mice results in almost complete impairment of pericyte recruitment to the retinal microvasculature, with severe defects in vascular patterning *(39)*. Detailed analysis of the microvasculature in PDGF-B and PDGFR-β knockout mice demonstrates abnormal capillary diameters, rupturing micro-aneurysms, endothelial hyperplasia, defects in endothelial junction formation, and formation of numerous cytoplasmic folds at the luminal surface of the endothelium *(23)*. Together with physiological signs of hypoxia in these knockout animals, such as upregulation of VEGF-A expression *(23)*, these observations indicate that pericytes control endothelial differentiation in vivo, have a profound role in sprouting angiogenesis in the retina, and have a major effect on capillary blood flow in general.

HUMAN MESENCHYMAL PRECURSOR CELLS AS PROGENITORS OF THE VASCULAR NETWORK

As with development of other organs in the embryo, establishment of the primitive marrow stroma involves a complex series of events that require vascular invasion of primitive bone rudiments *(40)*. The relevance of the vascular system persists in the postnatal skeleton, with the medullary vascular network consisting of a continuous layer of endothelial cells and subendothelial pericytes and being shared by bone and bone marrow *(41,42)*. Under normal steady-state conditions, human bone marrow expression of α-SMA is limited to vSMCs in the media of arteries, pericytes lining capillaries, and occasional flattened cells on the endosteal surface of bone *(43)*. Strikingly, pericytes in the arterial and capillary sections of the medullary vascular network co-express α-SMA and STRO-1, consistent with the identity and anatomical location of stromal/mesenchymal progenitors as vSMCs/pericytes *(18)*.

The perivascular in vivo location of human mesenchymal lineage precursors, together with their co-expression of markers of both endothelial and smooth muscle lineage cells and their multipotential capabilities, raise the intriguing possibility that mesenchymal lineage precursors may be true progenitors of the vascular tree. This possibility is supported by work with embryonic stem cells, where a common flk-1[+] precursor gives rise to cells of both endothelial and smooth muscle lineage, resulting in development of the embryonic vasculature *(44,45)*.

The intimate proximity of human perivascular mesenchymal lineage precursors to vascular endothelium suggests that each cell type influences the biology of the other. Migration of mesenchymal lineage precursors and formation of a pericyte coating in physical continuity with the nascent vascular network is dependent on production of EGF and PDGF-B by nascent endothelial tubes *(46)*. Conversely, maintenance of vessel integrity, stabilization, and prevention of vessel pruning is dependent on pericyte coating of the microvessel *(46)*.

During normal bone development, new bone formation occurs in a precise spatial and temporal sequence, best visualized in metaphyseal growth plates. Importantly, new bone cell growth accompanies endothelial cell growth, pericyte coverage, and active angiogenesis. Inhibition of angiogenesis results in blockade of both metaphyseal endochondral bone formation and related activities in the adjacent cartilage growth plates *(47)*.

Together, these observations suggest that STRO-1$^+$ mesenchymal lineage precursors serve as important regulators of new blood vessel formation in the bone marrow, in growing bone, and, in view of their ubiquitous expression throughout the body, perhaps in various tissues during periods of growth, damage, or remodeling.

NEW VASCULAR NETWORK FORMATION AND LONG-TERM SURVIVAL OF CARDIOMYOCYTE PRECURSORS IMPLANTED INTO ISCHEMIC MYOCARDIUM

A major limitation to successful cellular therapy in animal models of myocardial damage has been the inability of the introduced donor cells to survive in their host environment, whether such transplants have been congenic (analogous to the autologous scenario in humans) or allogeneic. One major reason for the poor survival of transplanted cardiomyocytes or skeletal myoblasts is that viability and prolonged function of transplanted cells requires an augmented vascular supply. Recent studies have shown that development of thin-walled capillaries in ischemic myocardium following transplantation of hematopoietic lineage endothelial precursors enhances survival of endogenous cardiomyocytes *(48)*. Moreover, transplanting cultured cardiomyocytes that incorporate more vascular structures in vivo results in significantly greater cell survival and protection against apoptosis *(49)*. Finally, in situations where transplanted cardiomyocyte precursors contained an admixture of cells also giving rise to vascular structures, survival and function of the newly formed cardiomyocytes has been significantly augmented *(50)*.

As a corollary of the above, it is reasonable to anticipate that cellular therapies for the treatment of ischemic cardiomyopathy will need to address two interdependent processes: (1) a renewable source of proliferating, functional cardiomyocytes and (2) development of a network of capillaries and larger blood vessels for supply of oxygen and nutrients to both the chronically ischemic, endogenous myocardium and to the newly implanted cardiomyocytes. To achieve these endpoints, a common cellular source for regenerating cardiomyocytes, vascular structures, and supporting cells such as pericytes and smooth muscle cells would be ideal. The mesenchymal lineage precursor cell would appear to be just such a cellular source.

MESENCHYMAL PRECURSOR CELLS AS CARDIOMYOCYTE PROGENITORS

Over the past several years, a number of studies have suggested that stromal or mesenchymal lineage stem cells can be used to generate cardiomyocytes ex vivo for potential use in a range of cardiovascular diseases *(51–54)*. The newly generated cardiomyocytes appear to resemble normal cardiomyocytes in terms of phenotypic properties, such as expression of actinin, desmin, and troponin I, and function, including positive and negative chronotropic regulation of contractility by pharmacological agents and production of vasoactive factors such as atrial and brain natriuretic peptides *(51,52)*. Moreover, in vivo transplantation of bone marrow-derived mesenchymal lineage stem cells has resulted in incorporation within endogenous heart tissue *(53)* and in cardiac muscle differentiaiton *(54)*.

However, significant and sustained functional cardiac improvement following in vivo transplantation of stromal/mesenchymal lineage stem cell-derived cardiomyocytes has been exceedingly difficult to show to date. In part this may be because the signals required for cardiomyocyte differentiation and functional regulation are complex and poorly understood. For example, phenotypic and functional differentiation of mesenchymal stem cells to cardiomyocyte lineage cells in vitro requires culture with exogenously added 5-azacytidine *(55)*. An alternative explanation is that xenogeneic components of the culture media, such as bovine calf serum, result in immunogenic modification of the cells during the ex vivo culture process, as has been shown for myocardial implantation of skeletal muscle. In the absence of tissue culture, skeletal myoblast implantation does not induce any adverse immune response and results in grafts showing excellent survival for up to 1 year, whereas injection of cultured isolated (congenic) myoblasts results in a massive and rapid necrosis of donor myoblasts, with more than 90% dead within the first hour after injection *(56–58)*. Rejection of the cells modified by tissue culture conditions is mediated by host natural killer cells, which recognize foreign proteins on the surface of the modified autologous or congenic cells. Other possible reasons for lack of sufficient engraftment and long-term survival of these cells include the lack of appropriate survival signals present in the ischemic myocardium or within the matrix/scaffolds in which the cells are delivered. Methods to increase endogenous expression of cell survival signals, such as by Akt genetic modification of stromal/mesenchymal lineage cells, can result in prolonged cellular survival in vivo and functional cardiac recovery *(59)*.

POTENTIAL FOR ALLOGENEIC USE OF MESENCHYMAL LINEAGE PRECURSOR CELLS

Some of the most exciting data generated recently relates to the ability of mesenchymal lineage stem cells to evade recognition by the immune cells of unrelated recipients, raising the possibility that they may potentially constitute a source of allogeneic cellular therapeutic products. Despite the expression of human leukocyte antigen molecules on their cell surface, these cells do not induce allogeneic mixed lymphocyte responses, even after being differentiated to bone, cartilage, or adipocytes *(60,61)*. Moreover, they suppress third-party mixed lymphocyte responses in vitro in a dose-dependent manner *(62)* and can suppress an ongoing immune response in vivo, as demonstrated in a recent study in which haploidentical mesenchymal stem cells inhibited a potentially fatal graft-vs-host response in a bone marrow transplant recipient *(63)*.

Allogeneic mesenchymal stem cells loaded on hydroxyapatite–tricalcium phosphate implants enhanced the repair of a critical-sized segmental defect in the canine femur without the use of immunosuppressive therapy, with no adverse immune responses detected for up to 4 months of follow-up *(64)*. These are the first animal studies that support the feasibility of using allogeneic mesenchymal lineage cells for tissue regeneration. If similar studies can be extended to large animal models of cardiovascular disease, they would open the exciting prospect of using well-regulated, centrally manufactured, allogeneic mesenchymal lineage cell therapy in patients with heart disease.

CONCLUSIONS

Adult bone marrow stromal or mesenchymal lineage precursors can be isolated to great purity by physical and immunological techniques, expanded easily by ex vivo culture techniques, and used to generate both vascular networks and new heart muscle when implanted into ischemic myocardium. However, challenges remain in optimizing the culture-expansion protocols and techniques for delivery of these cells before they can be considered ready for in vivo human transplantation. Specifically, their capacity for vascular network formation needs to be harnessed, conditions to direct their differentiaton to cardiomyocytes need to be defined, immunogenic factors in the culture media need to be eliminated, and biological matrices/scaffolds in which the cells are delivered in vivo need to be optimized for providing adequate cell survival signals.

REFERENCES

1. Friedenstein AJ, Chailakhyan RK, Lalykina KS. The development of fibroblast colonies in monolayer cultures of guinea pig bone marrow and spleen cells. Cell Tissue Kinet 1970;3:393–402.
2. Gronthos S, Simmons PJ. The growth factor requirements of STRO-1-positive human bone marrow stromal precursors under serum-deprived conditions in vitro. Blood 1995;85:929–940.
3. Kuznetsov SA, Krebsbach PH, Satomura K, et al. Single-colony derived strains of human marrow stromal fibroblasts form bone after transplantation in vivo. J Bone Miner Res 1997;12:1335–1347.
4. Satomura K, Krebsbach P, Bianco P, et al. Osteogenic imprinting upstream of marrow stromal cell differentiation. J Cell Biochem 2000;78:391–403.
5. Friedenstein AJ, Latzinik NW, Grosheva AG, et al. Marrowmicroenvironment transfer by heterotopic transplantation of freshly isolated and cultured cells in porous sponges. Exp Hematol 1982;10:217–227.
6. Ashton BA, Allen TD, Howlett CR, et al. Formation of bone and cartilage by marrow stromal cells in diffusion chambers in vivo. Clin Orthop 1980;151:294–307.
7. Pittenger MF, Mackay AM, Beck SC, et al. Multilineage potential of adult human mesenchymal stem cells. Science 1999;284:143–147.
8. Simmons PJ, Torok-Storb B. Identification of stromal cell precursors in human bone marrow by a novel monoclonal antibody, STRO-1. Blood 1991;78:55–62.
9. Haynesworth SE, Baber MA, Caplan AI. Cell surface antigens on human marrow-derived mesenchymal cells are detected by monoclonal antibodies. Bone 1992;13:69–80.
10. Joyner CJ, Bennett A, Triffitt JT. Identification and enrichment of human osteoprogenitor cells by using differentiation stage-specific monoclonal antibodies. Bone 1997;21:1–6.
11. Gronthos S, Graves SE, Ohta S, et al. The STRO-1+ fraction of adult human bone marrow contains the osteogenic precursors. Blood 1994;84:4164–4173.
12. Simmons PJ, Torok-Storb B. Identification of stromal cell precursors in human bone marrow by a novel monoclonal antibody, STRO-1. Blood 1991;78:55–62.
13. Gronthos S, Simmons PJ. The biology and application of human bone marrow stromal cell precursors. J Hematother 1996;5:15–23.
14. Simmons PJ, Gronthos S, Zannettino A, et al. Isolation, characterization and functional activity of human marrow stromal progenitors in hemopoiesis. Prog Clin Biol Res 1994;389:271–280.
15. Filshie RJ, Zannettino AC, Makrynikola V, et al. MUC18, a member of the immunoglobulin superfamily, is expressed on bone marrow fibroblasts and a subset of hematological malignancies. Leukemia 1998;12:414–421.
16. Gronthos S, Mankani M, Brahim J, et al. Postnatal human dental pulp stem cells (DPSCs) in vitro and in vivo. Proc Natl Acad Sci USA 2000;97:13,625–13,630.
17. Gronthos S, Zannettino AC, Hay SJ, et al. Molecular and cellular characterisation of highly purified stromal stems derived from human bone marrow. J Cell Sci 2003;116:1827–1835.
18. Shi S, Gronthos S. Perivascular niche of postnatal mesenchymal stem cells in human bone marrow and dental pulp. J Bone Miner Res 2003;18:696–704.
19. Galmiche MC, Koteliansky VE, Briere J, Herve P, Charbord P. Stromal cells from human long-term marrow cultures are mesenchymal cells that differentiate following a vascular smooth muscle differentiation pathway. Blood 1993;82:66–76.
20. Schor AM, Canfield AE. Osteogenic potential of vascular pericytes. In: Beresford JN, Owen ME, eds. Marrow Stromal Cell Culture. Cambridge University Press, Cambridge, UK, 1998, pp. 128–148.
21. Zuckerman KS, Wicha MS. Extracellular matrix production by the adherent cells of long-term murine bone marrow cultures. Blood 1983;61:540–547.

22. Gronthos S, Simmons PJ. The growth factor requirements of STRO-1+ human bone marrow stromal precursors under serum-deprived conditions. Blood 1995;85:929–940.
23. Hellstrom M, Kalen M, Lindahl P, Abramsson A, Betsholtz C. Role of PDGF-B and PDGFR-beta in recruitment of vascular smooth muscle cells and pericytes during embryonic blood vessel formation in the mouse. Development 1999;126:3047–3055.
24. Schor AM, Canfield AE, Sutton AB, Arciniegas E, Allen TD. Pericyte differentiation. Clin Orthop 1995;313:81–91.
25. Sims DE. The pericyte—a review. Tissue Cell 1986;18:153–174.
26. Diaz-Flores L, Gutiérrez R, Gonzales P, Varela H. Inducible perivascular cells contribute to the neo-chondrogenesis in grafted perichondrium. Anat Rec 1991;229:1–8.
27. Doherty MJ, Ashton BA, Walsh S, Beresford JN, Grant ME, Canfield AE. Vascular pericytes express osteogenic potential in vitro and in vivo. J Bone Miner Res 1998;13:828–838.
28. Doherty MJ, Canfield AE. Gene expression during vascular pericyte differentiation. Crit Rev Eukaryot Gene Exp 1999;9:1–17.
29. Brighton CT, Lorich DG, Kupcha R, Reilly TM, Jones AR, Woodbury, 2nd, RA. The pericyte as a possible osteoblast progenitor cell. Clin Orthop 1992;275:287–299.
30. Tavian M, Coulombel L, Luton D, San Clemente H, Dieterlen-Lievre F, Peault B. Aorta-associated CD34 hematopoietic cells in the early human embryo. Blood 1996;87:67–72.
31. Jaffredo T, Gautier R, Eichmann A, Dieterlen-Lievre F. Intraaortic hemopoietic cells are derived from endothelial cells during ontogeny. Development 1998;125:4575–4583.
32. Drake CJ, Hungerford JE, Little CD. Morphogenesis of the first blood vessels. Ann NY Acad Sci 1998;857:155–179.
33. Hungerford JE, Little CD. Developmental biology of the vascular smooth muscle cell: building a multilayered vessel wall. J Vasc Res 1999;36:2–27.
34. Bergwerff M, Verberne ME, DeRuiter MC, Poelmann RE, Gittenbergerde Groot AC. Neural crest cell contribution to the developing circulatory system: implications for vascular morphology? Circ Res 1998;82:221–231.
35. Etchevers HC, Couly GF, Le Douarin NM. Morphogenesis of the branchial vascular sector. Trends Cardiovasc Med 2002;12:299–304.
36. Vrancken Peeters MP, Gittenberger-de Groot AC, Mentink MM, Poelmann RE. Smooth muscle cells and fibroblasts of the coronary arteries derive from the epithelial-mesenchymal transformation of the epicardium. Anat Embryol (Berl) 1999;199:367–378.
37. D'Amore PA. Capillary growth: a two-cell system. Semin Cancer Biol 1997;3:49–56.
38. Gerhardt H, Wolburg H, Redies C. N-Cadherin mediates pericytic endothelial interaction during brain angiogenesis in the chicken. Dev Dyn 2000;218:472–479.
39. Uemura A, Ogawa M, Hirashima M, et al. Recombinant angiopoietin-1 restores higher-order architecture of growing blood vessels in mice in the absence of mural cells. J Clin Invest 2002;110:1619–1628.
40. Bianco P, Riminucci M. The bone marrow stroma in vivo: ontogeny, structure, cellular composition and changes in disease. In: Beresford JN, Owen M, eds. Marrow Stromal Cell Cultures. Cambridge University Press, Cambridge, UK, 1998, pp. 10–25.
41. Ascenzi A. Physiological relationship and pathological interferences between bone tissue and marrow. In: Bourne GH, ed. The Biochemistry and Physiology of Bone. Academic Press, New York, 1976, pp. 403–445.
42. Andreeva ER, Pugach IM, Gordon D, et al. Continuous subendothelial network formed by pericyte-like cells in human vascular bed. Tissue Cell 1998;30:127–135.
43. Bianco P, Riminucci M, Gronthos S, Robey PG. Bone marrow stromal stem cells: nature, biology, and potential applications. Stem Cells 2001;19:180–192.
44. Ema M, Faloon P, Zhang WJ, et al. Combinatorial effects of Flk1 and Tal1 on vascular and hematopoietic development in the mouse. Genes Dev 2003;17:380–393.
45. Yamashita J, Itoh H, Hirashima M, et al. Flk1-positive cells derived from embryonic stem cells serve as vascular progenitors. Nature 2000;408:92–96.
46. Benjamin LE, Hemo I, Keshet E. A plasticity window for blood vessel remodelling is defined by pericyte coverage of the preformed endothelial network and is regulated by PDGF-B and VEGF. Development 1998;125:1591–1598.
47. Gerber HP, Vu TH, Ryan AM et al. VEGF couples hypertrophic cartilage remodeling, ossification and angiogenesis during endochondral bone formation. Nat Med 1999;5:623–628.
48. Kocher AA, Schuster MD, Szabolcs MJ, et al. Neovascularization of ischemic myocardium by human bone-marrow-derived angioblasts prevents cardiomyocyte apoptosis, reduces remodeling and improves cardiac function. Nat Med 2001;7:430–436.

49. Klug MG, Soonpaa MH, Koh GY, Field LJ. Genetically selected cardiomyocytes from differentiating embryonic stem cells form stable intracardiac grafts. J Clin Invest 1996;98:216–224.
50. Hescheler J, Fleischmann BK, Wartenberg M, et al. Establishment of ionic channels and signalling cascades in the embryonic stem cell-derived primitive endoderm and cardiovascular system. Cells Tissues Organs 1999;165:153–164.
51. Makino S, Fukuda K, Miyoshi S, et al. Cardiomyocytes can be generated from marrow stromal cells in vitro. J Clin Invest 1999;103:697–705.
52. Tomita S, Li R-K, Weisel RD, et al. Autologous transplantation of bone marrow cells improves damaged heart function. Circulation 1999;100:II-247.
53. Liechty KW, MacKenzie TC, Shaaban AF, et al. Human mesenchymal stem cells engraft and demonstrate site-specific differentiation after in utero transplantation in sheep. Nat Med 2000;6:1282–1286.
54. Toma C, Pittenger MF, Cahill KS, Byrne BJ, Kessler, D. Human mesenchymal stem cells differentiate to a cardiomyocyte phenotype in the adult murine heart. Circulation 2003;105:93–96.
55. Beauchamp JR, Morgan JE, Pagel CN, Partridge TA. Dynamics of myoblast transplantation reveal a discrete minority of precursors with stem cell-like properties as the myogenic source. J Cell Biol 1999;144:1113–1122.
56. Smythe GM, Grounds MD. Exposure to tissue culture conditions can adversely affect myoblast behaviour in vivo in whole muscle grafts: implications for myoblast transfer therapy. Cell Transplant 2000;9:379–393.
57. Smythe GM, Hodgetts SI, Grounds MD. Problems and solutions in myoblast transfer therapy. J Cell Mol Med 2001;5:33–47.
58. Hodgetts SI, Beilharz MW, Scalzo T, Grounds MD. Why do cultured transplanted myoblasts die in vivo? DNA quantification shows enhanced survival of donor male myoblasts in host mice depleted of CD4+ and CD8+ or NK1.1+ cells. Cell Transplant 2000;9:489–502.
59. Mangi AA, Noiseux N, Kong D, et al. Mesenchymal stem cells modified with Akt prevent remodeling and restore performance of infarcted hearts. Nat Med 2003;9:1195–1201.
60. Di Nicola M, Carlo-Stella C, Magni M, et al. Human bone marrow stromal cells suppress T-lymphocyte proliferation induced by cellular or nonspecific mitogenic stimuli. Blood 2002;99:3838–3843.
61. Le Blanc K, Tammik C, Rosendahl K, Zetterberg E, Ringdén O. HLA expression and immunologic propertiesof differentiated and undifferentiated mesenchymal stem cells. Exp Hematol 2003;31:890–896.
62. Tse WT, Pendleton JD, Beyer WM, Egalka MC, Guinan E. Suppression of allogeneic T-cell proliferation by human marrow stromal cells: implications in transplantation. Transplantation 2003;75:389–397.
63. Le Blanc K, Rasmusson I, Sundberg B, et al. Treatment of severe acute graft-versus-host disease with third party haploidentical mesenchymal stem cells. Lancet 2004;363:1439–1441.
64. Arinzeh TL, Peter SJ, Archambault MP, et al. Allogeneic mesenchymal stem cells regenerate bone in a critical-sized canine segmental defect. J Bone Joint Surg Am 2003;85-A(10):1927–1935.

6

Umbilical Cord Blood Stem Cells for Myocardial Regeneration and Angiogenesis

Shyam Bhakta, MD and Mary J. Laughlin, MD

SUMMARY

Limitations of revascularization for ischemic heart disease include incompleteness of revascularization, even for surgical revascularization, especially for calcified lesions in distal segments of small-caliber vessels. Revascularization has not been shown to regenerate functional, viable myocardium from scarred and infarcted myocardium. Previous alternatives to revascularization such as transmyocardial laser revascularization, gene therapy, and orthotopic heart transplantation also have many disadvantages that limit their use in high-risk patients such as those with recent myocardial infarction and advanced heart failure.

Although preclinical and early clinical studies in cardiovascular disease of adult-derived stem cells have shown promise, many limitations remain. Umbilical cord blood (UCB)-derived stem cells have several advantages over adult stem cells, including ease of harvesting and storage and decreased risk for immune intolerance and transmission of infectious agents. Here we summarize our laboratory's preclinical in vitro and in vivo studies of UCB-derived stem cells: their phenotypic characterization, ability for neovascularization in a murine femoral artery ligation hindlimb ischemia model, reduced likelihood of stimulating an immune response, and interaction with stem cells of other origins.

Key Words: Umbilical cord blood hematopoietic stem cells; AC133[+] cells; vasculogenesis; coronary ischemia.

UMBILICAL CORD BLOOD-DERIVED STEM CELLS IN MYOCARDIAL REGENERATION AND VASCULOGENESIS

Umbilical cord blood (UCB) contains pluripotent stem cells, can be harvested after birth, and may have clinical and logistical advantages over individual patient adult-derived stem cells in potential application for therapeutic vasculogenesis *(1)*. These clinical advantages include UCB collection at no risk to the donor, greater accessibility for storage, immediate availability in a bank, wider availability of diverse human leukocyte antigen (HLA) genotypes, lower immune reactivity, and lower inherent pathogen transmission. UCB has a further advantage in that it is not subject to the social and political controversy related to embryonic stem cells. UCB is unique in that it is the

From: *Contemporary Cardiology: Stem Cells and Myocardial Regeneration*
Edited by: M. S. Penn © Humana Press Inc., Totowa, NJ

only tissue for which transplantation across HLA barriers has been successful *(2)*. UCB has been shown to be a prolific source of hematopoietic stem cells (HSCs). Single UCB units can reconstitute entire lympho-hematopoietic systems in adult patients *(3)*. UCB has significantly greater concentrations of HSCs, higher proliferation capacity, and longer telomeres than equivalent aliquots of adult peripheral blood or marrow. Current collection and banking practice limits units suitable for cryopreservation to those containing nucleated cell doses exceeding 900 million. HLA-matched UCB-derived HSCs therefore may have distinct advantages as a cell source including greater potential life span and greater reparative proliferation relative to existing models of therapeutic angiogenesis derived from patient peripheral blood or marrow.

UCB STEM CELLS AND VASCULOGENESIS

CD133+ Hemangioblasts

CD133+ HSCs are of particular interest in studies directed to therapeutic angiogenesis, as reports by Asahara and other groups indicate that these cells differentiate into endothelial cells after short-term culture *(4)*. HSCs are a heterogeneous cell population with varying proliferative and developmental capabilities. Of particular relevance to HSC studies in vasculogenesis is CD105 (endoglin) expression on HSCs and their responsiveness to exogenous vascular endothelial growth factor (VEGF) *(5)*. Our Case faculty group has previously reported that human mesenchymal stem cells (MSCs) also express CD105 *(6)*, rendering this cell population potentially responsive to VEGF elicited after vascular injury. Further relevant studies in HSC manipulation in vitro to optimize cellular infusion products for specific therapeutic applications in vasculogenesis include recent insights into HSC cycle regulation *(7)* as well as the critical role of specific regulatory proteins exemplified by EphB4 (HTK) and its ligand, ephrinB2, which have been shown to be critical for angiogenesis and result in fatal abnormalities of capillary formation in null mice. EphB4 has been shown to be expressed in erythroid progenitors, whereas its ligand ephrinB2 is expressed in bone marrow (BM) stromal cells, pointing to the important interplay between HSCs and MSCs in vasculogenesis and hematopoiesis *(8)*.

Hemangioblast and Stromal Cell Interactions

We have previously reported extensive research on methods to isolate, culture-expand, and phenotypically characterize human MSCs as well as their multilineage developmental potential and capacity to regulate a variety of other developmental events including angiogenesis *(6,9)*. Although MSCs are rare, comprising 0.01–0.0001% of the total nucleated cells of BM, we have perfected a cell culture methodology for their isolation from BM, purification to homogeneity from other BM cells, and mitotic expansion in culture without loss of their stem cell potential *(10)*. Human adult MSCs, although marrow derived, fail to express CD34 or CD45, but have been shown to express interleukin (IL)-6, -7, -8, -11, -12, -14, and -15, macrophage colony-stimulating factor, flt-3 ligand, and stem cell factor (SCF) in steady state but do not express IL-3 and transforming growth factor (TGF)-β. Exposure to dexamethasone results in decreased expression of leukocyte inhibitory factor, IL-6, and IL-11 *(11)*. Moreover, adhesion molecules expressed by stromal cells of importance in supporting early hemangioblasts include fibulin-1 and fibulin-2, tenascin-C, stromal cell-derived factor-1 (SDF-1), and collagen type VI.

Human MSCs home to sites of vascular injury and augment neovasculogenesis in concert with early hemangioblasts via secreted soluble factors and direct cell contact effects.

Vasculogenesis is a complex biological process requiring interaction of multiple cellular and cytokine factors. Few studies focus on interactions between mesenchymal and endothelial cells during the process of neovascularization. Induction of an angiogenic phenotype in microvascular endothelial cells in vitro and promotion of angiogenesis in vivo by cultured fibrocytes has been previously reported (12). In addition, vasculogenesis by early hemangioblasts has been shown to be augmented in the presence of mesenchymal cells (13). Mesenchymal cells constitutively secrete extracellular matrix-degrading enzymes, primarily matrix metalloproteinase 9, which promote endothelial cell invasion. In addition, mesenchymal cells secrete several pro-angiogenic factors, including VEGF, basic fibroblast growth factor (bFGF), IL-8, platelet-derived growth factor, and hematopoietic growth factors that promote endothelial cell migration, proliferation, and/or tube formation (12,14). Taken together, these reports point to potential synergy between endothelial and mesenchymal cells in mediating neovasculogenesis in response to vessel injury.

UCB-DERIVED STEM CELLS IN ACUTE MYOCARDIAL INFARCTION

The noncontroversial nature of umbilical cord blood stem cells has led several groups to study the effects of injection of UCB stem cells (UCBSCs) on cardiac function following acute myocardial infarction (MI). The first reported study was by Henning and colleagues, who studied the effects of 1 million mononuclear UCBSCs injected directly into the infarct border zone 1 hour after left anterior descending ligation in a rat model (15). Of note, these studies were performed without immunosuppression in immune-competent rats. They demonstrated that this strategy led to significant improvement in cardiac function and left ventricular wall thickness as measured by echocardiography and invasive hemodynamics. Furthermore, in response to phenylephrine, the human UCBSC-treated group had myocardial functional reserve similar to that in sham-infarcted animals (15).

Since the study by Henning et al., multiple groups have demonstrated that the delivery of UCBSCs has the potential to improve cardiac function in animal models (16–19). Leor and colleagues studied the intravenous infusion of approx 2 million CD133+ human UCBSCs into athymic nude mice 1 week after permanent left anterior descending artery (LAD) ligation (18). One month later, those animals that received UCBSCs had improved cardiac function of approx 42%; those that received saline 1 week after MI exhibited a 39% decline in function (18). Similar findings have been observed in an immunosuppressed porcine model using human unrestricted somatic stem cells isolated from umbilical cord (17). Ma and colleagues further demonstrated that UCBSCs will not enter the myocardium unless myocardial injury has occurred (18) and suggest that stem cell homing factors such as SDF-1 (20,21) are required to recruit UCBSCs to the myocardium. One of the difficulties of UCBSC-based therapies is the limited amount of cell material obtained from a single cord. To address this issue, Mal et al. studied the effects of culture-expanded UCBSC CD34+-derived cells in nude rats following LAD ligation. Whether these expanded cells were directly injected into the infarct zone (2 million cells) at the time of MI or infused via the tail vein 1 day after MI (4 million cells), shortening fraction was improved approx 97% compared to saline controls (22).

The exact mechanism for improvement in cardiac function with UCBSCs is unclear; however, there is little credible evidence for regeneration of cardiac myocytes. Consistent in all studies is evidence of angiogenesis or vasculogenesis (17,18) and improvement in left ventricular remodeling (16,18). Interestingly, there is a paucity of

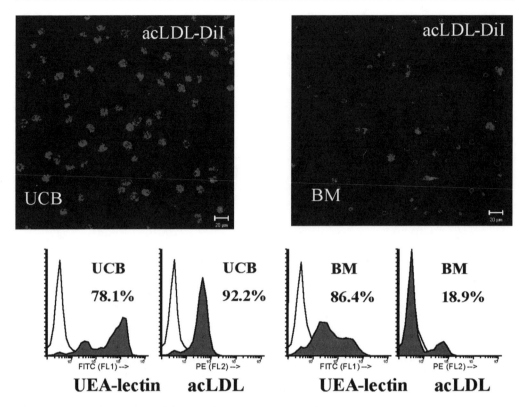

Fig. 1. Characteristics of umbilical cord blood (UCB)- and bone marrow (BM)-derived endothelial progenitor cells. Mononuclear cells from fresh UCB or BM were isolated and cultured under endothelial conditions for 7 d. Two principal cytochemical staining features of endothelial cells are the adherence of specific lectin proteins and the uptake of acetylated low-density lipoprotein (acLDL). Fluorescent microscopy of adherent cells was utilized to assess uptake of acLDL (red) and Ulex Europeas (UEA) lectin after 7 d of culture. Images shown here were representative and taken at 40x with a Zeiss LSM510 microscope. The cultures were then analyzed by flow cytometry to verify the results. (*See* color insert following p. 114.)

chimeric vessels or evidence of UCBSC differentiation into the endothelium of newly formed vessels, suggesting that the benefit of UCBSCs in myocardial function may be a result of paracrine effects. Consistent with this hypothesis is the observation that UCBSCs engineered to overexpress VEGF and angiotensin-1 demonstrated increased benefit when compared with control UCBSCs *(23)*.

ONGOING STUDIES AT CASE WESTERN RESERVE UNIVERSITY

Isolation and Characterization of Endothelial Progenitor Cells From UCB and Bone Marrow

Mononuclear cells (MNCs) from fresh UCB or BM were isolated by density-gradient centrifugation. Cells were plated on fibronectin-coated tissue culture flasks at a density of $4–6 \times 10^6$ cells/mL (UCB MNCs) or $1–2 \times 10^6$ cells/mL (BM MNCs) in EBM2 medium (Clonetics™) with 5% fetal bovine serum (FBS). In addition, the media was supplemented with standard SingleQuot™ additives that included VEGF, fibroblast growth factor, insulin-like growth factor, hydrocortisone, ascorbic acid, and heparin.

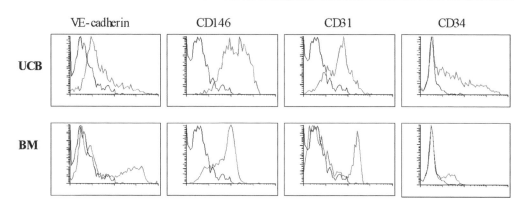

Fig. 2. Flow cytometric analysis of endothelial progenitor cells derived from umbilical cord blood (UCB) vs bone marrow (BM). UCB was cultured for 19 d, and BM for 12 d, in media, and adherent cells were trypsinized and stained for CD34 and the endothelial-specific markers VE-cadherin, CD146, and CD31. Nonstained control is shown in black; stained cells are shown in grey.

Nonadherent cells were removed after 4 days of culture, and medium was changed every fourth day thereafter. Adherent cell yield from UCB cultures was on average $2.5 \pm 0.4\%$ of initial MNC input compared to $21.5 \pm 3.7\%$ obtained from BM MNCs. Fluorescent microscopy of adherent cells revealed that the majority exhibited uptake of acetylated low-density lipoprotein. A smaller proportion exhibited positive staining for Ulex Europeas (UEA) lectin (Fig. 1).

Flow Cytometric Analysis of Endothelial Progenitor Cells Derived From UCB vs Bone Marrow

Further characterization was conducted of unselected UCB and BM MNCs cultured in endothelial progenitor cell (EPC) conditions. Adherent cells were trypsinized and stained for CD34 and mature endothelial-specific markers CD146 (P1H12, MUC18, or MCAM), CD31, and VE-cadherin, with more than 60% of the cultured adherent cells positive for CD146. CD31 expression was 25% in BM-derived EPCs compared with 50% in UCB-derived cells. However, CD31 staining was brighter in BM-derived EPCs. VE-cadherin was expressed in 10% of cells from BM compared to 24% in the cells from UCB. UCB-derived EPCs showed expression of CD34 in 25% of cells compared to 10% of the BM-derived EPCs (Fig. 2).

Functional Analysis of UCB-Derived and Bone Marrow-Derived Endothelial Progenitor Cells In Vivo

Severe Combined Immunodeficient–Nonobese Diabetic Murine Hindlimb Injury Model

EPCs (adherent cells only) were harvested at day 7, and 1×10^6 cells/mouse were injected into hind limb-injured mice after femoral artery ligation. Immediately after surgery and cell injection, baseline blood flow of both the ischemic right leg and the nonoperated left leg was measured by a laser Doppler flowmeter. Study mice were injected with EPCs derived from either UCB or BM. Control mice were injected with saline or complete EBM2 medium. Laser Doppler measurements of both hind limbs were taken on days 7, 14, and 28. A ratio of perfusion in the ischemic limb vs the healthy limb was used to compare neovascularization in the three study groups.

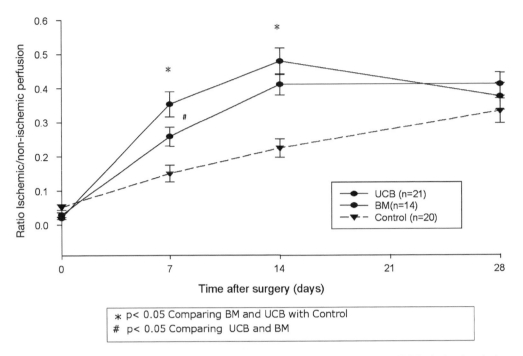

Fig. 3. Functional analysis of umbilical cord blood (UCB)- and bone marrow (BM)-derived endothelial progenitor cells in vivo in the nonobese (NOD)–severe combined immune-deficient (SCID) femoral artery ligation hindlimb injury model. NOD-SCID mice underwent femoral artery ligation and excision followed by intracardiac injection of saline, medium, or cells cultured for 7 d. Laser Doppler measurements were taken postoperatively and then at 7,14, and 28 days under the same conditions. Depicted is a comparison of the perfusion ratios between the ischemic and nonischemic legs.

Immediately following femoral ligation, the perfusion ratios were 0.057 ± 0.011 (control group), 0.029 ± 0.007 (UCB-derived EPCs), and 0.020 ± 0.004 (BM-derived EPCs), showing reduced perfusion in all groups (Fig. 3). After 14 d there was a statistically significant higher blood flow in the injured leg in study groups receiving UCB-derived EPCs between the control group ($p < 0.05$) and between the BM-derived EPC group and the control group ($p < 0.001$). Perfusion ratios in the control group remained low, with 0.24 ± 0.032 ($n = 14$) compared to 0.41 ± 0.031 ($n = 22$) in the group receiving UCB-derived EPCs ($p = 0.0008$) and 0.48 ± 0.039 ($n = 14$) in the group receiving BM-derived EPCs. Importantly, at day 14 there was no significant difference between the two sources of EPCs ($p = 0.18$). Subsequent measurements at 28 days was notable for improvement in Doppler blood flow in control animals, rendering perfusion ratios equalized when comparing the control group to mice receiving cell infusions.

HISTOLOGY CONFIRMATION STUDIES

Tissue from the lower calf muscle of both hind limbs was harvested at day 28 for histological evaluation. Samples were fresh-frozen in liquid nitrogen and fixed in formalin. Frozen sections of 6-μm thickness were mounted on saline-coated glass slides and stained using immunohistochemistry technique to identify incorporation of EPCs derived from human cells by staining with human anti-CD31 antibody. Specimens from mice injected with EPCs showed positive staining for CD31, whereas control mice injected with complete EBM2 medium did not. Healthy limbs of all groups did not show positive CD31 staining (data not shown). Further histological analyses included assessment of capillary density by alkaline phosphatase staining. Animals treated with EPCs derived from either marrow or UCB demonstrated significantly higher capillary density at 28 days compared with saline/cytokine controls. Taken together, these results support the hypothesis that UCB demonstrates equivalent biological effect in the in vivo model to that exerted by EPCs derived from BM sources.

Selection of AC133+ Cells From UCB and Characterization of Early Events During Vascular Endothelial Differentiation

Our initial studies demonstrated that nonselected UCB cells proliferate rapidly and expand in endothelial cell culture conditions. These UCB-derived EPCs exhibited multiple endothelial characteristics and functionality. Our next experiments included cell selection of CD133+ from UCB. Selected CD133+ cells were characterized by flow cytometry and staining for CD34 and CD133 (Fig. 4). Distinct populations of CD133+/CD34− and CD133+/CD34+ cells were identified. For isolation and purification, CD133+ cells from UCB MNCs were labeled with CD133-conjugated magnetic beads followed by automated sorting through magnetic columns (Automacs, Miltenyi). By passaging the labeled cells through one column, routine yield was 1.6% of MNCs, with a purity ranging between 75 and 85%.

Differential Expression of CD45, CD34, BCL-2, and p21 in Purified CD133+ Cells After 24 Hours of Culture

Purified CD133+ cells from UCB were cultured in conditions described below in hematopoiesis-driving cytokines as well as in cytokines reported to generate endothelial cells from CD133+ cells (31). After 24 hours of incubation, cells were analyzed by flow cytometry for CD34 and CD45, as well as for expression of BCL-2 and p21 (Fig. 5). CD45 and CD34 expression was strongly increased after 24 hours of culture in hematopoiesis lineage-specific cytokines. CD45 expression was entirely lost after culture in endothelial cytokines, suggesting that the cells had already started differentiation away from hematopoietic lineage.

Further analysis included expression of the cell cycle and apoptosis-regulating proteins p21$^{cip1/waf}$ and BCL-2, which have been shown to play a role in regulation of HSC fate. p21$^{cip1/waf1}$, an inhibitor of cyclin-dependent kinases, mediates cell cycle arrest in G1. It has been shown that in p21$^{cip1/waf1}$-deficient mice there is increased proliferation of HSCs under normal homeostatic conditions and exhaustion of the stem cell pool. This suggests that p21$^{cip1/waf1}$ may be a molecular switch governing the entry of HSCs into the cell cycle (24). Overexpression of the antiapoptotic protein BCL-2 in the hematopoietic compartment of transgenic mice has been shown to improve numbers of HSC as well as in vitro plating capacity and to maintain HSCs in a more quiescent cell cycle status. Expression of both p21 and BCL-2 proteins was increased in hematopoietic cytokine conditions. Interestingly, however, expression of both proteins decreased significantly in vascular endothelial cytokine conditions, again suggesting that the two AC133 cell populations have initiated differential gene expression at this early (24-hour) time point.

Cell Cycle Analysis of Cultured CD133+ Cells

Further analysis included measurement of cell cycle stages in freshly isolated CD133+ cells as well as in CD133+ cells after 24 hours of culture in either medium (IMDM, 2% FBS) or hematopoietic or endothelial cytokines. As expected, freshly isolated CD133+ cells were resting in G_0 phase (99%). Interestingly, after 24 hours of culture in cytokines, we did not observe significant cellular division in hematopoietic

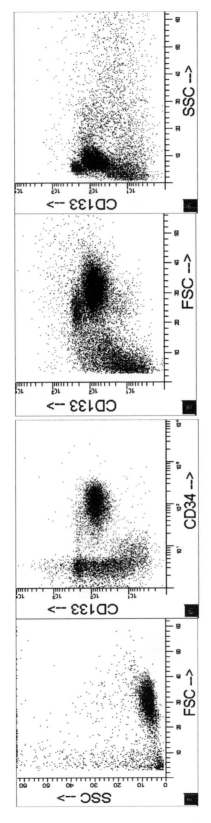

Fig. 4. Selection of AC133+ cells from UCB and characterization of early events during vascular endothelial differentiation.

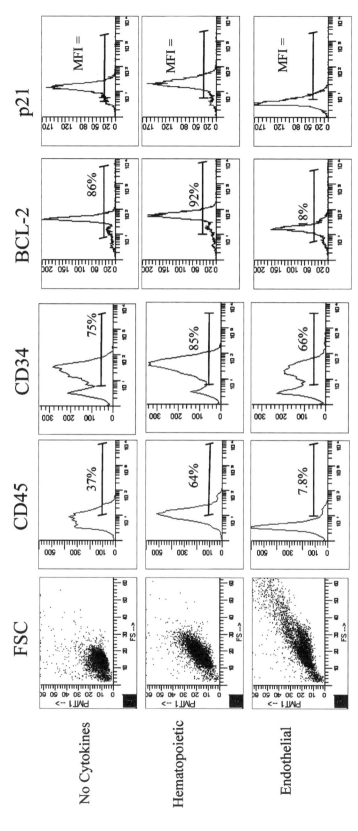

Fig. 5. Differential expression of CD45, CD34, BCL-2, and p21 in purified CD133$^+$ cells after 24 h of culture. CD133$^+$ cells were selected as above, and 0.2 × 10^6 cells/well/condition were plated on a 96-well plate and incubated for 24 h in either medium alone (IMDM) with 2% FBS, in hematopoietic conditions (IMDM, 30% FBS, 50 ng/mL of SCF, 20 ng/mL of GM-CSF, G-CSF, IL-3, IL-6, 3U/mL of EPO) or endothelial conditions (IMDM, 10% FBS, 10% horse serum, 1 mM hydrocortisone, 100 ng/mL of SCGF, 50 ng/mL of VEGF). Cells were surface stained for CD45 and CD34 and permeabilized and stained for BCL-2 and p21 expression. Percentages are out of total cells analyzed.

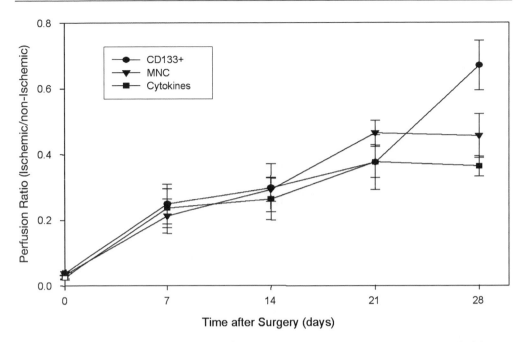

Fig. 6. Neovascularization by purified CD133$^+$ cells vs mononuclear stem cells (MNCs). Purified CD133 cells (0.5×10^6) from umbilical cord blood ($n = 3$) were injected intracardiac after femoral artery ligation. Comparison groups included crude MNCs (1.0×10^6) ($n = 5$) and cytokines alone ($n = 4$). Blood flow measured by Doppler over time is expressed as ratio of the injured leg to the noninjured leg.

or endothelial conditions, with the majority of the cells (93–94%) remaining in G_0 phase at that point. These preliminary data of differential protein expression after only 24 hours of incubation in hematopoietic vs vascular endothelial specific cytokines indicate that although no significant cell division has yet taken place, the CD133$^+$ cell has already progressed along differential gene expression programs. More importantly, with no cellular division having occurred, cells cultured in hematopoietic cytokine conditions remain, in effect, the same cells as plated, with only changes in gene expression patterns. The same is valid for the cells plated in endothelial conditions.

Neovascularization by Endothelial Progenitor Cells Derived From Purified CD133$^+$ Cells

After hindlimb femoral artery ligation, 0.5×10^6 selected CD133$^+$ cells, 1×10^6 MNCs, or cytokines (EGM2 medium) were given via intracardiac injection. Data from this limited set ($n = 3$) showed significantly increased blood flow in mice receiving CD133$^+$ cells 28 days after surgery when compared to MNCs or control cytokines ($p = 0.03$) (Fig. 6).

Mixed Lymphocyte Culture: Adult Lymphocyte Proliferative Response to Umbilical Cord Blood CD133$^+$ Stem Cells

One important concern with the use of UCB as source material for AC133$^+$ for vasculogenesis therapeutic intent is the potential alloreactivity exerted by patient immune cells in response to the intracoronary infusion of HLA-mismatched UCB AC133$^+$-selected cells. To determine whether AC133$^+$-selected cells from UCB elicit robust

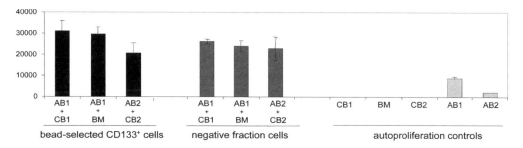

Fig. 7. Proliferation elicited by purified CD133+ in standard MLR. CD133+ cells were magnetic bead-selected from 2 UCB units (CB1, CB2) and 1 BM, irradiated and 0.1×10^6 cells were presented as stimulators to 0.3×10^6 responder MNC from 2 different adults (AB1, AB2), incubated for 72 h, labeled with ^{3}H-thymidine for an additional 18 h, harvested and thymidine incorporation analyzed. Proliferation was compared to the response elicited by the cells of the negative fraction, i.e., the cells not retained on the magnetic column.

lymphocyte response in normal adults, we performed mixed lymphocyte culture to measure the degree of proliferation of adult blood (AB) lymphocytes in the presence of selected AC133± stimulator cells from HLA-disparate UCB. Cells were cultured at a 3:1 stimulator (UCB AC133) to responder (AB) ratio. Responder AB lymphocytes were stained with carboxyfluorescein diacetate succinimidyl ester (CFSE) and cultured for 24, 72, and 120 hours with AC133 stimulator cells selected from UCB using an automated magnetic column (AutoMACS, Miltenyi). Appropriate passive hemagglutination (PHA) controls were run concomitantly (Fig. 7).

As can be seen in Fig. 7 both BM- and UCB-derived CD133+ cells elicit in vitro proliferation of allogeneic MNCs derived from healthy adults. This proliferation response is comparable in amplitude to that elicited by the CD 133-negative fractions containing MNCs from which CD133+ cells were selected. These results suggest that allogeneic CD133+ cell transplantation may elicit an immune response in an immunocompetent adult.

When UCB-derived CD133+ cells stimulated healthy adult-derived CFSE-labeled MNCs (AB), proliferation above autoproliferation of adult-derived MNCs (Fig. 8, AB alone panel) was visible.

In conclusion, our preliminary data showing HLA expression on UCB-derived CD133+ cells and the immune proliferation elicited by them strongly suggests that selected CD133+ cells may elicit an immune response when transplanted into immunocompetent patients.

UCB-CD133+ Ex Vivo Expansion

Potential clinical application of UCB-derived CD133 progenitors is limited by the small cell content of collected UCB. We anticipate this significant problem and have established a collaboration with Takayuki Asahara at Tokai University School of Medicine, Tokyo, Japan. Dr. Asahara has studied an ex vivo serum-free expansion culture system consisting of UCB-derived CD133+ cells.

UCB-CD133+ cells isolated by AutoMACS were expanded for 14 d with serum-free culture medium including recombinant human (rh) VEGF, rhSCF, rhFlt-3 ligand, rhTPO (thrombopoietin), rhIL-6, and TGF-α inhibitor (SB-431542). The total expanded cells (Ex-CB133+) increased without firm adhesion, compared to pre-expanded CD133+ cells (x-fold on day 7 = x*54.7 ± 7.8, day 14 = x*696.2 ± 163.0 vs day 0; *$p < 0.05$).

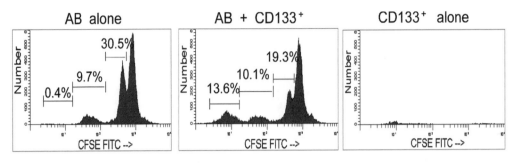

Fig. 8. Proliferation induced by selected CD133⁺ cells from UCB. UCB CD133⁺ and healthy adult CSFE-labeled MNC were mixed in an MLR at a ratio of 1:3 respectively, the cells incubated for 72 h and stained for CD3. CSFE expression was measured on gated CD3⁺ cells and CSFE fluorescence plotted vs cell numbers. Upon proliferation of the CSFE-labeled cells, the dye dilutes at each cellular division, the fluorescence diminishes and the peaks move out to the left side of the histogram.

Table 1
Effects on Ejection Fraction and Fractional Shortening Following UCB-Derived AC133⁺
Cell Transplantation in Nude Rat Ischemic Myocardium After Left Coronary Artery Ligation

	Control group	1×10^5 cells/rat	5×10^5 cells/rat
EF% (mean ± SE)	36.9 ± 3.2	53.6 ± 3.4	66.9 ± 4.3
FS% (mean ± SE)	20.1 ± 0.6	27.5 ± 0.6	31.2 ± 0.9

UCB, umbilical cord blood; EF, ejection fraction; FS, fractional shortening; SE, standard error. $p < 0.05$ for comparison between both cell therapy groups and control group for both EF and FS.

Enriched progenitor cells in Ex-CB133⁺ were evaluated by vasculogenic methylcellulose culture (vascMCC), where progenitor cells were detected as doubly stained cells with FITC-UEA-1 lectin and acLDL-DiI. The frequency of progenitor colonies increased (percentage of progenitor colony no./total colony no. per 1×10^3 cells = day 7, *52.3 ± 4.4; day 14, *68.4 ± 5.8; vs day 0, 25.0 ± 4.8; *$p < 0.05$), although the number per 1×10^3 cells was not changed. Progenitor colonies per total expanded cells drastically increased (colony no. = day 7, *5.58 × 10⁴; day 14, *3.19 × 10⁵ vs day 0; 1.04 × 10³; *$p < 0.05$).

After 14 days of expansion, Ex-CB133⁺ were transplanted into ischemic myocardium of nude rats following left coronary artery ligation. Ex-CB133⁺-transplanted ischemic myocardium was assessed functionally by echocardiography and immunohistochemically by CD31 or anti-smooth muscle actin antibodies combined with HLA class I. Cardiac function improved after 28 days following cell transplantation (*see* Table 1). Immunohistochemical analysis demonstrated that Ex-CB133⁺ contributed not only to neovessel formation but also to myocardiogenesis by themselves in ischemic sites via differentiation into endothelial cells, pericytes, and cardiomyocytes.

Comparison of Mesenchymal Stem Cells Alone, UCB Alone, and Their Combination in Perfusion Ratios

We next performed a series of experiments to test whether stromal elements (hMSC) added to UCB-derived EPCs might augment neovascularization in the in vivo model. Injection of UCB-derived EPCs in combination with hMSC into mice

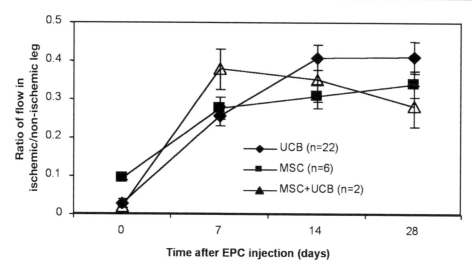

Fig. 9. Comparison of mesenchymal stem cells (MSCs), umbilical cord blood (UCB), and the combination of UCB and human MSC perfusion ratios. Shown are the perfusion ratios between the ischemic and nonischemic limbs of nonobese diabetic–severe combined immunodeficient mice injected with MSCs, UCB, and the combination after ligation of femoral artery in one hindlimb.

after hindlimb injury resulted in improved Doppler flow at day 7 compared with mice infused with EPCs alone (Fig. 9). However, this improvement was not significantly higher than that observed in mice infused with EPCs alone, and the augmentation effect of concurrent hMSC infusion did not persist at later time points. To date, only a small number of mice have been studied, and there are insufficient data to generate appropriate statistical analysis. Further studies of the effect of hMSC alone and in combination with EPC are ongoing.

SUMMARY

Current revascularization therapies for coronary artery disease including percutaneous transluminal coronary angioplasty and coronary artery bypass graft have limited efficacy in patients with diffuse small vessel disease. Bench-to-bedside studies to determine the safety and efficacy of UCB-derived CD133[+] selected progenitor cells infused by intracoronary injection as adjunct to percutaneous transluminal coronary angioplasty will attempt to augment postnatal vasculogenesis in coronary artery disease patients. Crude MNC preparations from adult BM or mobilized peripheral blood have been isolated and culture-expanded to generate EPCs for clinical use in therapeutic angiogenesis *(24,25)*. Little is known about EPC ontogeny. Murine studies included infused culture-expanded EPCs, which are notably heterogeneous and include immature EPCs derived from early hemangioblasts and myeloid progenitors, mesenchymal cells, as well as endothelial cells at various stages of maturation. What specific cell population within these heterogeneous cell cultures homes to sites of vascular injury and promote neovascularization is not known.

Moreover, the role of stromal cell populations including marrow-derived mesenchymal cells, which may facilitate neovascularization, either by direct cellular interactions and/or secondary paracrine effects, is not well delineated *(26,27)*. Because angiogenesis is rapidly initiated during wound healing, we have utilized a skin organotypic study model in an attempt to gain a further understanding of this process, which is regulated by multiple cell populations, including endothelial cells, fibroblasts, hematopoietic cells, and epidermal cells. These studies of the regulation of angiogenesis show that this process depends not only on the production and release of signaling factors such as VEGFs and FGF-2 but also on the production of suitable extracellular matrix elicited by mesenchymal and endothelial cell–cell interactions.

Our Case Western Reserve University collaborative group includes faculty of diverse backgrounds who have designed and evaluated results of these studies from the perspectives of cardiovascular disease, endothelial and stromal cell biology, and stem cell hematology/immunology. These differing faculty perspectives provide both an in-depth evaluation of UCB as a potential stem cell source for hemangioblasts as well as an interpretation of studies to further understand the cellular interactions between hemangioblasts and mesenchymal cells and their secreted factors in neovasculogenesis. UCB is chosen as a stem cell source because of its high content of early CD133[+] stem cells as well as its robust proliferative capacity, low immunogenicity, low infectious contamination, including virions, and off-the-shelf clinical application potential, with diverse representation of HLA genotypes present in unrelated banked UCB. UCB procurement poses no imposition on the normal birthing process and is not associated with ethical concerns in the arena of use of embryonic stem cells. UCB stem cell infusion has been routinely performed for hematology clinical use in approx 3000 procedures. To date, no malignant transformation has been observed in any study patient. This potential risk in humans is a concern in the use of embryonic stem cells, which are known to generate teratomas in animal study models.

Our laboratory has compared isolated CD133[+] stem cell populations and culture-expanded EPCs from UCB and adult marrow using standard in vitro and in vivo readouts. EPCs generated from UCB are comparable to adult marrow in mediating neovascularization, despite differing CD133[+] and stromal cell populations. Further, our studies point to cell–cell and conditioned media interactions between human mesenchymal cells and endothelial cells, as well as in vitro organotypic studies utilizing skin wound healing as a paradigm for study of postnatal vasculogenesis. The hypothesis underlying this work is that early CD133[+]-selected hemangioblasts is a crucial cell population that migrates to sites of vascular injury and mediates new vessel formation in vivo. We further hypothesize that mesenchymal cells augment CD133[+] stem cell homing and neovasculogenesis at sites of vascular injury either by direct cell–cell contact and/or secreted factors.

REFERENCES

1. Fredrickson JK. Umbilical cord blood stem cells: my body makes them, but do I get to keep them? Analysis of the FDA proposed regulations and the impact on individual constitutional property rights. J Contemp Health Law Policy 1998;14:477–502.
2. Rubinstein P, Carrier C, Scaradavou A, et al. Outcomes among 562 recipients of placental-blood transplants from unrelated donors. N Engl J Med 1998;339:1565–1577.
3. Laughlin MJ, Barker, Bambach B, et al. Hematopoietic engraftment and survival in adult recipients of umbilical-cord blood from unrelated donors. N Engl J Med 2001;344:1815–1822.
4. Gehling UM, Ergun S, Schumacher U, et al. In vitro differentiation of endothelial cells from AC133-positive progenitor cells. Blood 2000;95:3106–3112.
5. Pierelli L, Bonanno G, Rutella S, Marone M, Scambia, Leone G. CD105 (endoglin) expression on hematopoietic stem/progenitor cells. Leuk. Lymphoma 2001;42:1195–1206.

6. Barry FP, Boynton RE, Haynesworth S, Murphy M, Zaia J. The monoclonal antibody SH-2, raised against human mesenchymal stem cells, recognizes an epitope on endoglin (CD105). Biochem Biophys Res Commun 1999;265:134–139.
7. Cheng T, Scadden DT. Cell cycle entry of hematopoietic stem and progenitor cells controlled by distinct cyclin-dependent kinase inhibitors. Int J Hematol 2002;75:460–465.
8. Wang Z, Miura N, Bonelli A, et al. Receptor tyrosine kinase, EphB4 (HTK), accelerates differentiation of select human hematopoietic cells. Blood 2002;99:2740–2747.
9. Fleming E, Jr, Haynesworth SE, Cassiede P, Baber MA, Caplan AI. Monoclonal antibody against adult marrow-derived mesenchymal stem cells recognizes developing vasculature in embryonic human skin. Dev Dyn 1998;212:119–132.
10. Haynesworth SE, Goshima J, Goldberg VM, Caplan AI. Characterization of cells with osteogenic potential from human marrow. Bone 1992;13:81–88.
11. Haynesworth SE, Baber MA, Caplan AI. Cytokine expression by human marrow-derived mesenchymal progenitor cells in vitro: effects of dexamethasone and IL-1 alpha. J Cell Physiol 1996;166:585–592.
12. Hartlapp I, Abe R, Saeed RW, et al. Fibrocytes induce an angiogenic phenotype in cultured endothelial cells and promote angiogenesis in vivo. FASEB J 2001;15:2215–2224.
13. Alessandri G, Girelli M, Taccagni G, et al. Human vasculogenesis ex vivo: embryonal aorta as a tool for isolation of endothelial cell progenitors. Lab Invest 2001;81:875–885.
14. Ankoma-Sey V, Matli M, Chang KB, et al. Coordinated induction of VEGF receptors in mesenchymal cell types during rat hepatic wound healing. Oncogene 1998;17:115–121.
15. Henning RJ, Abu-Ali H, Balis JU, Morgan MB, Willing AE, Sanberg PR. Human umbilical cord blood mononuclear cells for the treatment of acute myocardial infarction. Cell Transplant 2004;13:729–739.
16. Leor J, Guetta E, Feinberg MS, et al. Human umbilical cord blood-derived CD133+ cells enhance function and repair of the infarcted myocardium. Stem Cells 2005;
17. Kim BO, Tian H, Prasongsukarn K, et al. Cell transplantation improves ventricular function after a myocardial infarction: a preclinical study of human unrestricted somatic stem cells in a porcine model. Circulation 2005;112:196–104.
18. Ma N, Stamm C, Kaminski A, et al. Human cord blood cells induce angiogenesis following myocardial infarction in NOD/scid-mice. Cardiovasc Res 2005;66:45–54.
19. Hirata Y, Sata M, Motomura N, et al. Human umbilical cord blood cells improve cardiac function after myocardial infarction. Biochem Biophys Res Commun 2005;327:609–614.
20. Askari A, Unzek S, Popovic ZB, et al. Effect of stromal-cell-derived factor-1 on stem cell homing and tissue regeneration in ischemic cardiomyopathy. 2003;697–703.
21. Abbott JD, Huang Y, Liu D, Hickey R, Krause DS, Giordano FJ. Stromal cell-derived factor-1alpha plays a critical role in stem cell recruitment to the heart after myocardial infarction but is not sufficient to induce homing in the absence of injury. Circulation 2004;110:3300–3305.
22. Mal R, Deluca K, Liebmann-Vinson A, et al. Intravenous infusion of human umbilical cord stem cells one day after myocardial infarction leads to neovascularization and improves cardiac function. Proc Miami Nat Biotechnol Winter Symp 2006;17:(abstr).
23. Chen HK, Hung HF, Shyu KG, et al. Combined cord blood stem cells and gene therapy enhances angiogenesis and improves cardiac performance in mouse after acute myocardial infarction. Eur J Clin Invest 2005;35:677–686.
24. Shi Q, Rafii S, Wu MH, et al. Evidence for circulating bone marrow-derived endothelial cells. Blood 1998;92:362–367.
25. Asahara T, Masuda H, Takahashi T, et al. Bone marrow origin of endothelial progenitor cells responsible for postnatal vasculogenesis in physiological and pathological neovascularization. Circ Res 1999;85:221–228.
26. Asahara T, Takahashi T, Masuda H, et al. VEGF contributes to postnatal neovascularization by mobilizing bone marrow-derived endothelial progenitor cells. EMBO J 1999;18:3964–3972.
27. Majka M, Janowska-Wieczorek A, Ratajczak J, et al. Numerous growth factors, cytokines, and chemokines are secreted by human CD34(+) cells, myeloblasts, erythroblasts, and megakaryoblasts and regulate normal hematopoiesis in an autocrine/paracrine manner. Blood 2001;97:3075–3085.

7

Endogenous Cardiac Stem Cells

Elisa Messina, MD, PhD,
Alessandro Giacomello, MD, PhD,
and Eduardo Marbán, MD, PhD

SUMMARY

In recent years, the evidence of myocardial regeneration in animal models as well as in humans has produced a paradigm shift in scientific opinion: cardiomyocytes can be generated *ex novo* in the adult heart. The origin of these dividing myocytes is still the subject of scientific debate. In fact, following the first observations of chimerism in transplanted heart and myocyte growth in cardiac hypertrophy and failure, studies of different groups pointed to the existence of local primitive stem (or progenitor) cells, which are able to proliferate and differentiate during the entire cardiac cell lineage.

This chapter will focus on those resident cardiac cells claimed to be local sources of myocardial regeneration (endogenous cardiac stem cells). Different isolation procedures, characterization, and potential clinical application will be discussed.

Key Words: Adult cardiac stem cells; myocardial regeneration; chimera.

INTRODUCTION

Until recently, the heart has been considered a terminally differentiated organ, incapable of self-regeneration after injury. The major response to myocardial damage was thought to be hypertrophy of still viable cardiomyocytes that have exited the cell cycle *(1–3)*. This dogma has been challenged by recent findings of cycling myocytes undergoing mitosis and cytokinesis under both physiological and pathological conditions *(4–7)*. That would imply that there is a population of stem cells or cardiac progenitor cells (CSCs) either resident in the mammalian heart or recruited from noncardiac sources from which new myocytes can be derived.

Recent studies reveal that the heart contains a reservoir of small cells expressing stem cell markers (c-kit, MDR-1, Sca-1) and harboring telomerase activity, which is only present in replicating cells. The in vivo relevance of these cardiac stem cells was emphasized by the fact that their number increased more than 13-fold in the hypertrophied myocardium of aortic stenosis patients. The cell clusters revealed stem cell markers on cells in different stages of cardiomyocyte differentiation, which was determined by both early and late cardiac markers. This suggests the existence of a lineage commitment of resident cardiac stem cells toward becoming cardioblasts and then cardiomyocytes in the heart.

From: *Contemporary Cardiology: Stem Cells and Myocardial Regeneration*
Edited by: M. S. Penn © Humana Press Inc., Totowa, NJ

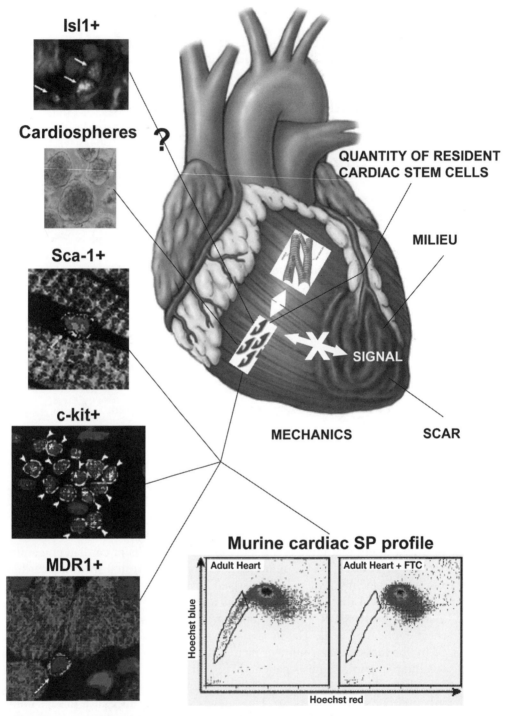

Fig. 1. Resident cardiac stem cells and obstacles for myocardial regeneration. In the adult heart resident cardiac stem cells and perhaps cardioblasts (isl1+ cells) generate new cardiac myocytes and contribute in the renewal of individual cells within this tissue. Yet new myocytes are not normally generated in large enough numbers to fully repair a severely damaged myocardium. Limited numbers of cardiac stem cells, scar formation, an unfavorable milieu associated with the injured tissue (inflammatory environment or lack of vascular supply), and continuous contractile activity of the injured heart may all limit myocardial repair and regeneration. Scar formation may serve as an anatomical boundary to limit the release of

Table 1
Properties of Resident Populations of Cardiac/Progenitor Stem Cells

CSC	Source	Cardiac	Clonogenic	Multipotent	Other markers	Ref.
Side population	Mouse	Yes Co-culturing	ND	Yes	Yes	(+) Sca-1[a] (−) CD31[a]	11
Abcg2	Mouse	Yes Co-culturing	ND	Yes	Yes	(+) Sca-1 (high), c-Kit (low), CD34 (low), CD45 (low)	12
C-Kit	Rat, human, dog	Yes Spontaneous	Yes	Yes	Yes	(−) CD34, CD45, Lin skeletal markers (!) GATA4, Nkx2.5, MEF2	13
Sca-1	Rat	Yes 5-Azacytidine	ND	?	Yes	(−) C-Kit, CD34, CD45, Lin, Nkx2.5, sarcomeric proteins	14
	Mouse	Oxytocin				(+) SP, GATA4, MEF2, CD45 (40%), CD34 and c-Kit (10%)	15
Cardio-spheres	Mouse, man guinea pig, pig	Yes Spontaneous Co-culturing	Yes	Yes	Yes	(+) C-kit (20–30%), cardiac and vascular markers	16
Islet-1	Rat, mouse, human	Yes Co-culturing	ND	Yes	Yes	(−) Sca-1, c-Kit, sarcomeric proteins (+) Nkx2.5, GATA4	17

[a]From ref. 18.
ND, not determined.

The recognition of the existence of CSCs rationalizes the much older observation of mitotic events interspersed in adult myocardium, events which are dramatically increased in frequency under stress (e.g., heart failure or hemodynamic overload) (8). Such mitotic events likely represent replication and differentiation of resident CSCs, rather than cell divisions of adult myocytes. The presence of CSCs has challenged the paradigm that the heart is a postmitotic organ characterized by a predetermined number of parenchymal cells, which is defined at birth and preserved throughout life until death of the organ and organism. Thus, the heart belongs to the group of constantly renewing tissues, in which the capacity to replace cells depends on the persistence of a stem cell compartment (9,10). Under these conditions, regeneration conforms to a hierarchical archetype in which slowly dividing stem cells give rise to highly proliferating lineage-restricted progenitor cells that become committed precursors and, eventually, reach growth arrest and terminal differentiation.

Fig. 1. (Continued) recruitment signals from the injured tissue, or the scar may prevent the mobilization of resident stem cells to the area of injury. SP, side population; FTC, Fumitremorgin C.

Stem cells have a high capacity for cell division, and this property is preserved throughout the lifetime of an organism. Conversely, the less primitive cells have a limited proliferative capacity but represent the largest group of dividing cells. This forms the basis of a new paradigm for the heart in which multipotent CSCs are implicated in the normal turnover of myocytes, endothelial cells, smooth muscle cells, and fibroblasts.

Seven separate studies (11–17) have independently described a CSC or progenitor cell population that may participate in limited myocardial regeneration in response to an injury (Table 1; Fig. 1).

In these studies, three approaches yielded CSCs from heart: (1) isolation based on the ability to efflux Hoescht dye (side population [SP]) or on the presence of cell-surface stem cell markers (either c-kit or Sca-1) that allows for the identification and isolation of the respective cell populations using magnetic cell sorting or flow cytometry; (2) tissue culture of cardiac explants with spontaneous shedding of CSCs in vitro; and (3) expression of the islet-1 gene (isl1[POS] cells in the adult heart are remnants of a cardiac progenitor cell population from the heart of the developing fetus).

The relationship among CSCs isolated using different methods is at present unknown. An important emerging consensus is the observation that more than one stem cell may be present in a particular tissue (19).

RESIDENT CARDIAC STEM CELL ISOLATION

Isolation Based on the Presence of Stem Cell-Like Properties or Cell-Surface Proteins

RESIDENT CARDIAC SIDE POPULATION

Most adult tissues contain a stem cell or progenitor cell population (SP) characterized by its ability to efflux metabolic markers such as rhodamine and Hoechst 33342 on the basis of high expression of membrane pumps encoded by the multiple drug-resistance genes (20). Hoechst dyes intercalate into the cellular DNA and are slightly toxic. The ability to efflux the fluorescent dyes depends on the cell cycle status of the cells (21).

Megeney and colleagues (11) presented the first evidence for the existence of a putative cardiac progenitor cell population in the adult heart. They showed that postnatal mouse heart contains a resident Hoechst dye-excluding, verapamil-sensitive SP (approx 1% of the total cell number) with stem cell-like activity: in methylcellulose, stem cell medium gave rise to cell colonies (approx 1 colony per 50,000 cells plated) and were capable of differentiating into the cardiomyocyte lineage in co-culture experiments with primary cardiomyocytes. This myocardial SP cell population changed with altered physiological demands. When growth of the postnatal heart was attenuated through overexpression of a dominant-negative cardiac transcription factor (MEF2C), the resident SP cell population was subject to activation, followed by a consequent depletion. In addition, cardiac SP cells were capable of fusion with other cell types, but did not adopt the corresponding gene expression profile.

The ability of SP cells to efflux rhodamine and Hoechst 33342 dye appears to be dependent on the expression of ABCG2 (also known as Bcrp1 for breast cancer resistance protein), a member of the family of ATP-binding cassette (ABC) transporters. The continued presence of SP cells in an ABCG2 knockout mouse implies that more than one drug efflux pump is responsible for the SP phenotype. Furthermore, ABCG2 does not efflux the Hoechst dye in actively dividing stem cells (22). However its presence can certainly serve as a marker specific for stem cells.

Garry and colleagues *(12)* examined ABCG2 expression during murine embryogenesis and observed robust expression in the blood islands of the E8.5 yolk sac and in developing tissues including the heart. During the latter stages of embryogenesis, ABCG2 identifies a rare cell population in the developing organs. They further established that the adult heart contains an ABCG2-expressing SP cell population, distinct from endothelial cells, and these progenitor cells are capable of proliferation (forming hematopoietic colonies after 14 days into methylcellulose media) and differentiation into α-actinin-positive cells (after 14 days of co-culture with primary cardiomyocytes). Increased numbers of ABCG2-expressing cells have been observed in the border zone following myocardial infarction (MI). Cardiac ABCG2 expressing SP cells included $Sca1^{high}$, $cKit^{low}$, $CD34^{low}$, and $CD45^{low}$. An alternative analysis revealed that cardiac SP cells were $Sca1^+$, $cKit^+$, $CD34^+$, and $CD45^-$.

The ability of this resident cardiac SP cell group to differentiate into contracting cardiac myocytes or to contribute to functional repair of damaged heart muscle has not yet been extensively evaluated.

C-KIT^{POS} RESIDENT CARDIAC STEM CELLS

Anversa and colleagues *(13)* reported the discovery of a distinct resident population of cardiac stem cells. These cells are negative for blood lineage markers CD34, CD45, CD20, CD45RO, and CD8 (Lin^-) and positive for c-kit (c-kit^{POS}), the receptor for stem cell factor. In the adult (20–23 months of age) rat myocardium, Lin^- c-kit^{POS} cells are relatively rare (~1 per 10^4 myocytes). The cells are roughly one-tenth the size of cardiac myocytes.

Cardiac c-kit^{POS} cells isolated by fluorescence-activated cell sorting (FACS) are heterogeneous, with rare (7–10%) cells expressing Nkx2-5, GATA4, and Mef2, and fewer still (0.5%) expressing genes encoding sarcomeric proteins. These cells retain these characteristics with passage in culture and can be expanded. Cardiac c-kit^{POS} cells were self-renewing (expanded in culture after plating 1 cell per well) and multipotential (generating cardiac myocytes, smooth muscle cells, and endothelial cells). However, in culture, the "differentiated" cells had an immature phenotype. When placed in differentiation medium, c-kit^{POS} clones differentiate into cells that biochemically (but not phenotypically) resemble cardiac myocytes. Sarcomeres or striations and/or contractile activity are not observed.

To test whether these cells could achieve full mature differentiation in vivo, they were labeled and injected into the border zone of hearts of syngeneic rats after experimental myocardial infarction. A band of labeled regenerating myocardium was observed in 19 of 20 treated infarcts. The labeled cells expressing sarcomeric proteins were small relative to mature cardiac myocytes, but these cells exhibited visible striations and expressed connexin 43, a component of the fascia adherens of intercalated discs. An increase in capillary and arteriole density and contribution of labeled cells to blood vessels was also observed, as was a marked improvement in multiple indices of cardiac performance. However, the average infarct size was greater in the treated animals than in the controls, most likely because untreated animals did not survive with infarcts as large as those in the treated group.

One potential caveat for these findings would be if the stem cells had fused with existing host cells. This might appear to be differentiation when, in fact, it would be hybrid cells giving the appearance of differentiation. However, the Anversa study *(13)* ruled this out by a number of criteria, including showing that the number of new myocytes is orders of magnitude higher than the number of injected cells and stating that the DNA content of the new cells is diploid and not tetraploid. Results with clonally derived cardiac c-kit^{POS} cells were equivalent to those with the initial cardiac c-kit^{POS} population, which suggests that an expandable source from within the heart might be applied to cardiac repair.

The capacity of cardiac c-kit^{POS} cells to home to the heart and engraft following intravascular (aortic root) injection was tested in rats subjected to ischemia–reperfusion injury *(23)*. Echocardiographic analysis showed that injection of c-kit^{POS} cells attenuated the increase in left ventricular (LV) end-diastolic dimensions and impairment in LV systolic performance at 5 weeks after MI. Pathological analysis showed that treated hearts exhibited a smaller increase in LV chamber diameter and volume and a higher wall thickness-to-chamber radius ratio and LV mass-to-chamber volume ratio. C-kit^{POS} cells induced myocardial regeneration, decreasing infarct size by 29%. A diploid DNA content and only two copies of chromosome 12 were found in new cardiomyocytes, indicating that cell fusion did not contribute to tissue reconstitution *(23)*.

A subsequent preliminary report from the Anversa lab extended the isolation and expansion of ckit^{POS} cells to human heart tissue, using surgical specimens of human myocardium, specifically cultured slices of human atrial and ventricular myocardium *(13a)*. C-kit^{POS} cells were found in 1.8 ± 1.7% of the unsorted myocardial cell population and included lineage negative (52 ± 12%) and early committed cells (48 ± 12%). After plating, c-kit^{POS} cells attached rapidly and continued to grow up to P8 undergoing approx 25 population doublings. Ki67 labeling showed that the number of cycling cells remained constant from P1 to P8 (48 ± 10%). Human c-kit^{POS} cells were clonogenic. Doubling time was approx 28 h, and approx 90% of cells were labeled by BrdU after 5 days of exposure. In differentiation medium, clonogenic cells gave rise to myocytes, endothelial cells, and vascular smooth muscle cells. When human c-kit^{POS} cardiac progenitor cells were locally injected in the infarcted myocardium of immunodeficient rats and mice, they regenerated myocytes and coronary vessels of human origin. This repair process resulted in an improvement in cardiac function.

Resident stem cells in other tissues are dependent upon appropriate local environments, or niches, to maintain viability, but detailed information regarding a cardiac resident stem cell niche is lacking. Preliminary results indicate that c-kit^{POS} CSCs are stored in niches that are preferentially located in the atria and apex but are also detectable in the ventricle. The niches have an ellipsoid shape and are composed of undifferentiated and early committed cells nested within interstitial fibronectin. The peculiar topographical distribution of c-kit^{POS} CSCs in the heart suggests that a relationship may exist between the function of CSCs and level of hemodynamic stress. C-kit^{POS} CSCs accumulate in niches located in the atria and apex that are anatomical areas exposed to low levels of wall stress. The preferential localization of CSCs in zones where physical forces are modest is consistent with the common sites of storage of stem cells in self-renewing organs: c-kit^{POS} CSCs occupy the most protected areas of the heart.

Sca-1^{POS} Cardiac Progenitor Cells

Schneider and colleagues *(14)* reported a resident population of cardiac progenitor cells that copurifies with the nonmyocyte fraction and is characterized by expression of stem cell antigen 1 (Sca-1^{POS}). Cardiac-resident Sca-1^{POS} cells lack the hematopoietic stem cell (HSC) markers CD45 and CD34 (also a marker of EPCs), lack hematopoietic transcription factors (Lmo2, Gata2, Tal), and thus are readily distinguished from bone marrow HSCs. These cells express telomerase reverse transcriptase, which has been associated with self-renewal potential. Although they do express the early cardiac markers

GATA4, Mef2, and Tef1, they do not express Nkx2-5 or genes encoding cardiac sarcomeric proteins. Although these cells do not spontaneously differentiate in vitro, when exposed to the cytosine analog 5-azacytidine *(14)* or to oxytocin *(15)*, a small subpopulation of cells started to express cardiac transcription factors, showed sarcomeric structures, and formed spontaneously beating cardiomyocytes with spontaneous calcium transients. Various agonists and antagonists could affect the beating rate of the differentiated cells. Clearly, the majority of cells do not differentiate into cardiac progenitors under the conditions tested, raising the question of what other cell fates, if any, were induced following prolonged exposure to oxytocin or 5-azacytidine. Sca-1[POS] cells may possess multipotency; however, multipotency needs to be proven in the progeny of single cells.

When freshly isolated Sca-1[POS] cells were injected intravenously into mice after ischemia-reperfusion, they were shown to target the border zone of the injured myocardium and differentiate into cardiomyocytes, expressing sarcomeric α-actin, cTnI, and connexin-43, with and without fusing with host cells. No functional assessment was made. Further studies will be required to determine whether a subpopulation of cardiac Sca-1[POS] cells exists with restricted developmental potential to differentiate (at high frequency) into cardiac progenitors or cardiac myocytes.

Isolation From Tissue Culture of Cardiac Explants With Spontaneous Shedding In Vitro (Cardiospheres)

The first report that CSCs can be clonally expanded from human myocardial biopsies was from the Giacomello lab *(16)*. In that study we reported that these cells are spontaneously shed from human surgical specimens and murine heart samples in primary culture. This heterogeneous population of cells expresses stem cell and endothelial progenitor cell markers. At day 0, roughly 10% of these cells derived from the mouse express either c-Kit, Sca-1, CD34, or CD31. These cells form multicellular clusters, dubbed cardiospheres (CSps), in suspension culture. CSps express the c-Kit marker in roughly 30% of the cells by day 6 with no significant upregulation of the other three markers examined. We have demonstrated that cardiospheres are composed of clonally derived cells, consist of proliferating c-Kit-positive cells primarily in their core and differentiating cells expressing cardiac and endothelial cell markers on their periphery.

CSps become partially differentiated toward the cardiac lineage. These show *lacZ*-stained images of CSps from transgenic mice expressing nuclear *lacZ* driven by the MLC3 or cTnI promoter, both of which are cardiac lineage markers. Nuclear *lacZ* expression is mainly localized in the external layers of the CSps; internal structures often stain positive for endothelial or smooth muscle markers. Immunohistochemistry of a mouse CSp reveals expression of cTnI in association with obvious sarcomeres. By video microscopy, we have demonstrated "beating" of CSC-derived CSps in vitro, either in co-culture with neonatal rat myocytes (human CSCs) or spontaneously (CSCs from embryonic mouse heart).

We have evaluated the response of human CSps after their intramyocardial delivery into the severe combined immunodeficient mouse model. Functional studies in vivo to date have focused on the implantation or infusion of undifferentiated CSCs. Our work, in which CSps were injected into the peri-infarct zone of mice, represents one exception. Despite the fact that only approx 10 CSps were injected, in contrast to more than 10,000 CSCs in the work of Anversa and colleagues *(13)*, functional improvement was comparable (fractional shortening 37% in the CSp-injected group vs 18% in the control

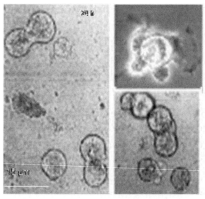

Human cardiospheres in culture

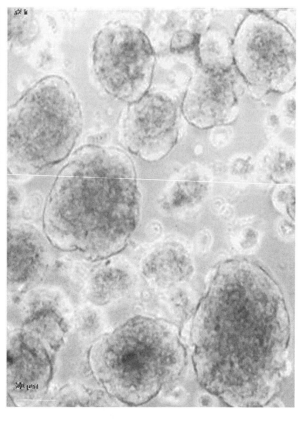

Fig. 2. Human cardiospheres in culture. Phase micrograph of floating cardiac stem cells (cultured from <24 hours to >48 hours) derived from primary culture of a human bioptical sample. Time course observations of cells derived from human explants showed that, early after their seeding (30 minutes), some of these cells began to divide while still in suspension; most cells became loosely adherent, others remained in suspension, and some contaminating fibroblast-like cells attached firmly to the poly-D-lysine coat. Cellular divisions were evident also from the loosely adherent cell population and produced clusters of small, round phase-bright cells (cardiospheres).

group; $p < 0.05$) with vigorous engraftment and cardiogenesis. It is also noteworthy that cryopreserved human CSps were used in our work and resulted in vigorous engraftment in post-MI mice.

We have shown that CSCs can be harvested from surgically obtained human cardiac specimens (left atrial appendages or open ventricular biopsies). Such human CSCs have full cardiogenic potential. The collaboration of Marbán's team at Johns Hopkins University allowed us to extend these data to show that CSCs can be harvested from routine endomyocardial biopsy specimens from humans or pigs, opening the prospect for autologous therapy without thoracotomy *(16a)*. In the Cardiology Division at Johns Hopkins, endomyocardial biopsies were obtained using standard clinical procedures, which can be completed in 15 minutes. The human samples we are working with are approx 25 mg wet weight on average and are obtained from transplant or heart failure patients. Samples are kept on ice in heparinized cardioplegic solution until processing occurs within 1–2 hours.

Processing (Fig. 2) consists of partial enzymatic digestion of the minced sample, plating and cultured as explants. When maintained in primary culture for 2–7 days for pigs and 14–24 days for humans, explants begin to produce a carpet of migratory cells. Small, round cells can be seen budding off from the explant and dividing in suspension. Cells are then harvested by gentle enzymatic digestion. The explants are left behind to regenerate cardiac stem cells. These cells could be isolated at repeated intervals from the same biopsy specimen. They are then grown in suspension culture in differentiation media to form CSps within 3–6 days for pigs and 12–18 days for humans. Cardiospheres, as depicted in Fig. 2, grow primarily in suspension.

In an effort to improve our cell yield given such a small amount of starting material, we have tried expanding these cardiospheres as single cells on a monolayer. Those cardiospheres that are floating in culture are selected for expansion.

Floating cardiospheres, 100–1000 cells in size, can then be expanded as monolayers with a doubling time of approx 18 hours for pigs and approx 24 hours for humans. Cells expanded in this manner can then be used to regenerate cardiospheres, verified up to passage four in humans. CSCs grown in this manner from adult human ventricular biopsies can be expanded to upwards of 7–70 million cells in about a month and a half from a single endomyocardial biopsy specimen.

One of the most critical features of cell coupling in the heart is the expression of connexin 43 (the mean gap-junction protein in this organ). Both CSs growing on three-dimensional suspension culture, rather than single cells growing as a monolayer, show connexin 43 expression, confirming what was hown in the cited paper *(16)*. The finding suggests that these cells could show very efficient electrical and metabolic coupling within them and with the cardiac syncytium.

Roughly 20% of co-cultured CSp-derived cells demonstrate the ability to beat spontaneously. We have found *(16a)* that spontaneous repetitive action potentials could be recorded from pig CSp-derived cells after 6 days in co-culture, and the action potentials are reminiscent of nodal cell activity. These recordings confirm that CSp-derived cells can become spontaneously excitable when co-cultured for 1 week. Spontaneous calcium transients have been observed in a small percentage of CSp-derived cells out to day 10 in co-culture. So, CSCs (or cells with the function of these in the feature of CSs) can be isolated from routine biopsy specimens, even those taken from abnormal patients, and can be expanded to obtain clinically relevant numbers of cells in a short period of time, making autologous cardiac regeneration therapy a distinct possibility.

CSps are an interesting in vitro model of partial cardiogenic differentiation. The spontaneous formation of spheres is a known prerogative of neural stem cells, some tumor cell lines (LIM) *(24)*, endothelial cells *(25)*, and fetal chicken cardiomyocytes *(26)*. All these models (the cardiospheres included) mimic the true three-dimensional architecture of tissues. They consist of spheroids of aggregated cells, which develop a two-compartment system composed of a surface layer of differentiated cells and a core of unorganized cells that first proliferate and thereafter disappear over time (perhaps through apoptotic cell death). Moreover, as is well documented in fetal chick cardiomyocytes and endothelial cell spheroid culture, three-dimensional structure affects the sensitivity of cells to survival and growth factors. In contrast to monolayer cultures, three-dimensional cultivation technologies have been reported to mimic cardiac tissue-like morphologies and provide a suitable environment for coordination of cell–cell interaction, self-organization, differentiation, and electrical properties, all of which are essential qualities for the identity and integrity of heart structures *(21)*. Therefore, cell–cell contact and membrane-associated factors could be already involved in the cardiosphere system: in this structure, as in the "niche," stem cells (or cells with stem-cell function) may only retain their potency within an appropriate environment.

Isolation Based on the Expression of the Islet-1 Gene (Postnatal isl^{POS} Cardioblasts)

Chien and coworkers *(17)* argued that there are progenitor cells in the heart that might be able to engage in repair. These cells are distinguished by their expression of the islet-1 gene (that is, they are isl1^{POS}).

The LIM homeodomain transcription factor islet-1 (isl1) marks a cell population that makes a substantial contribution to the embryonic heart, comprising most cells in the right ventricle, both atria, the outflow tract, and specific regions of the left ventricle *(28)*. This population of cells, called the secondary or anterior heart field, originates near the cardiac crescent, migrates to the anterior pharynx, and infiltrates the rostral and caudal poles (the outflow region) of the looped primary heart tube. Cells in the secondary heart field express Nkx2-5 and GATA4, as do the cells of the primary heart fields, but they remain undifferentiated until later in development, and they express some additional markers. Expression of isl1 is lost when these cells differentiate into cardiac myocytes. Interestingly, some isl1^{POS} cells can be identified in the mature hearts of newborn rodents and humans, where they remain undifferentiated. They are found most commonly in the outflow tract, the atria, and the right ventricle, in agreement with the embryonic contribution of the secondary heart field.

Unlike some other putative resident cardiac progenitor populations, these cells fail to express Sca-1, CD31, or c-kit, although they do express Nkx2-5 and GATA4. Importantly, Laugwitz and co-workers have shown that these cells can differentiate into cardiac myocytes both in vivo, using an inducible *cre–lox* system, and in vitro. Isl1^{POS} cells from hearts can be expanded in culture. Co-culture with cardiac myocytes leads to expression of terminal differentiation markers and electrophysiological characteristics of fully differentiated cardiac myocytes, including responsiveness to β-adrenergic agonists. The resident population of isl1^{POS} cells in the heart probably represents specified cardiac progenitors or cardioblasts.

Isl1^{POS} cells have been isolated only from very young animal and human specimens, and the number of progenitor cells falls rapidly over the first few weeks of life. Most of the ex vivo studies were performed on cells taken from 1- to 5-day -old animals, where only 500–600 isl1^{POS} cells were identified per rat heart.

It remains to be determined whether isl1^{POS} cells exist in the adult heart beyond the early postnatal period. The rare isl1^{POS} cells identified at later times were not evaluated for their ability to expand or differentiate. Importantly, isl1^{POS} cells were identified in multiple organisms, including humans, but the single human sample examined beyond 8 days of age (at 148 days) failed to reveal any isl1 progenitors. Furthermore, although a high percentage (25%) of cultured cells expressed troponin T under differentiation conditions, only 2.3% displayed calcium transients characteristic of cardiac myocytes. The degree to which significant and meaningful expansion is possible, including expansion from a single isolated cell, is at present unknown. The capacity of isl1^{POS} cardiac progenitors to engraft in the heart and to regenerate myocardium, to electrically couple, and to contribute to cardiac work has not been tested.

OTHER LOCAL SOURCES OF POTENTIAL CARDIAC STEM CELLS

A stem function has been assigned to some of the committed (or differentiated) cell lineages forming the heart: the epicardium and the epicardially derived cardiac stem cells, the smooth muscle cells, and the neural crest stem cells.

A series of studies reviewed by Wessels and Perez-Pomares *(29)* has demonstrated that a subset of epicardially derived cells can differentiate into multiple cardiac cell types. Many of these studies are focused on the analysis of the mechanisms that control the conversion of the epicardial epithelial (mesothelial) cells into a population of pluripotent epicardially derived cells (EPDCs) that contributes to many cardiac tissues. Others are looking at different aspects of EPDC development, including the regulatory role of EPDCs in myocardial proliferation and the involvement of EPDCs in endocardial cushion morphogenesis. EPDCs, in fact, have been suggested to have a role in the differentiation of endothelial/smooth muscle cell lineage, cardiac fibroblasts, valvuloseptal mesenchyme, and, under certain in vitro conditions, cardiomyocytes.

Studies elucidating the pathways that control epicardial differentiation will help us better understand normal heart morphogenesis, the mechanisms underlying the etiology of congenital heart disease, and the potential of EPDC usefulness and applicability.

In the adult, vascular smooth muscle cells must continually repair arterial injuries and maintain functional mass in response to changing demands upon the vessel wall. Recent evidence *(30)* suggests that this is accomplished, in part, by recruiting multipotential vascular progenitors from bone marrow-derived stem cells as well as from less well-defined sources within adult tissues themselves. The smooth muscle progenitors cells within skeletal muscle (referred to as non-SP cells) *(31,32)* exhibit a phenotype reminiscent of embryonic mesenchymal cells (they are adherent and express smooth muscle antibody and platelet-derived growth factor receptor). Furthermore, they also express c-met (receptor for hepatocyte growth factor), a marker of satellite cells that regenerating skeletal muscle. Whether the same progenitor cells within skeletal muscle are capable of regenerating multiple muscle types remains to be conclusively demonstrated. Furthermore, vascular smooth muscle cells of infiltrating host cell origin can be found in human cardiac allograft. However, the results regarding the evidence that chimerism is present in cardiac myocytes are controversial *(33)*.

Cardiac neural crest cells participate in the septation of the cardiac outflow tract into aorta and pulmonary artery. The migratory cardiac neural crest consists of stem cells, fate-restricted cells, and cells that are committed to the smooth muscle cell lineage. During their migration within the posterior branchial arches, the developmental potentials of pluripotent neural crest cells become restricted. Conversely, neural crest stem cells persist at many locations, including in the cardiac outflow tract.

Many aspects of neural crest cell differentiation are driven by growth factor action *(34)*. Neural crest stem cells persist in target locations. However, during advanced migration, the developmental potentials of neural crest cells become increasingly more restricted. For instance, cultured cardiac neural crest stem cells at the onset of migration can give rise to at least six phenotypes: smooth muscle cells, fibroblasts, chondrocytes, sensory neurons, autonomic neurons, and pigment cells *(35)*. In contrast, once they have migrated through the posterior branchial arches and have arrived in the cardiac outflow tract, they can no longer generate sensory neurons or melanocytes *(36,37)*. Together with the neural tube segment from the midotic placoide to somite 3 axial level (where cells forming cardiac outflow tract and proximal great vessels originate), another distinct population of neural crest cells enters the heart at the venous pole. In addition to the fact that the conduction system is derived from cardiac miogenic precursors *(38)*, this second cell population may play an important role in the development of the conduction system *(39)*.

Some features of neural crest stem cells in the heart seem to match those of the cardioblast population described by Laugwitz and co-workers (cardiac distribution, isl1 expression, disappearance with age) *(17)*. However, the potential correlation between these two cell populations has not yet investigated.

Many features of these potential sources of cardiac stem cells could also be interpreted as manifestations of cell plasticity and transdifferentiation or fusion phenomena. In fact, in addition to the fusion mechanism involved in the acquisition of the cardiac fate by some of the published CSCs *(14)*, cardiomyocytes themselves have been reported *(40)* to have fusogenic activity with many different types of cells (such as cardiac fibroblasts or smooth muscle cells) and obtain proliferative ability after fusion with somatic cells without losing their phenotypes in vitro and in vivo.

In this regard, plasticity (i.e., the nonrestricted potential of adult stem cells to adopt phenotypes different from those of the original tissue source) and transdifferentiation (the acquisition by a differentiated cell of a new phenotype different from the committed one, mostly in defined in vitro conditions) will be discussed here.

WHERE, WHEN, AND HOW DO CARDIAC RESIDENT STEM/PROENITOR CELLS ARISE IN THE HEART?

The origin of CSCs is still unclear; in principle, they can be either cells that have existed from fetal life onwards, or they could come from extracardiac sources. CSCs can arise in the heart early during embryogenesis and cardiogenesis: SP cells are present early during embryogenesis *(12)*, and postnatal isl1[POS] cardioblasts *(17)* appear to result from persistence as undifferentiated remnants of heart-forming tissue.

The first indication that there is a circulating pool of stem cells that participate in the regeneration of cardiac muscle came from analyzing posttransplant organs of sex-mismatched heart transplantations. Examination of the female donor hearts revealed cardiomyocytes and vascular cells derived from the male recipients *(7)*. These cells presumably derived from extracardiac sources of the heart transplantation recipient and may embody a population of endogenous circulating stem cells. Although considerable controversy exists regarding the frequency of extracardiac stem cells, which migrate and repopulate the myocardium in adult *(41)*, these results suggest that extracardiac stem cells give rise to cardiomyocytes to participate in myocardial repair. A population of early tissue committed stem cells (TCSCs) has been recognized in the circulating pool of mononuclear cells *(42)*. TCSCs express nuclear proteins of skeletal muscle cell lineage—Myf5, MyoD, and myogenin—and transcription factors that drive the cardiac commitment during heart development—GATA4, Mef2C, and Nkx2.5. The expression of endothelial cell mRNAs in the TCSC pool was also documented by real-time reverse transcriptase polymerase chain reaction. TCSCs seem to correspond to circulating cells that carry the surface antigens CD34, CXCR4, CD117, and c-Met, although this has not been proven conclusively. The possibility that TCSCs are a subset of the cells positive for these membrane epitopes is supported by the similarity in their responses in patients with myocardial infarction and ST-segment elevation. These cell classes increase synchronously, and their changes in number are paralleled by increases in the plasma concentration of several growth factors and cytokines with chemoattractant properties.

The origin of circulating cardiac progenitor cells is unknown. Because definitive proof of the source of these circulating cells is lacking, it is tempting to suggest that tissue-specific stem/progenitor cells migrate between the organ of origin and the blood. The recently published finding that macrophages invading myocardial tissue can contribute to the formation of new myocytes *(43)* is in agreement with the hypothesis that the circulating pool of mononuclear cells might contribute to cardiac repair.

For the origin of Sca-1^{POS} cells, a mechanism involving ingrowth of the developing coronary vasculature has been suggested (44) given the cells' striking similarities to the mesangioblasts (45), which include surface labeling, microarray findings, and the earliest sites of marker expression.

CSCs could also arise from dedifferentiated adult cardiac myocytes. In mammals, epimorphic regeneration is largely limited by an irreversible differentiation process, and neither transdifferentiation nor dedifferentiation has been identified as a naturally occurring process. However, urodele amphibians uniquely use a cellular dedifferentiation mechanism at damaged sites to form a blastema that contains dedifferentiated progenitor cells. These cells can then proliferate and reifferentiate to regenerate a variety of tissues incuding limb, tail, and lens (46). Recent in vitro studies suggest that terminally differentiated C2C12 myotubes can be induced to undergo dedifferentiation into mesenchymal progenitor cells by ectopic expression of Msx1 (47), addition of extracts form regenerating newt limb (48), or by treatment with reversine (49), a 2,6-disubstituted purine analog.

Intriguingly, a recent publication (50) has shown that adult mammalian cardiomyocytes can divide. One important mechanism used by mammalian cardiomyocytes to control cell cycle is p38 mitogen activated protein kinase activity. p38 regulates expression of genes required for mitosis in cardiomyocytes, including cyclin A and cyclin B. The authors demonstrated that activation of p38 in vivo reduces fetal cardiomyocyte proliferation, whereas inhibition of p38 in cardiomyocytes promotes cytokinesis. Finally, mitosis in adult cardiomyocytes is associated with transient dedifferentiation of the contractile apparatus. These results indicate that the inhibitory effects of p38 on cardiomyocyte proliferation are reversible and that postmitotic differentiated cells are capable of proliferation. Interestingly, the authors provocatively argue that cardiac regeneration could involve, as occurs in the liver, proliferation of differentiated cells and not stem cells.

In other stem cell populations (19), stem cells isolated from an adult organ and then incorporated into blastocysts or injected into irradiated adult animals were able to contribute to multiple lineages in vivo, including lineages derived from a different embryonic germ layer than the donor cell. These studies suggest that many or all tissues contain a population of pluripotent stem cells and challenge the widely held view that tissue-specific stem cells are predetermined, i.e., monopotential, or able to give rise only to a particular cell type. In fact, these stem cells appear to be pluripotential or even totipotent, possessing the ability to activate various genetic programs when exposed to the appropriate environment. Thus, such pluripotential stem cells must differentiate as a function of the growth factors and signals provided by their host tissue. However, skeletal myoblasts and bone marrow cells do not appear to transdifferentiate into cardiomyocytes. This limitation has always been clear for myoblasts (51). For bone marrow cells, the issue remains more controversial (52–55), although their alleged developmental plasticity (52,55) has been seriously challenged by studies that have used unambiguous genetic tracking methods to show that what was mistakenly interpreted as transdifferentiation may have corresponded to fusion events or to immunohistochemical artifacts (53,54).

RESIDENT CARDIAC STEM CELLS AND HEART FAILURE: A PARADOX

An apparent paradox exists when considering the availability of stem cells in the heart and the prevalence of heart failure. Stem cells provide regenerative potential and should influence the status of the heart, thereby decreasing the incidence of heart failure. So why is heart failure so prevalent? Why, in infarction, do regenerative processes fail to complete the repair?

Primitive and early committed cells accumulate acutely in the region bordering the infarct in humans and animals. After homing, these cells grow and differentiate in new myocytes and coronary vessels. However, a block exists at the sharp boundary that separates the viable myocardium of the border zone from the dead tissue of the infarct. CSCs; progenitors and precursors may not cross this boundary because their translocation to the dead myocardium is impeded. Such an obstruction hampers the reconstitution of infarcted myocardium and the recovery of function. The entire phenomenon is obscure and of great clinical relevance for its impact on all organs. The number of resident myocardial stem cells might be inadequate to repopulate injured tissue after a large MI. Alternatively, the fibroproliferative response after a myocardial injury produces a fibrotic scar. This scar may function to limit the access of resident stem cells to the area of injury, or it may limit the release (or serve as an anatomical barrier) of signals (growth factors such as hepatocyte growth factor, insulin growth factors, stromal-derived growth factor, etc.) that recruit stem cells to the site of injury. Additionally, the milieu of the injured myocardium may have a negative (i.e., inflammatory environment or lack of vascular supply) effect on stem cell viability and differentiation. Finally, an active working contracting heart may have a limited regenerative response compared with a resting, unloaded heart (Fig. 1).

Heart failure and the unpredictable path of the disease may influence the CSC compartment and, thereby, cardiac reserve. Depletion of the CSC pool in the chronically decompensated heart may involve the expression of genes that inhibit cell replication and activate CSC death. Whether the CSC pool is worn out in end-stage failure and/or the growth reserve of the remaining CSCs is exhausted remains an important question.

RESIDENT CARDIAC STEM CELLS AND AUTOLOGOUS CARDIOMYOPLASTY

Recently, the technique of cardiac cell therapy (CCT) has been developed. This method consists of transplanting cells into the infarcted area of the myocardium to (1) increase or to preserve the number of cardiomyocytes, (2) improve vascular supply, and (3) augment the contractile function of the injured myocardium. Animal and clinical studies clearly show that stem cells may improve cardiac function after a heart attack, but we still not have identified the optimal population of cells to use *(56,57)*.

Embryonic stem cells (ESCs) replicate indefinitely and are able to differentiate into cardiomyocytes. There are several difficulties in using human ESCs. The first is the ethical issue surrounding the use of human ESCs derived from products of conception. Second, ESCs are allogeneic, and immunosuppressive therapy might be needed. Third, increased cell death resulting from ischemia has been observed when ESC-derived cardiomyocytes were grafted into a normal myocardium. Finally, human ESCs have also been shown to have the potential to form teratomas. These drawbacks have led researchers to seek alternative undifferentiated cells for CCT.

Recently, there has been major interest in the use of adult stem cells because they can be used in an autologous setting, and many reports highlight their plasticity. However, there is still a great deal of controversy surrounding these claims *(52–55)*. These include failures to reproduce results, contamination of donor samples by other rare stem cells, and the possibility that cell fusion accounts for apparent lineage-switching and transdifferentiation.

Multiple cell types of myocardial infarction have been tested experimentally in animal models, with functional improvement as the primary endpoint *(44,51,56,57)*. So far, safety and practicality considerations have dictated the use of autologous skeletal myoblasts and bone marrow-derived cells as the first cell types to be tested in patients. Several trials have been completed or are underway. Their results, although often reported as positive, should be interpreted cautiously because most of these trials involve small numbers of patients and often lack randomization, double-blinding, and traditional placebo-controlled groups.

No matter the ultimate results, it now seems clear that skeletal myoblasts and bone marrow cells share a fundamental limitation: an inability to convert into true cardiomyocytes that could replace those irreversibly injured by heart attack(s). This limitation has always been clear for myoblasts, which, once engrafted, remain committed to their skeletal muscle phenotype.

For bone marrow cells, the issue remains more controversial. There is little doubt that bone marrow cells and their derivatives can acquire a cardiomyogenic phenotype, but the extent to which such differentiation occurs in vivo for the cell types in clinical use needs to be better defined. Mesenchymal stem cells have clearer potential than hematopoetic cells to form cardiomyocytes upon injection into the heart *(44,57)*. Even if skeletal myoblasts and bone marrow cells cannot transdifferentiate, they may still have functional benefits, mediated by a limitation of ventricular dilatation or paracrine induction of angiogenesis. Yet it is increasingly clear that these cells fail to satisfy the two major prerequisites for cardiac regeneration: an electrical coupling of the grafted cells with host cardiomyocytes and the subsequent generation of an active mechanical force.

The difficulty of inducing adult stem cells to cross their lineage boundaries gives new impetus to the intuitively appealing idea that the most appropriate cells for replacing dead cardiomyocytes might turn out to be cardiomyocytes. This view is supported by groundbreaking proof-of-principle experiments showing that transplanted fetal cardiac cells successfully engrafted into myocardial scars, connected with their host neighbors, and improved function. However, the ethical, availability, scalability, and immunological issues associated with fetal material make it unlikely that these cells could be used for large-scale clinical myocardial replacement therapy.

The limitations of both fetal cells and ESCs highlight the potential of a third source of cardiac cells: resident cardiac stem cells. They offer many advantages for regenerative therapy: (1) CSCs, if harvested and grown in vitro for later transplantation in the same patient, are autologous and thus unlikely to trigger infectious or immunological complications; (2) CSCs are more cardiogenic than other adult stem cells; (3) CSCs trigger robust angiogenic responses after myocardial transplantation. Most importantly, cardiosphere-forming cells can be harvested using standard methods (endomyocardial biopsy or surgery) and can be expanded to obtain clinically relevant numbers of cells in a short period of time. Furthermore, partially differentiated cells present in cardiospheres may enhance engraftment, cardiogenesis, and functional improvement. Percutaneous injection of autologous CSCs may enable the reconstitution of dead or scarred myocardium and halt the inevitable unfavorable evolution of the infarcted heart. Moreover, the replacement of poorly functional, markedly hypertrophied myocytes of the severely decompensated heart with new, younger, more powerful muscle cells and coronary resistance and nonresistance vessels may positively interfere with the onset of terminal failure and death.

However, we will ultimately need to gain a more fundamental understanding of CSC proliferation and differentiation to control it both in vitro and in vivo. Timing of the delivery, routes of application, the capacity of engrafted cells to differentiate and maintain a mature cardiac phenotype while at the same time integrating with the host myocardium and contributing to contractile function, the longevity of intracardiac grafts, and the response of engrafted cells to physiological and pathological stimuli are all issues that require optimization or definition before this strategy can be applied in the clinical setting. More research is needed to determine the long-term outcome and assess the potential associated risks.

REFERENCES

1. Soonpaa MH, Field LJ. Survey of studies examining mammalian cardiomyocyte DNA synthesis. Circ Res 1998;83:15–26.
2. MacLellan WR, Schneider MD. Genetic dissection of cardiac growth control pathways. Annu Rev Physiol 2000;62:289–319.
3. Chien KR, Olson EN. Converging pathways and principles in heart development and disease. Cell 2002;110:153–162.
4. Anversa P, Kajstura J. Ventricular myocytes are not terminally differentiated in the adult mammalian heart. Circ Res 1998;83:1–14.
5. Nadal-Ginard B, Kajstura J, Leri A, Anversa P. Myocyte death, growth, and regeneration in cardiac hypertrophy and failure. Circ Res 2003;92:139–150.
6. Beltrami AP, Urbanek K, Kajstura J, et al. Evidence that human cardiac myocytes divide after myocardial infarction. N Engl J Med 2001;344:1750–1757.
7. Quaini F, Urbanek K, Beltrami AP, et al. Chimerism of the transplanted heart. N Engl J Med 2002;346:5–1.
8. Urbanek K, Quaini F, Tasca G, et al. Intense myocyte formation from cardiac stem cells in human cardiac hypertrophy. Proc Natl Acad Sci USA 2003;100:10,440–10,445.
9. Sussman MA, Anversa P. Myocardial aging and senescence: where have the stem cells gone? Annu Rev Physiol 2004;66:29–48.
10. Anversa P, Sussman MA, Bolli R.Molecular genetic advances in cardiovascular medicine: focus on the myocyte. Circulation 2004;109(23):2832–2838.
11. Hierlihy AM, Seale P, Lobe CG, Rudnicki MA, Megeney LA. The post-natal heart contains a myocardial stem cell population. FEBS Lett 2002;530(1–3):239–243.
12. Martin CM, Meeson AP, Robertson SM, et al. Persistent expression of the ATP-binding cassette transporter, Abcg2, identifies cardiac SP cells in the developing and adult heart. Dev Biol 2004;265(1):262–275.
13. Beltrami AP, Barlucchi L, Torella D, et al. Adult cardiac stem cells are multipotent and support myocardial regeneration. Cell 2003;114(6):763–776.
13a. Bearzi C, Cascapera S, Nascimbene A, et al. Characterization and growth of human cardiac stem cells. Late-breaking developments in stem cell biology and cardiac growth regulation. Circulation 2005;111(13):1720.
14. Oh H, Bradfute SB, Gallardo TD, et al. Cardiac progenitor cells from adult myocardium: homing, differentiation, and fusion after infarction. Proc Natl Acad Sci USA 2003;100(21):12,313–12,318.
15. Matsuura K, Nagai T, Nishigaki N, et al. Adult cardiac Sca-1-positive cells differentiate into beating cardiomyocytes. J Biol Chem 2004;279:11,384–11,391.
16. Messina E, De Angelis L, Frati G, et al. Isolation and expansion of adult cardiac stem cells from human and murine heart. Circ Res 2004;95(9):911–921. Epub 2004 Oct 7.
16a. Smith RR, Abraham MR, Messina E, Cho HC, Giacomello A, Marbán E. Electrophysiology of human and porcine adult cardiac stem cells isolated from endomyocardial biopsies. Late-breaking developments in stem cell biology and cardiac growth regulation. Circulation. 2005;111(13):1720.
17. Laugwitz KL, Moretti A, Lam J, et al. Postnatal isl1+ cardioblasts enter fully differentiated cardiomyocyte lineages. Nature 2005;433(7026):647–653.

18. Pfister O, Mouquet F, Jain M, et al. CD31– but Not CD31+ cardiac side population cells exhibit functional cardiomyogenic differentiation. Circ Res 2005;97(1):52–61.
19. Cai J, Weiss ML, Rao MS. In search of "stemness." Exp Hematol 2004;32(7):585–598.
20. Goodell MA, Brose K, Paradis G, et al. Isolation and functional properties of murine hematopoietic stem cells that are replicating in vivo. J Exp Med 1996;183:1797–1806.
21. Bonde J, Hess DA, Nolta JA. Recent advances in hematopoietic stem cell biology. Curr Opin Hematol. 2004;11(6):392–398.
22. Sarkadi B, Ozvegy-Laczka C, Nemet K, Varadi A. ABCG2—a transporter for all seasons. FEBS Lett. 2004;567:116–120.
23. Dawn B, Stein AB, Urbanek K, et al. Cardiac stem cells delivered intravascularly traverse the vessel barrier, regenerate infarcted myocardium, and improve cardiac function. Proc Natl Acad Sci USA 2005;102(10):3766–3771.
24. Bates RC, Edwards NS, Yates JD. Spheroids and cell survival. Crit Rev Oncol Hematol 2000;36: 61–74.
25. Korff T, Augustin HG. Integration of endothelial cells in multicellular spheroids prevents apoptosis and induces differentiation. J Cell Biol 1998;143:1341–1352.
26. Armstrong MT, Lee DY, Armstrong PB. Regulation of proliferation of the fetal myocardium. Dev Dyn 2000;219:226–236.
27. Kelm JM, Ehler E, Nielsen LK, et al. Design of artificial myocardial microtissues. Tissue Eng 2004;10(1/2):201–214.
28. Cai CL, Liang X, Shi Y, Chu PH, Pfaff SL, Chen J, Evans S. Isl1 identifies a cardiac progenitor population that proliferates prior to differentiation and contributes a majority of cells to the heart. Dev Cell 2003;5:877–889.
29. Wessels A, Pe' Rez-Pomares JM. The epicardium and epicardially derived cells (Epdcs) as cardiac stem cells. Anat Rec 2004;276a(pt A):43–57.
30. Hirschi KK, Majesky MW. Smooth muscle stem cells. Anat Rec 2004;276a(pt A):22–33.
31. Asakura A, Seale P, Girgis-Gabardo A, Rudnicki M. Myogenic speci.cation of side population cells in skeletal muscle. J Cell Biol 2002;159:123–134.
32. Majka S, Jackson K, Kienstra K, Majesky M, Goodell M, Hirschi K. Distinct progenitor populations in skeletal muscle are bone marrow derived and exhibit different cell fates during vascular regeneration. J Clin Invest 2003;111:71–79.
33. Glaser R, Lu MM, Narula N, Epstein JA. Smooth muscle cells, but not myocytes, of host origin in transplanted human hearts Circulation 2002;106:17–19.
34. Sieber-Blum M. Cardiac neural crest stem cells. Anat Rec 2004;276a(pt A):34–42.
35. Ito K, Sieber-Blum M. In vitro clonal analysis of quail cardiac neural crest development. Dev Biol 1991;148:95–106.
36. Ito K, Sieber-Blum M. Pluripotent and developmentally restricted neural-crest-derived cells in posterior visceral arches. Dev Biol 1993;156:191–200.
37. Sieber-Blum M, Ito K, Richardson MK, Langtimm CJ, Duff RS. Distribution of pluripotent neural crest cells in the embryo and the role of brain-derived neurotrophic factor in the commitment to the primary sensory neuron lineage. J Neurobiol 1993;24:173–184.
38. Cheng G, Litchenberg WH, Cole GJ, Mikawa T, Thompson RP, Gourdie RG. Development of the cardiac conduction system involves recruitment within a multipotent cardiomyogenic lineage. Development 1999;126:5041–5049.
39. Poelman RE, Gittenberger-de Groot AC. A subpopulation of apoptosis-prone cardiac neural crest cells targets the venous pole: multiple functions in heart development? Dev Biol 1999;207:271–286.
40. Matsuura K, Wada H, Nagai T, et al. Cardiomyocytes fuse with surrounding noncardiomyocytes and reenter the cell cycle J Cell Biol 2004;167:351–363.
41. Laflamme MA, Myerson D, Saffitz JE, Murry CE. Evidence for cardiomyocyte repopulation by extracardiac progenitors in transplanted human hearts. Circ Res 2002;90:634–640.
42. Wojakowski W, Tendera M, Michalowska A, et al. Mobilization of CD34/CXCR4+, CD34/CD117+, c-met+ stem cells, and mononuclear cells expressing early cardiac, muscle, and endothelial markers into peripheral blood in patients with acute myocardial infarction. Circulation 2004;110:3213–3220.
43. Eisenberg LM, Eisenberg CA. Adult stem cells and their cardiac potential. Anat Rec A Discov Mol Cell Evol Biol 2004;276:103–112.
44. Dimmeler S, Zeiher AM, Schneider MD. Unchain my heart: the scientific foundations of cardiac repair. J Clin Invest 2005;115:572–583.

45. Sampaolesi M, Torrente Y, Innocenzi A, et al. Cell therapy of alpha-sarcoglycan null dystrophic mice through intra-arterial delivery of mesoangioblasts. Science 2003;301:487–492.
46. Brockes JP. Amphibian limb regeneration: rebuilding a complex structure. Science 1997;276:81–87.
47. Odelberg SJ, Kollhoff A, Keating MT. Dedifferentiation of mammalian myotubes induced by msx1. Cell 2000;103:1099–1109.
48. McGann CJ, Odelberg SJ, Keating MT. Mammalian myotube dedifferentiation induced by newt regeneration extract. Proc Natl Acad Sci USA 2001;98:13,699–13,704.
49. Chen S, Zhang Q, Wu X, Schultz PG, Ding S. Dedifferentiation of lineage-committed cells by a small molecule. J Am Chem Soc 2004;126:410, 411.
50. Engel FB, Schebesta M, Duong MT, et al. MAP kinase inhibition enables proliferation of adult mammalian cardiomyocytes.Genes Dev 2005;19:1175–1187.
51. Menasche P. Skeletal myoblast for cell therapy. Coron Artery Dis 2005;16:105–110.
52. Orlic D, Kajstura J, Chimenti S, et al. Bone marrow cells regenerate infarcted myocardium. Nature 2001;410:701–705.
53. Balsam LB, Wagers AJ, Christensen JL, Kofidis T, Weissman IL, Robbins RC. Haematopoietic stem cells adopt mature haematopoietic fates in ischaemic myocardium. Nature 2004;428:668–673.
54. Murry CE, Soonpaa MH, Reinecke H, et al .Haematopoietic stem cells do not transdifferentiate into cardiac myocytes in myocardial infarcts. Nature 2004;428(6983):664–668.
55. Kajstura J, Rota M, Whang B, et al. Bone marrow cells differentiate in cardiac cell lineages after infarction independently of cell fusion. Circ Res 2005;96:127–137.
56. Davani S, Deschaseaux F, Chalmers D, Tiberghien P, Kantelip JP. Can stem cells mend a broken heart? Cardiovasc Res 2005;65:305–316.
57. Smits AM, van Vliet P, Hassink RJ, Goumans MJ, Doevendans PA. The role of stem cells in cardiac regeneration. J Cell Mol Med 2005;9(1):25–36.

8

Embryonic Stem Cells for Myocardial Repair

Lior Gepstein, MD, PhD

SUMMARY

Cell replacement therapy is emerging as a novel therapuetic paradigm for restoration of the myocardial electromechanical properties. This innovative strategy has been significantly hampered by the paucity of cell sources for human heart cells. The recent establishment of the human embryonic stem cell (hESC) lines may provide a possible solution for this cell-sourcing problem. These unique pluripotent cell lines can be propagated in the undifferentiated state in culture and coaxed to differentiate into cell derivatives of all three germ layers, including cardiomyocytes. This chapter will focus on the derivation and properties of hESC and their cardiomyocyte cell derivatives. The potential applications of this unique differentiating system in several research areas will be discussed, with special emphasis on the steps required to fully harness their unique potential in the emerging field of cardiovascular regenerative medicine.

Key Words: Embryonic stem cells; stem cells; cell therapy; tissue engineering; cardiac development; cardiomyocytes.

The adult heart lacks effective repair mechanisms, and therefore any significant cell loss or dysfunction, such as occurs during myocardial infarction, is mostly irreversible and may lead to the development of progressive heart failure. Chronic heart failure is currently a growing epidemic that results in significant disability and mortality while placing a heavy burden on health care systems *(1,2)*. Despite advances in pharmacological, interventional, and surgical therapeutic measures, the prognosis for patients with this disease remains poor. With chronic lack of donors limiting the number of patients who can benefit from heart transplantations, development of new therapeutic paradigms has become imperative.

The recent advances in the areas of stem cell biology and tissue engineering coupled with parallel achievements in molecular and cell biology have paved the way to the development of a new field in biomedicine, regenerative medicine. This approach seeks to develop new biological solutions to replace or modify the function of diseased, absent, or malfunctioning tissue. The heart represents an attractive candidate for these new therapeutic paradigms, and molecular manipulation of the myocardial tissue and

From: *Contemporary Cardiology: Stem Cells and Myocardial Regeneration*
Edited by: M. S. Penn © Humana Press Inc., Totowa, NJ

cell transplantation represents exciting new possibilities for assisting the failing myocardium. The rationale behind the cell replacement approach is based on the assumption that myocardial function may be improved by repopulating diseased areas with a new pool of functional cells *(3–5)*. Based on this assumption, a variety of different cell types have been suggested as potential sources for tissue grafting. Recent animal studies have shown that cells derived from some of these sources may survive to a certain degree, differentiate within the host myocardium, and improve cardiac function *(3–5)*.

Although a number of cell types have been suggested as possible cell candidates for myocardial repair, the inherent electrophysiological, structural, and contractile properties of cardiomyocytes (CMs) strongly suggest that they may be the ideal donor cell type. In early studies, fetal CMs transplanted into healthy mice hearts were demonstrated to survive, align, and form cell-to-cell contacts with host CMs *(6)*. Interestingly, early-stage CMs (fetal and neonatal) were demonstrated to show superior engraftment results in both healthy and infarcted rat hearts when compared to more mature cardiac cells *(7)*. More recently it was demonstrated that these cells could survive and improve cardiac function for up to 6 mo in a rat model of chronic infarction *(8)*. CM transplantation was associated with smaller infarcts *(9)*, prevented cardiac dilatation and remodeling following infarction *(10)*, and improved ventricular function in some of the studies *(11)*.

Despite these encouraging results, the clinical utility of this approach is significantly hampered by the paucity of cell sources for human CMs, by the high degree of donor cell death following cell grafting *(12,13)*, and by the limited evidence for direct functional integration of grafted and host cells. A possible solution to the above-mentioned cell-sourcing problem may be the use of the recently described human embryonic stem cell (hESC) lines *(14,15)*, because these unique cells can be propagated in vitro in large quantities and coaxed to differentiate into the desired cardiac lineage *(16–18)*. The current chapter will therefore focus on describing the unique properties of the hESC lines and on the establishment of a reproducible CM differentiating system using these cells. The possible role of hESC-derived CMs (hESC-CMs) in cardiovascular regenerative medicine will be discussed as well as the steps required to fully harness their potential.

HUMAN EMBRYONIC STEM CELLS

All stem cells, whether from adult or embryonic sources, share a number of properties *(19)*. First, they are capable of self-renewal, meaning that they can divide and give rise to stem cell progeny with similar properties. Second, the stem cells are clonogenic, meaning that each cell can form a colony in which all the cells are derived from this single cell and have identical genetic constitution. Third, they are capable of differentiation into one or more mature cell types. The different stem cells can be categorized anatomically, functionally, or by different cell surface markers, transcription factors, and the proteins they express. One clear division of the stem cell family is between those present in adult somatic tissue, known as adult stem cells, and those isolated from the embryo, known as embryonic stem cells (ESCs).

Although adult stem cells have been found to be more versatile than originally believed, they typically can differentiate into a relatively limited number of cell types. In contrast, the early preimplantation mammalian embryo (at the blastocyst stage) contains a group of cells (inner cell mass [ICM] cells) that will eventually give rise, through specialized progenitor cells, to all the tissues in the body. In 1981 ICM cells isolated from mouse blastocysts were used to generate pluripotent stem cell lines (ESCs) *(20,21)*.

Given the unique properties of mouse ESCs and the large impact that they had on modern biology during the last 20 years, it is not surprising that much effort has been spent on the development of similar human pluripotent lines. Similar to the mouse and rhesus ESC systems, the origin of the hESC lines is from the preimplantation embryo produced by in vitro fertilization for clinical purposes and donated by individuals after informed consent. The hESC lines were established by isolating the ICM cells using specific antibodies (immuno-surgery) to remove an outer cell layer called the trophoectoderm. The ICM cells were then plated on a feeder layer of mitotically inactivated mouse embryonic fibroblasts (MEFs). The resulting colonies were selected, passaged, and expanded for the creation of the hESC lines (Fig.1).

hESCs have been demonstrated to fulfill all the criteria defining ESCs, namely: derivation from the pre- or peri-implantation embryo, prolonged undifferentiated proliferation under special conditions in culture, and the capacity to form derivatives of all three germ layers. Hence, when cultured on the MEF feeder layer, hESCs could be maintained in the undifferentiated state for prolonged periods. When removed from the feeder layer and allowed to spontaneously differentiate, hESCs form three-dimensional differentiating cell clusters termed embryoid bodies (EBs) containing cell derivatives of all three germ layers (Fig. 1). The undifferentiated hESCs were also shown to possess high levels of telomerase activity, to retain a normal karyotype for several passages, and to express specific cell surface markers such as the stage-specific embryonic antigens 3 and 4 (SSEA3, SSEA4), Tra-1-60, Tra-1-81, and the embryonic transcription factor Oct-4.

CARDIOMYOCYTE DIFFERENTIATION OF hESC LINES

Since the initial report of derivation of the hESC lines, a variety of studies have established in vitro spontaneous and directed differentiation systems to several cell lineages, including neuronal tissue *(22,23)*, β islet pancreatic cells *(24)*, hematopoietic progenitors *(25)*, endothelial cells *(26)*, and hepatocytes *(27)*. Recently we were also able to establish a reproducible spontaneous CMs differentiating from hESCs (Fig. 1) *(16)*. Undifferentiated hESCs of the single-cell clone H9.2 were propagated on top of the MEF feeder layer. The hESCs were then removed from the feeder layer, dissociated into small clumps of 3–20 cells, and grown in suspension for 7–10 days, where they formed EBs. The EBs were then plated on gelatin-coated culture dishes. Rhythmically contracting areas appeared 4–22 days later in about 10% of the EBs.

Several lines of evidence confirmed the CM nature of the cells within the beating EBs (Fig. 2) *(16)*. Reverse transcriptase–polymerase chain reaction studies demonstrated the expression of cardiac specific transcription factors (such as GATA4 and Nkx2.5) and cardiac-specific structural genes (cTnI, cTnT, ANP, MLC-2V, MLC-2a). Initial analysis of gene expression pattern during in vitro CM differentiation of hESCs revealed a reproducible developmental temporal pattern. This was manifested initially by a gradual decrease during differentiation in the expression of undifferentiated stem cell markers, such as OCT-4, coupled with an early increase, during the suspension phase, in the expression of cardiogenic-inducing growth factors such as Wnt11 and BMP-2. This was followed by expression of cardiac specific transcription factors (Nkx2.5, Mef2c, and GATA4) and finally by the expression of cardiac specific structural genes such as ANP and myosin heavy chain major histo-compatibility complex (MHC).

Immunostaining studies of cells isolated from the contracting areas within the EBs confirmed the presence of cardiac specific proteins (myosin heavy chain, sarcomeric α-actinin, desmin, cTnI, and ANP). These studies also demonstrated the presence of early cardiac morphology with a typical early striated staining pattern. Ultrastructural analysis of the differentiating CMs demonstrated that these cells were mainly mononuclear, contained varying degrees of myofibrillar bundle organization, and exhibited nascent intercalated discs. Transmission electron microscopy of EBs at varying developmental stages showed the progressive ultrastructural maturation from an irregular myofilament distribution to a more mature sarcomeric organization in late-stage EBs *(28)*. Interestingly, in parallel to this ultrastructural maturation process we also observed a reproducible temporal pattern of early CM cell proliferation (using [^{3}H]thymidine incorporation and immunostaining for Ki67, a marker of cycling cells), cell-cycle withdrawal, and cellular hypertrophy and maturation.

Several functional assays including extracellular and intacellular electrophysiological recordings, calcium imaging, and pharmacological studies clearly demonstrated that the contracting areas within the EBs display functional properties consistent with an early-stage human cardiac phenotype *(16,29,30)*. These studies also revealed important insights into the mechanism of automaticity, excitability, and repolarization in these developing CMs as well as calcium handling and electromechanical coupling *(29)*.

Extracellular electrophysiological recordings using microelectrodes demonstrated a sharp and a slow component, consistent with a relatively long action potential duration characteristic of CMs (Fig. 2). The contracting EBs also displayed appropriate chronotropic responses to adrenergic and cholinergic stimulation indicating functional receptors and signaling pathways.

Whole cell patch-clamp recording from hESC-CMs demonstrated the presence of cardiac-specific action potentials and ionic currents (Fig. 2). These studies also provided mechanistic insights for the basis for spontaneous excitability in early human cardiac cells, namely a high-input resistance as a result of low expression of the Ik_1 current coupled with a prominent sodium current and the presence of the hyperpolarization activated pacemaker current (I_f) *(29)*.

Our next step was to determine whether the hESC differentiating system is limited to the creation of isolated CMs or whether a functional cardiac tissue is generated. In order to answer this question, we microdissected the spontaneously contracting areas within the EBs and plated them on top of a unique microelectrode array (MEA) mapping technique. This allowed long-term, high-resolution electrophysiological recordings from the

---

Fig. 1. *(Opposite page)*   Early embryonic development, derivation of the human embryonic stem cell (hESC) lines and in vitro differentiation. (**A**) The hESC lines were generated from the early-stage embryo at the blastocyst stage. At this stage the embryo is composed of the trophectoderm and the inner cell mass (ICM), which will eventually give rise to all tissue types in the embryo. (**B, C**) ICM cells isolated by immunosurgery and plated on the mouse embryonic fibroblast (MEF) feeder layer were used for the generation of the hESC lines. The resulting colonies were propagated and expanded. Following establishment of the hESC lines, they can be propagated continuously in the undifferentiated state when grown on top of the MEF feeder layer. When removed from these conditions and grown in suspension, they form embryoid bodies (EBs). This in vitro differentiating system can be used to generate a plurality of tissue types, including cardiomyocytes.

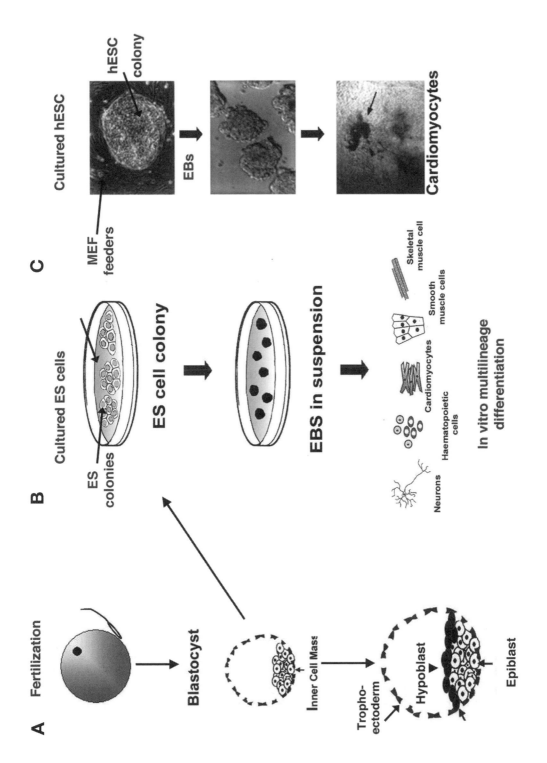

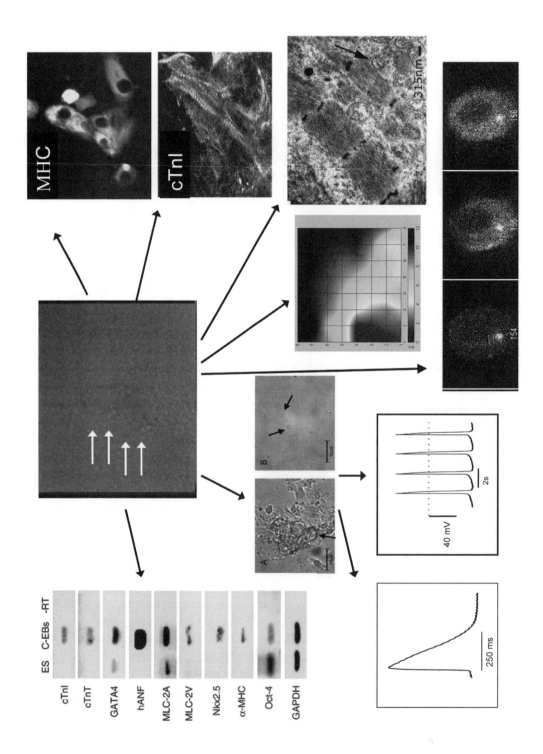

EBs. These measurements demonstrated the presence of a functional syncytium with stable spontaneous pacemaking activity and synchronous action-potential propagation *(30)*.

POSSIBLE RESEARCH AND CLINICAL APPLICATIONS OF hESCs

The absence of in vitro sources for human cardiac tissue imposes significant limitations on cardiovascular research. Therefore, the ability to generate CM tissue from the hESC lines may, for the first time, provide researchers with a unique tool for the investigation of the mechanisms involved in early human cardiac lineage commitment, differentiation, and maturation. In addition, the generation of a long-term in vitro model to study human cardiac tissue may also be used for several pathophysoiological studies, for functional genomics, drug and growth factor discovery, drug testing, and reproductive toxicology. Finally, the ability to generate ex vivo human cardiac tissue may bring a unique value to the developing field of cardiovascular regerative medicine.

MYOCARDIAL REGENERATION STRATEGIES USING hESC-CMs

Myocardial cell replacement therapy is emerging as an innovative therapeutic approach to degenerative heart diseases. Although a number of cell types have been suggested for tissue grafting, the ideal donor cell should probably display the electrophysiological, structural, and contractile properties of CMs and should be able to integrate structurally and functionally with host tissue. In addition, this ideal cell should preferably retain an initial proliferative potential that may enable improved colonization of the scar. The ability to screen the phenotypic properties or to engineer the desired properties of the cells prior to cell grfating may be another advantage of such an ideal cell type. Finally, the optimal candidate cell should be autologous or display minimal immunogenicity and should be readily available in large quantities for transplantation.

Although none of the suggested cell sources can fulfill all the aforementioned criteria, the derivation of the hESC lines offers a number of potential advantages. hESCs are currently the only cell source that can provide, ex vivo, a potentially unlimited number of human CMs for cell transplantation, and because of their inherent cardiac phenotype, these cells are more likely to achieve functional connections with host myocardium. Another possible advantage of hESCs is their ability to differentiate into a plurality of cell lineages such as endothelial progenitor cells for induction of angiogenesis *(26,31)* and even specialized CMs subtypes (pacemaking cells, atrial, ventricular, etc.) tailored for specific applications. hESC-CMs could also lend themselves to extensive characterization and genetic manipulation to promote desirable characteristics such as resistance to ischemia and apoptosis, improved contractile function, and specific electrophysiological

---

Fig. 2. *(Opposite page)* The contracting areas within the embryoid bodies displayed molecular, structural, and functional properties of early-stage human cardiomyocytes. These properties include expression of cardiac-specific genes and transcription factors and positive immunocytochemical staining for cardiac specific proteins (such as major histocompatibility complex and cTnI). Transmission electron microscopy studies demonstrated the presence of early sarcomeric ultrastructural pattern and intercalated discs typical of cardiomyocytes. Finally, the cells were also demonstrated to display cardiac specific action potentials, ionic transients, and intracellular calcium transients at the cellular level during patch-clamp recordings and calcium imaging and spontaneous pacemaker activity and electrical conduction at the tissue level using multielectrode recordings (*see* color-coded activation map). (*See* color plate following p. XX)

properties. Finally, the ability to generate potentially unlimited numbers of CMs ex vivo may also bring a unique value to tissue engineering approaches.

Nevertheless, despite the enormous potential of the hESC-CMs and the important progress achieved so far, several obstacles must be overcome before this strategy can become a clinical reality. These include the need to study the mechanisms underlying hESC cardiomyogenesis in order to generate a directed and more efficient differentiating system, the need to establish selection protocols to derive pure populations of cardiac cells, the need to upscale the entire process to derive clinically relevant numbers of cells, the need to develop methods for in vivo cell grafting and to improve the engraftment, survival, function, and regenerative properties of these cells in healthy and diseased hearts, and the need to counter immune rejection. Similarly, the ability of donor cells to integrate structurally and functionally with host cells should be evaluated, as should their ability to improve myocardial performance in disease hearts. Finally, care should be taken to prevent possible adverse effects such as the possible generation of teratomas or ventricular arrhythmias.

FUNCTIONAL INTEGRATION OF hESC-CM GRAFTS

Optimal functional improvement following cell grafting would require structural, electrophysiological, and mechanical coupling of donor cells to the existing network of host CMs. For example, although transplantation of skeletal myoblasts was shown to improve myocardial performance, gap junctions were not observed between graft and host tissues *(32)*. Yet even the presence of such gap junctions between host and donor CM tissues, as observed in some studies, does not guarantee functional integration. For such integration, currents generated in one cell passing through gap junctions must be sufficient to depolarize neighboring cells.

In a recent study we tested the ability of hESC-CMs to integrate structurally and functionally with host cardiac tissue both in vitro and in vivo *(33)*. Initially, the ability of the hESC-CMs to form electromechanical connections with primary cardiac cultures was assessed using a high-resolution in vitro co-culturing system. Primary cultures were created from neonatal rat ventricular myocytes. The contracting areas within the EBs were then mechanically dissected and added to the co-cultures. Within 24 hours postgrafting, we could detect synchronous contraction in the co-cultures that persisted for several weeks. To further elucidate the functional interaction within the co-cultures, we utilized the MEA mapping technique and documented synchronous activity and tight electrophysiological coupling between the two tissue types. Immunostaining studies demonstrated that this coupling was the result of the generation of gap junctions between the human and rat CMs.

To demonstrate the ability of the hESC-CMs to survive, function, and integrate in the in vivo heart, we assessed their ability to pace the heart and to function as a "biological pacemaker" in an animal model of slow heart rate (the pig complete heart block model, generated by catheter ablation of the atrioventricular [AV] node). Following creation of an AV block, we injected spontaneously contracting EBs into the posterolateral left ventricular wall. A few days following cell grafting, we could begin to detect, in some of the animals, episodes of a new ectopic ventricular rhythm. Three-dimensional electrophysiological mapping revealed that this ectopic ventricular rhythm originated from the area of cell transplantation. Pathological studies validated the presence and integration of the grafted hESC-CMs at the site of earliest electrical activation.

CARDIOMYOCYTE ENRICHMENT, PURIFICATION, AND UPSCALING STRATEGIES

Although CMs can be reproducibly generated from hESCs using the EB differentiating system, these cells typically account for only a minority of the cells within the EBs. Similarly, spontaneously contracting areas were observed in only 10–20% of all EBs. Consequently, developing strategies to augment CM differentiation as well as methods for the selection of the generated CMs should have an important impact on the ultimate success of these cells in myocardial repair.

Directing Cardiac Differentiation

The current CM differentiation system of hESCs is spontaneous and is characterized by a relatively low CM yield. The development of a directed and more efficient differentiation system is hampered, however, by the relative paucity of data regarding the inductive clues that lead to commitment and differentiation of early cardiac tissue in humans. Thus, strategies for directed differentiation should undoubtedly follow research conducted in a number of model organisms, most notably the chick, amphibians, zebrafish, and mouse *(34–37)*.

The heart arises from cells in the anterior lateral plate mesoderm of the early embryo. The endoderm that is in direct contact with the cardiac crescent is considered to have an obligatory role in cardiac fate induction *(38)*. Experimental results from a variety of in vitro and in vivo models suggest that bone morphogenic proteins (BMPs), expressed in the endoderm adjacent to the heart-forming region, may play an important instructive role in cardiogenic induction as well as in maintaining the cardiac lineage *(39)*.

Studies from the xenopus and chick models suggest that the boundaries of the heart-forming region (the cardiac crescent) are also delineated by repressive signals mediated by members of the Wnt family *(36)*. These proteins are secreted from the underlying neural tube and notochord and inhibit cardiomyogenesis in the posterior mesoderm. Coordination of these signaling gradients is further accomplished by secretion of the Wnt-binding proteins (Crescent and Dkk-1) in the anterior endoderm, inhibiting Wnt activity and thereby defining the heart field in an area of low Wnt activity and high BMP strength signals. However, two recent articles suggest that the role of the Wnt family in cardiomyogenesis is more complex then previously thought. Pandur et al. demonstrated that Wnt-11, an activator of the noncanonical Wnt/JNK pathway, is required for cardiogenesis in the xenopus model and the pluripotent mouse embryonic carcinoma stem cell line *(40)*. Nakamura et al., using the P19 cell line as well, revealed that the canonical β-catenin pathway of Wnt signaling is actually activated early during mammalian cardiogenesis *(41)*.

Possible strategies for increasing CM yield during hESC differentiation may include the use of different growth factors, overexpression of cardiac transcription factors, co-culturing with feeder layers, and mechanical factors. Directed differentiation of ESCs to the cardiac lineage in the murine model was achieved using a variety of soluble factors including dimethysulfoxide (DMSO), retinoic acid (RA), and, more recently, BMP-2, transforming growth factor-β, and ascorbic acid. Xu et al. demonstrated enhancement of cardiac differentiation in the hESC model by using 5-Aza-2′-deoxycytidene but, surprisingly, not by DMSO or RA *(18)*.

There is also evidence to suggest that lessons learned from early cardiac differentiation in the model systems, described above, may also be applicable to the hESC system. The cardiogenic inductive role of the primitive visceral endoderm (VE) was demonstrated to play a role in hESC-CM differentiation in an elegant study conducted by Mummery et al. Co-culturing of the hESC line (hES2) that does not regularly differentiate spontaneously to CMs with END-2 cells (a VE-like cell line) provided the missing trigger for cardiac differentiation *(17)*.

Purification of hESC-CMs

Although CM differentiation may be enhanced by one of the possible directed differentiation approaches described above, it is unlikely that the degree of purity that will be achieved would be sufficient for clinical purposes. Given the heterogeneous mixture of differentiating cells within the EB, achieving the goal of obtaining pure cultures of CMs would probably require some form of selection. This selection strategy is required to increase the number of CMs and to avoid the presence of other cell derivatives or remaining pluripotent stem cells in the graft. The latter is crucial to prevent the generation of hESC-related teratomas.

A relatively simple and elegant strategy for CM selection during hESC differentiation was previously reported in the mouse model by Field's group *(42)*. In this approach a cardiac-restrictive promoter is used to drive a selection marker such as an antibiotic-resistance gene (Neo^R). Once a clone that stably expresses the vector is isolated, undifferentiated genetically modified ES cells could be propagated and expanded. The ES cells are then allowed to differentiate in vitro and are subjected to selection with the appropriate antibiotic. Using this selection process during in vitro differentiation, Klug et al. showed that more than 99% pure CM cultures could be generated in the murine model *(42)*. The selected CMs were further demonstrated to form stable grafts following in vivo transplantation.

Using a slightly different approach, researchers have transfected murine ES cells with a construct encoding a cytomegalovirus enhancer and a ventricular specific (MLC-2V) promoter, driving the green fluorescent protein (GFP) product *(43)*. The use of Percoll gradient centrifugation and subsequent fluorescent-activated cell sorting (FACS) yielded 97% pure CM fractions. Approximately 80% of these CMs displayed a typical ventricular action potential.

Upscaling

It is estimated that hundreds of millions of CMs are typically lost in a large myocardial infarction that results in heart failure. Moreover, transplantation of an even a greater number of cells may be required to replace this cell loss because of the relatively low percentage of cells surviving following engraftment. Therefore, a major barrier for the clinical use of hESC-CMs is the generation of sufficient numbers of CMs.

Strategies to increase the number of CMs generated during hESC differentiation may theoretically be employed at several levels: (1) by increasing the initial number of undifferentiated hESC used, (2) by increasing the percentage of hESCs differentiating to the cardiac lineage, (3) by increasing the ability of the cells to proliferate following CM differentiation, and (4) by upscaling the entire process using bioreactors and related technologies.

PREVENTION OF IMMUNE REJECTION

A major obstacle in the utilization of hESC derivatives in the regeneration of different tissue types is the prevention of their immune rejection. A detailed discussion of this issue is beyond the scope of this chapter; it is discussed in detail in a number of excellent reviews (44), and we will briefly discuss some of the strategies suggested to deal with this problem.

The first question to be contended with is precisely how immunogenic are tissues derived from the hESC. Initial characterization of the immunogencity of the hESC was conducted by Drukker et al.(45). hESCs were shown to express relatively low levels of human leukocyte antigen (HLA) class I molecules. This expression was only moderately increased after differentiation in vitro (to EBs) and in vivo (to teratoma cells) but was significantly augmented following interferon-γ treatment. No expression of HLA class II molecules and the ligands for natural killer cell receptors was detected on hESCs or their differentiated products. This may provide an inherent immune advantage to hESC-derived grafts, theoretically requiring milder immunosuppressive regimens. In addition, strategies aimed at reducing the mass of alloreactive T-cells are being developed, and these and other novel therapies with particular relevance to the anticipated immune response mounted against hESC transplants will probably be employed (46).

Other approaches for reducing graft rejection may be the establishment of banks of MHC antigen typed hESCs, establishment of hematopoeitic chimerism using different cell products of hESC-CMs, or the generation of universal donor hESC lines (44). The latter could be achieved by silencing genes associated with the assembly or transcriptional regulation of MHCs or by inserting or deleting other genes that can modulate the immune response.

SUMMARY

The development of hESC lines and their ability to differentiate into CM tissue holds great promise for several cardiovascular research and clinical areas. Research based on the cells may help to elucidate the mechanisms involved in early human cardiac lineage commitment, differentiation, and maturation. Moreover, this research may promote the discovery of novel growth and transcriptional factors using gene-trapping techniques, functional genomics and proteomics, as well as providing a novel in vitro model for drug development and testing. Finally, the ability to generate, for the first time, human cardiac tissue provides an exciting and promising cell source for the emerging discipline of regenerative medicine, tissue engineering, and myocardial repair. Nevertheless, as described above, several milestones have to be achieved in order to fully harness the enormous research and clinical potential of this unique technology.

REFERENCES

1. Cohn JN, Bristow MR, Chien KR, et al. Report of the National Heart, Lung, and Blood Institute Special Emphasis Panel on Heart Failure Research. Circulation 1997;95(4):766–770.
2. Eriksson H. Heart failure: a growing public health problem. J Intern Med 1995;237(2):135–141.
3. Lee MS, Makkar RR. Stem-cell transplantation in myocardial infarction: a status report. Ann Intern Med 2004;140(9):729–737.
4. Mathur A, Martin JF. Stem cells and repair of the heart. Lancet 2004;364(9429):183–192.
5. Reinlib L, Field L. Cell transplantation as future therapy for cardiovascular disease?: A workshop of the National Heart, Lung, and Blood Institute. Circulation 2000;101(18):E182–E187.
6. Soonpaa MH, Koh GY, Klug MG, Field LJ. Formation of nascent intercalated disks between grafted fetal cardiomyocytes and host myocardium. Science 1994;264(5155):98–101.
7. Reinecke H, Zhang M, Bartosek T, Murry CE. Survival, integration, and differentiation of cardiomyocyte grafts: a study in normal and injured rat hearts. Circulation 1999;100(2):193–202.

8. Muller-Ehmsen J, Peterson KL, Kedes L, et al. Rebuilding a damaged heart: long-term survival of transplanted neonatal rat cardiomyocytes after myocardial infarction and effect on cardiac function. Circulation 2002;105(14):1720–1726.

9. Li RK, Mickle DA, Weisel RD, et al. Natural history of fetal rat cardiomyocytes transplanted into adult rat myocardial scar tissue. Circulation 1997;96(9 Suppl):II-179–187.

10. Etzion S, Battler A, Barbash IM, et al. Influence of embryonic cardiomyocyte transplantation on the progression of heart failure in a rat model of extensive myocardial infarction. J Mol Cell Cardiol 2001;33(7):1321–1330.

11. Scorsin M, Hagege AA, Marotte F, et al. Does transplantation of cardiomyocytes improve function of infarcted myocardium? Circulation 1997;96(9 suppl):II-188–193.

12. Zhang M, Methot D, Poppa V, Fujio Y, Walsh K, Murry CE. Cardiomyocyte grafting for cardiac repair: graft cell death and anti-death strategies. J Mol Cell Cardiol 2001;33(5):907–921.

13. Muller-Ehmsen J, Whittaker P, Kloner RA, et al. Survival and development of neonatal rat cardiomyocytes transplanted into adult myocardium. J Mol Cell Cardiol 2002;34(2):107–116.

14. Thomson JA, Itskovitz-Eldor J, Shapiro SS, et al. Embryonic stem cell lines derived from human blastocysts. Science 1998;282(5391):1145–1147.

15. Reubinoff BE, Pera MF, Fong CY, Trounson A, Bongso A. Embryonic stem cell lines from human blastocysts: somatic differentiation in vitro. Nat Biotechnol 2000;18(4):399–404.

16. Kehat I, Kenyagin-Karsenti D, Snir M, et al. Human embryonic stem cells can differentiate into myocytes with structural and functional properties of cardiomyocytes. J Clin Invest 2001;108(3):407–414.

17. Mummery C, Ward-van Oostwaard D, Doevendans P, et al. Differentiation of human embryonic stem cells to cardiomyocytes: role of coculture with visceral endoderm-like cells. Circulation 2003;107(21): 2733–2740.

18. Xu C, Police S, Rao N, Carpenter MK. Characterization and enrichment of cardiomyocytes derived from human embryonic stem cells. Circ Res 2002;91(6):501–508.

19. Weissman IL, Anderson DJ, Gage F. Stem and progenitor cells: origins, phenotypes, lineage commitments, and transdifferentiations. Annu Rev Cell Dev Biol 2001;17:387–403.

20. Evans M, Kaufman M. Establishment in culture of pluripotent cells from mouse embryos. Nature 1981;292:154–156.

21. Martin G. Isolation of a pluripotent cell line from early mouse embryos cultured in medium conditioned by teratocarcinoma stem cells. Proc Natl Acad Sci USA 1981;78:7635.

22. Reubinoff BE, Itsykson P, Turetsky T, et al. Neural progenitors from human embryonic stem cells. Nat Biotechnol 2001;19(12):1134–1140.

23. Zhang SC, Wernig M, Duncan ID, Brustle O, Thomson JA. In vitro differentiation of transplantable neural precursors from human embryonic stem cells. Nat Biotechnol 2001;19(12):1129–1133.

24. Assady S, Maor G, Amit M, Itskovitz-Eldor J, Skorecki KL, Tzukerman M. Insulin production by human embryonic stem cells. Diabetes 2001;50(8):1691–1697.

25. Kaufman DS, Hanson ET, Lewis RL, Auerbach R, Thomson JA. Hematopoietic colony-forming cells derived from human embryonic stem cells. Proc Natl Acad Sci USA 2001;98(19):10,716–10,721.

26. Levenberg S, Golub JS, Amit M, Itskovitz-Eldor J, Langer R. Endothelial cells derived from human embryonic stem cells. Proc Natl Acad Sci USA 2002;99(7):4391–4396.

27. Lavon N, Yanuka O, Benvenisty N. Differentiation and isolation of hepatic-like cells from human embryonic stem cells. Differentiation 2004;72(5):230–238.

28. Snir M, Kehat I, Gepstein A, et al. Assessment of the ultrastructural and proliferative properties of human embryonic stem cell-derived cardiomyocytes. Am J Physiol Heart Circ Physiol 2003;285(6): H2355–2363.

29. Satin J, Kehat I, Caspi O, et al. Mechanism of spontaneous excitability in human embryonic stem cell derived cardiomyocytes. J Physiol 2004;559(Pt 2):479–496.

30. Kehat I, Gepstein A, Spira A, Itskovitz-Eldor J, Gepstein L. High-resolution electrophysiological assessment of human embryonic stem cell-derived dardiomyocytes: a novel in-vitro model for the study of conduction. Circ Res 2002;91(8):659–661.

31. Levenberg S, Rouwkema J, Macdonald M, et al. Engineering vascularized skeletal muscle tissue. Nat Biotechnol 2005;23(7):879–884.

32. Reinecke H, MacDonald GH, Hauschka SD, Murry CE. Electromechanical coupling between skeletal and cardiac muscle. Implications for infarct repair. J Cell Biol 2000;149(3):731–740.

33. Kehat I, Khimovich L, Caspi O, et al. Electromechanical integration of cardiomyocytes derived from human embryonic stem cells. Nat Biotechnol 2004;22(10):1282–1289.

34. Cripps RM, Olson EN. Control of cardiac development by an evolutionarily conserved transcriptional network. Dev Biol 2002;246(1):14–28.

35. Harvey RP. Patterning the vertebrate heart. Nat Rev Genet 2002;3(7):544–556.

36. Olson EN. Development. The path to the heart and the road not taken. Science 2001;291(5512): 2327–2328.

37. Zaffran S, Frasch M. Early signals in cardiac development. Circ Res 2002;91(6):457–469.

38. Nascone N, Mercola M. An inductive role for the endoderm in Xenopus cardiogenesis. Development 1995;121(2):515–523.

39. Monzen K, Nagai R, Komuro I. A role for bone morphogenetic protein signaling in cardiomyocyte differentiation. Trends Cardiovasc Med 2002;12(6):263–269.

40. Pandur P, Lasche M, Eisenberg LM, Kuhl M. Wnt-11 activation of a non-canonical Wnt signalling pathway is required for cardiogenesis. Nature 2002;418(6898):636–641.

41. Nakamura T, Sano M, Songyang Z, Schneider MD. A Wnt- and beta-catenin-dependent pathway for mammalian cardiac myogenesis. Proc Natl Acad Sci USA 2003;100(10):5834–5839.

42. Klug MG, Soonpaa MH, Koh GY, Field LJ. Genetically selected cardiomyocytes from differentiating embronic stem cells form stable intracardiac grafts. J Clin Invest 1996;98(1):216–224.

43. Muller M, Fleischmann BK, Selbert S, et al. Selection of ventricular-like cardiomyocytes from ES cells in vitro. FASEB J 2000;14(15):2540–2548.

44. Bradley JA, Bolton EM, Pedersen RA. Stem cell medicine encounters the immune system. Nat Rev Immunol 2002;2(11):859–871.

45. Drukker M, Katz G, Urbach A, et al. Characterization of the expression of MHC proteins in human embryonic stem cells. Proc Natl Acad Sci USA 2002;99(15):9864–9869.

46. Strom TB, Field LJ, Ruediger M. Allogeneic stem cells, clinical transplantation, and the origins of regenerative medicine. Transplant Proc 2001;33(7–8):3044–3049.

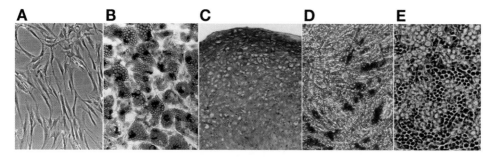

Color Plate 1. Mesenchymal stem cells growing culture. (Chapter 3, Fig. 1; *see* full caption on p. 32.)

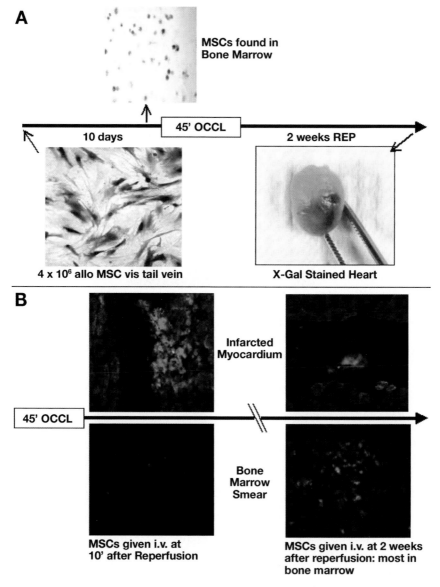

Color Plate 2. Mesenchymal stem cells transduced in vitro with the β-galactosidase reporter gene. (Chapter 3, Fig. 3; *see* full caption on p. 36.)

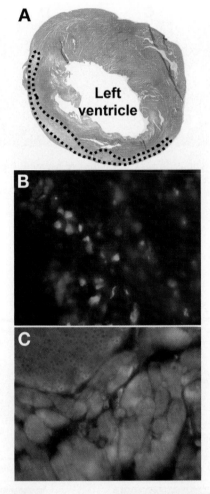

Color Plate 3. Analysis of myocardial infarct induction and multipotent adult progenitor cell engraftment. (Chapter 4, Fig. 5; *see* full caption on p. 54.)

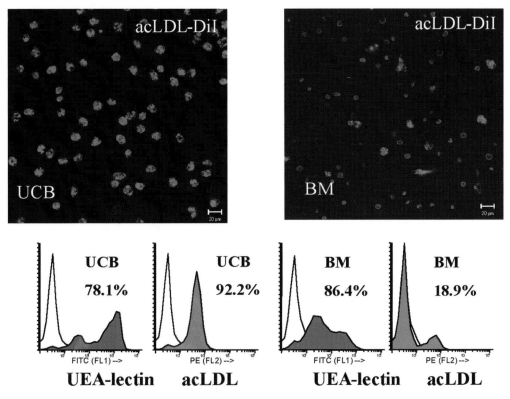

Color Plate 4. Characteristics of umbilical cord blood- and bone marrow-derived endothelial progenitor cells. (Chapter 6, Fig. 1; *see* full caption on p. 70.)

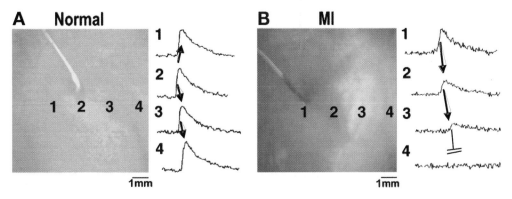

Color Plate 5. Myocardial infarction is associated with conduction block and a lack of significant electrical viability in the infarct border zone as determined by optical mapping. (Chapter 12, Fig. 4; *see* full caption on p. 164.)

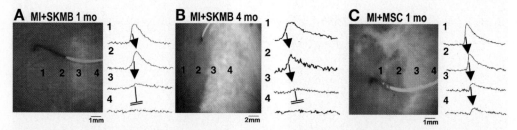

Color Plate 6. Mesenchymal stem cell, but not skeletal muscle myoblast, therapy associated with enhanced electrical viability. (Chapter 12, Fig. 5; *see* full caption on p. 165.)

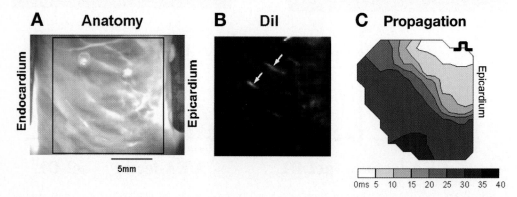

Color Plate 7. The transmural surface of the left ventricular wedge preparation. (Chapter 12, Fig. 6; *see* full caption on p. 166.)

II MECHANISMS AND CRITICAL PATHWAYS INVOLVED IN MYOCARDIAL REPAIR

9

Chemokine and Homing Factor Expression in Acute Myocardial Infarction and Chronic Heart Failure

Arman T. Askari, MD
and Marc S. Penn, MD, PhD

SUMMARY

Acute myocardial infarction (MI) remains a leading cause of morbidity and mortality despite advances in treatment that have resulted in the lowest mortality rate to date. However, a significant proportion of patients do not receive these beneficial therapies because they are deemed ineligible or they present outside the window of opportunity for benefit. Thus, the prevalence of heart failure continues to rise. Although the treatments for heart failure have advanced tremendously, they simply focus on attenuating hemodynamic stimuli that induce deranged remodeling. The limitations of these therapies have prompted the search for additional treatments that may improve the outcomes experienced by patients stricken with an acute MI as well as those who have developed heart failure.

Central to the development of novel therapeutic strategies to treat these two manifestations of ischemic heart disease is an understanding of the different goals for treatment in each situation as well as the differences in the molecular milieu present in each. Whereas targeting preservation of injured tissue and restoration of ample blood flow may be targets in the acute setting, restoring the deranged infrastructure as well as regenerating myocardium may be targets in the failing myocardium.

Potent molecular signaling processes are present that respond to the initial insult of an acute MI and facilitate the initiation of the repair process. However, overactive or persistent expression of these factors may lead to altered myocardial matrix and, ultimately, facilitate the development of heart failure. This chapter will serve to expose the reader to this molecular signaling focusing on the acutely infarcted myocardium and the failing heart.

Key Words: Myocardium; cytokines; growth factors; chemokines; heart failure; myocardial infarction.

INTRODUCTION

Ischemic heart disease, ranging from acute myocardial infarction (MI) to established heart failure, remains the leading cause of morbidity and mortality worldwide. Through

From: *Contemporary Cardiology: Stem Cells and Myocardial Regeneration*
Edited by: M. S. Penn © Humana Press Inc., Totowa, NJ

rigorous research and advances in management strategies, patients have enjoyed the lowest mortality rate associated with acute ischemic syndromes to date. Nevertheless, a substantial proportion of patients are ineligible for acute therapies established to improve outcomes following acute ischemic syndromes, fail to achieve optimal left ventricular (LV) preservation after receiving acute therapy, or present years after their event with an already established cardiomyopathy. Ultimately, a sizable number of patients will be stricken with LV dysfunction and the syndrome of heart failure.

The detrimental effects of an ischemic event do not cease after the acute insult. Progressive expansion of the initial infarct territory, dilatation of the LV cavity, and replacement of cardiomyocytes with fibrous tissue characterizes the untoward reactions following an acute MI *(1)*. Both inflammation and a limited vascular supply seem to facilitate this ventricular remodeling *(2)*, a process that is inversely related to cardiac output, pressure-generating capacity, and, ultimately, increased morbidity and decreased survival following ana acute MI *(3)*. Currently available therapies for heart faliure remain limited, and death rates from heart failure continue to rise *(4)*, which heightens the potential for stem cells in the treatment at the time of acute MI and in patients with chronic heart failure.

THE ACUTELY INFARCTED MYOCARDIUM

The Inflammatory Response to Myocardial Injury

POSTINFARCTION CYTOKINE RELEASE

The inflammatory response is particularly active after an MI, the degree of which is an important determinant of the extent of cardiac remodeling and, ultimately, outcomes *(2)*. Elevated serum levels of markers of inflammation have predicted short- and long-term outcomes in patients with unstable coronary artery disease (CAD) *(5,6)*. In addition, elevation in the white blood cell count following acute MI is an independent predictor of adverse prognosis *(7)*. However, emerging data suggest that a specific faction of mononuclear cells, the hematopoietic stem cell (HSC), may also be mobilized in response to an ischemic stimulus and that this response could be integral to and/or exploited as an adaptive mechanism following an MI resulting in neovascularization and tissue preservation/regeneration *(8–10)*. Although elevations in endothelial progenitor cells have been demonstrated in patients following acute MI *(11)*, a comprehensive understanding of the time course and stimuli of mobilization of HSCs remains in its infancy. Enhanced understanding of the integral components of HSC mobilization, homing, and differentiation may facilitate improved long-term outcomes for this population of patients.

Cytokines released following the acute ischemic insult play an integral role in modulation of tissue repair. The elaboration of cytokines and various growth factors represents an innate response to myocardial injury (Table 1) *(12)*. Increased expression of pro-inflammatory cytokine mRNA, including tumor necrosis factor (TNF)-α, interleukin (IL)-1β, and IL-6, seen in the infarct area (up to 50-fold), as well as in the non-infarcted myocardium (up to 15-fold), generally occurs within 24 hours following an MI and may be transient or more sustained depending on the infarct size *(13,14)*. Acutely, this leads to further local oxidative stress and remodeling but also initiates the processes of wound healing. Chronically, sustained presence of cytokines leads to myocyte phenotype transition and activation of matrix metalloproteinases, which

Table 1
Selected Cytokines and Growth Factors Elaborated After an Acute MI

Cytokine, growth factor, chemokine	Source	Effects on myocardium	Hazardous effects	Comment
TNF-α[a]	Monocytes/macrophages Mast cells Cardiac fibroblasts Cardiac myocytes	High levels in ischemic myocardium modulates inflammatory response Acute–may increase inotropy Regulates apoptosis May induce CM resistabce to hypoxia Modulates LV remodeling	Chronic–heart failure	TNF has also been shown to have chemoattractive properties but also antiproliferative properties on BMSC Facilitates LV remodeling
IL-1[a]	Monocytes/macrophages	High levels in ischemic myocardium modulates inflammatory response stimulates production of acute phase reactants Modulates LV remodeling	Heart failure	Plays an important role in wound healing in the acute phase after an MI
IL-6[a]	Monocytes/macrophages	Regulates myocyte survival/apoptosis Modulates LV remodeling Attenuates myocardial contractility	Potent negative inotrope	Rapidly elaborated soon after MI in ischemia/reperfusion models
MCP[b]	Monocytes/macrophages	Promotes transmigration of macrophages into injured myocardium	Amplification of the inflammatory response to injury	An additional source of local cytokine production and amplification of inflammation
G-CSF[a,b]	Monocytes/macrophages Exogenous	Mobilization of stem cells	Neutrophil attractant	Pro-angiogenic Induces BMSC mobilization Facilitates LV remodeling
HIF-1α[a,c]	Cardiomyocytes Interstitial cells Endothelial cells	Induce secretion of VEGF and EPO Balances oxygen demand and supply	ND	Transcription regulator of response to hypoxia Facilitates LV remodeling

(Continued)

119

Table 1 (Continued)

Cytokine, growth factor, chemokine	Source	Effects on myocardium	Hazardous effects	Comment
VEGF[a,b,c]	Monocyte/macrophages Cardiomyocytes Interstitial cells Endothelial cells	Endothelial cell migration, proliferation, differentiation Induction of cardiomyocyte proliferation Mobilizes BMSC	Increased vascular permeability	Group of secreted proteins Induce BMSC recruitment Facilitates LV remodeling
HGF[c]	Fibroblasts Smooth muscle cells Mast cells Macrophages Endothelial cells Leukocytes Kidneys	Cardiogenesis Enhances cardiomyocyte survival in ischemic Antiapoptotic	ND	Expression induced by IL-1, PDGF, G-CSF Suppressed by TGF and GCC Promotes adhesion, proliferation, and survival of HSC
EPO[c]	Activated macrophages	Cardiomyocyte mitogen Stimulates cardiac angiogenesis	Excess promotes MI	EPOR expressed in epicardium, pericardium, endothelial cells, cardiomyocytes Involved in proliferation and mobilization of BMSC
TGF-β[b,c]	Fibroblasts Smooth muscle cells Platelets Endothelial cells	Cardiac myocyte differentiation Angiogenesis: EC and SMC migration/proliferation ECM production Antiapoptotic Monocyte chemoattractant	Myocardial fibrosis	Up-regulated in response to MI Combined with stem cell transplantation promotes cardiac differentiation Suppresses HGF expression

IL-8 (CXCL8)[a,b,c]	Monocytes Endothelial cells	Regulates neutrophil recruitment and activation Mobilizes BMSC Involved in LV remodeling	Neutrophil attractant	Pro-angiogenic
IP-10[a]	Endothelial cells	Inhibits angiogenesis Involved in LV remodeling	ND	Induced by TNF-α Downregulated by TGF-β
SDF-1[b,c]	Cardiac fibroblasts	Cardiogenesis and vasculogenesis Regulates cardiac myocyte apoptosis Involved with vasculogenesis Mobilizes BMSC	ND	Potent stem cell chemoattractant

[a]Signaling factors that are expressed after myocardial infarction involved in the patho-physiological healing process.
[b]Signaling factors known for their mobilizing and chemotactic abilities.
[c]Signaling factors that are involved in cardiogenesis and neo-angiogenesis.
BMSC = bone marrow stem cell; EC = endothelial cell; ECM = extracellular matrix; EPO = erythropoietin; EPOR = erythropoietin receptor; GCC = glucocorti-coids; G-CSF = granulocyte colony stimulating factor; HGF = hepatocyte growth factor; HIF = hypoxia inducible factor; HSC = hematopoietic stem cell; IL = inter-leukin; IP-10 = interferon-inducible protein-10; LV = left ventricular; MCP = monocyte chemoattractant protein; MI = myocardial infarction; ND = not described; PGDF = platelet derived growth factor; SDF-1 = stromal cell-derived factor 1; SMC = smooth muscle cell; TGF = transforming growth factor; TNF = tumor necrosis factor; VEGF = vascular endothelial growth factor.

Table 2

Triggers of Cytokine Release Following Acute Myocardial Infarction

Trigger	*Effect of stimulus*
Mechanical stress	Most severe at infarct border zone
	Triggers TNF-α and IL-6 production within 30 min
	Acts through stimulation of mechanosensors
	Upregulates Nf-κB
Acute ischemia	Upregulates stress-induced transcription factors
	Increased expression of PPARs
	Sets into motion stimuli that regulate cellular proliferation and the inflammatory response
ROS	Induce and are induced by cytokines
	H_2O_2 increases TNF production through p38/MAPK pathway
	Participate in several myocardial signaling events
Cytokine self-amplification	Self-amplification through feedback loop targeting Nf-κB
	Facilitated through recruitment of inflammatory cells
	High levels of pro-inflammatory cytokines seen in uninfarcted myocardium

TNF, tumor necrosis factor; IL, interleukin; NF-κB, nuclear factor κB; PPAR, peroxisome proliferation-activated receptor; ROS, reactive oxygen species; MAPK, mitogen-activated protein kinase.

modifies the interstitial matrix, further augmenting the remodeling process *(15)*. This in turn alters the local collagen composition and also the integrins that constitute the interface between myocytes and the matrix. These processes ultimately, when favorable, pave the way for angiogenesis and cellular regeneration.

STIMULI FOR POSTINFARCTION CYTOKINE RELEASE

The triggers of cytokine release in the acute postinfarction period include mechanical deformation *(16)*, the ischemic stimulus *(17)*, reactive oxygen species *(18–20)*, and cytokine self-amplification pathways *(21)* (Table 2). Mechanical stress associated with MI leads to the prompt production of TNF-α and IL-6 in the myocardium through stimulation of potential mechanosensors. These pathways activate related downstream nuclear transcription factors, such as nuclear factor (NF)-κB and activating protein (AP)-1, which are required for the induction of most cytokine genes, including TNF-α and IL-6 *(22)*. Similarly, the ischemic stress is a potent stimulus for the transient induction of stress-induced transcription factors, culminating in the expression of cytokines and regulators of cellular proliferation and apoptosis *(23,24)*. These signaling pathways are upregulated in response to diverse stimuli such as hypoxia, free radical excess, osmotic dysregulation, and early membrane injury.

Acute and appropriate cytokine activation in the postinfarct myocardium is fundamentally protective for the host. TNF-α, IL-1β, IL-6, and transforming growth factor (TGF)-β appear to facilitate wound healing, a process that includes phagocytosis and resorption of the necrotic tissue, survival, and hypertrophy of the surviving myocytes, degradation and synthesis of matrix support, such as collagens and integrins, proliferation of the myofibroblasts and angiogenesis/vasculogenesis, and, to a limited extent, progenitor cell proliferation *(13,25,26)*. That inhibition of IL-1β early postinfarction leads to poor wound healing and delayed collagen deposition further supports the role of these inflammatory cytokines in wound healing *(27)*.

Transmigration of macrophages from the blood, in response to the ischemic induction of monocyte chemoattractant protein (MCP), provides a supplementary source of cytokine production and amplification of the local inflammatory response. Participating in this cellular amplification are additional inflammatory cells. For example, mast cells accumulate within infarcted myocardium in response to macrophage-secreted stem cell factor and secrete preformed TNF-α, leading to further localization of mononuclear cells.

Growth Factors, Chemokines, and Myocardial Regeneration

GROWTH FACTORS AND ACUTE ISCHEMIA

Along the continuum of ventricular remodeling following an MI exists the possibility of myocardial regeneration. Resulting from both angiogenesis and myogenesis, this process has been shown to occur naturally and can be augmented in order to improve outcomes. Although tissue injury and inflammation are considered essential for the induction of angiogenesis, the molecular controls of this cascade are mostly unknown. Angiogenic factors, chemokines, and inflammatory cells all play a role in mediating myocardial repair following an MI. In addition, the expression of these mediators of repair may be dictated by the time from the initial insult. For example, expression of vascular endothelial growth factor (VEGF) 120 was found at days 1 and 4 after MI, whereas VEGF164 and VEGF188 along with expression of TNF-α and inducible nitric oxide synthase were noted for a much longer period of time in a postinfarction model *(28)*.

Several growth factors, including IL-3, IL-6, granulocyte–colony-stimulating factor (G-CSF), hepatocyte growth factor (HGF), hypoxia-inducible factor-1-α (HIF-1α), VEGF, erythropoietin (EPO), and TGF-β, have been reported to facilitate HSC mobilization and/or to minimize myocardial cell loss following an ischemic insult. The ability of G-CSF to attenuate LV remodeling through the mobilization of HSC *(29)* and through Akt-induced inhibition of apoptosis *(30)* has been suggested. Based on these mechanisms of benefit, the effects of G-CSF administration were recently assessed in patients with an ST-segment-elevation MI receiving primary percutaneous coronary intervention (PCI) *(31)*. Postreperfusion G-CSF administration over 6 d exposed postischemic human myocardium to approx 2.8×10^{10} mobilized CD34$^+$ cells with potential for homing to necrotic areas and documented improvement of both regional and global myocardial function with sustained functional benefit over 1 year. This benefit was without associated accelerated restenosis post-PCI.

HGF is a multifunctional factor implicated in tissue regeneration, wound healing, and angiogenesis. Circulating HGF is reportedly elevated during the early stage of myocardial infarction. The significance of this rests in its ability to facilitate endothelial cell regeneration *(32)* as well as mesenchymal stem cell (MSC) proliferation, migration, and differentiation *(33)*. The increase in HGF following an acute coronary syndrome also has been correlated with clinical outcomes *(34)*.

HIF-1α is a hypoxia-sensitive transcription factor, which is able to orchestrate and activate many factors and pathways following an ischemic insult. Early overexpression of HIF-1α can result in an increased transcriptional response of factors, such as VEGF and EPO, involved in pathways that increase oxygen delivery and promote adaptive pro-survival responses *(35)*. The release of these factors has been correlated with the increase in circulating HSCs following an MI *(11)* and has been shown to induce the differentiation of these cells into the endothelial cells essential for neovascular tissue formation. After permanent coronary artery ligation in rats, HIF-1α accumulates at the infarct border zone and in the nuclei of cardiomyocytes, interstitial cells, and endothelial cells. This persists for 4 weeks and is co-localized with transcriptional target gene expression *(36)*.

VEGF also plays a role in attenuating LV remodeling in response to an acute MI. VEGF is involved in several pathophysiological processes in response to an acute MI *(37)*. In addition to its role in the healing process and neo-angiogenesis, VEGF possesses CD34+-mobilizing and chemotactic abilities, with the time course of VEGF elevation following an acute MI correlating with the peak in mobilized CD34+ cells *(11)*. Furthermore, myocardial stimulation with MSC transplantation 1 week after an acute MI induced the expression of VEGF, supporting its important role following myocardial injury *(38)*.

Similar to its ability to mediate tissue regeneration in models of nervous system injury *(39,40)*, EPO has demonstrated significant benefit in models of acute myocardial ischemia *(41–43)*. The physiological functions of EPO are mediated by its specific cell-surface receptor, which has been shown to be expressed in the adult heart. In one model of myocardial ischemia and infarction, the administration of EPO imparted significant benefit by preventing myocyte apoptosis and attenuating deterioration in hemodynamic function *(44)*. This benefit may also accrue from the mobilization of circulating stem cells, as observed in brain injury.

TGF-β is a growth factor that possesses a myriad of functions that facilitate healing in response to an MI, not the least of which is limiting infarct size through the attenuation of myocardial apoptosis during reperfusion following an MI *(45,46)*. In addition, TGF-β has been shown to facilitate cardiac myocyte differentiation of CD117+ stem cells transplanted into infarcted myocardium following ex vivo preprogramming with this growth factor *(47)*. The ability of TGF-β to facilitate cardiac commitment of various populations of stem cells makes it an attractive target for the purposes of myocardial regeneration *(48)*.

From the description of the various activities/properties of the above-mentioned growth factors, it can be seen that they play an important role in the response to acute MI and provide potential targets for future therapeutics within the field of myocardial regeneration.

GROWTH FACTORS AND BONE MARROW-DERIVED CELLS

That inflammatory cells such as macrophages participate in angiogenesis has also been suggested. The macrophage-derived peptide PR39 was shown to inhibit the ubiquitin proteasome-dependent degradation of HIF-1α, resulting in accelerated formation of vascular structures in vitro, and increased the production of functional blood vessels in mice *(49)*. These findings suggest that PR39-induced inhibition of HIF-1α degradation may contribute to inflammation-induced angiogenesis. Furthermore, macrophages secrete additional proteases and growth factors necessary for neovascularization.

Additional bone marrow cells with phenotypic and functional characteristics of embryonic hemangioblasts can be used to directly induce new blood vessel formation in the infarct bed and proliferation of preexisting vasculature after experimental MI *(10)*. This neoangiogenesis has been shown to contribute to decreased apoptosis of hypertrophied myocytes in the peri-infarct region, long-term salvage and survival of viable myocardium, reduction in collagen deposition, and sustained improvement in cardiac function. These cells can be recruited in response to the secretion of various chemokines in the acute infarct period *(50).*

CHEMOKINES AND ACUTE ISCHEMIA

Myocardial infarction is associated with an inflammatory response leading to leukocyte recruitment, healing, and formation of a scar. Chemotactic cytokines, members of the chemokine superfamily, are rapidly induced in the infarcted myocardium and may critically regulate the postinfarction inflammatory response. Unlike cytokines, which have pleiotropic effects, chemokines have more specific cellular targets. A CXC chemokine, CXCL8/IL-8, is upregulated in the infarcted area and may induce neutrophil infiltration. In addition, mononuclear cell chemoattractants, such as the CC chemokines CCL2/MCP-1, CCL3/macrophage inflammatory protein (MIP)1α, and CCL4/MIP-1β are expressed in the ischemic area and may regulate monocyte and lymphocyte recruitment following an ischemic insult.

Chemokines may have additional effects on healing infarcts beyond their chemotactic properties. The CXC chemokine CXCL10/interferon-γ inducible protein (IP)-10, a potent angiostatic factor with antifibrotic properties, is induced in the infarct and may prevent premature angiogenesis and fibrous tissue deposition until the infarct is debrided and the provisional matrix necessary to support granulation tissue in-growth is formed. Subsequently, TGF-β-mediated downregulation of IP-10 may shift the balance towards angiogenesis. In addition, TGF-β potently upregulates b-FGF and VEGF expression in endothelial cells and smooth muscle cells, thus enhancing angiogenic activity.

The transient expression of chemokines in recently infarcted myocardium orchestrates the response to injury and induces the inefficient repair processes that have been shown to occur. A key component of the repair process involves stem cell homing to infarcted myocardium. Although the mechanisms involved are incompletely understood, "homing" of stem cells to injured myocardium is essential because it concentrates bone marrow stem cells in a milieu conducive for their engraftment, expansion, and differentiation. That G-CSF-mobilized stem cells fail to engraft in already remodeled myocardium suggests that whatever homing signal may be present in the early postinfarct period is present transiently. Stromal cell-derived factor(SDF)-1 (CXCL12) is known to be a mediator of stem cell homing to the bone marrow, and knockout animals of SDF-1 and its receptor CXCR4 are not viable due to abnormal hematopoietic trafficking *(51,52).* We and others have demonstrated the transient nature of SDF-1 expression following an acute MI *(50,53).* Coupled with the expression of VEGF *(11),* this may provide another link between the response to an MI and the possibility of regeneration of myocardium, especially because SDF-1 overexpression has been shown to induce mobilization of hematopoietic and mesenchymal stem cells.

The complex interactions between growth factors, chemokines, and stem cells discussed above suggest that in order for myocardial regeneration to become a feasible treatment goal following an MI, a multifaceted approach harnessing each of these components may be necessary. In the early post-MI period, focusing on signaling factors known for their mobilizing and chemotactic abilities, signaling factors expressed after MI involved in the pathophysiological healing process and signaling factors involved in cardiogenesis and neo-angiogenesis may afford the best opportunity for myocardial preservation and/or regeneration (Table 1).

THE MYOCARDIUM IN CHF

Once believed to result from an aberrant response to hemodynamic loading following an MI, heart failure appears to be the phenotypic expression of an equally dynamic interplay of inflammation, alterations in the myocyte infrastructure, and the perpetuation of stimuli known to facilitate negative remodeling. The complexity of the myocardium in heart failure cannot be understated, especially in light of the paradoxical worsening of heart failure with the administration of anti-TNF agents *(54,55)*. Furthermore, the myocardium in heart failure does not secrete agents known to facilitate stem cell homing, engraftment, and improved function unless provoked to do so *(50)*. An understanding of these components may potentially facilitate the development of targeted therapeutics in order to improve the dismal outcome destined for these patients.

Inflammation and the Failing Heart

Whereas the inflammatory response to an acute MI facilitates the response to injury and initiates the healing process, unregulated or continuous production of cytokines contributes to the progression to heart failure via their known biological effects (Table 3). TNF-α *(56)*, IL-1 *(57)*, and IL-6 *(58)* all produce deleterious effects on LV function and have been correlated with the progression to heart failure and adverse outcomes *(59)*. Although the expression of pro-inflammatory cytokines peaked at 1 week in infarcted tissue, persistent gene expression was noted in noninfarcted tissue *(17)*. The level of one of these cytokines, IL-1, was correlated with the amount of collagen deposition supporting the role in pathological remodeling.

The pro-inflammatory cytokines impart their deleterious effects through several mechanisms, including depression of LV systolic function, pathological LV remodeling, and deleterious effects on the endothelium. Nitric oxide (NO) appears to mediate, at least in part, the negative inotropic effects of these cytokines *(60)*. Cytokine-induced NO mediates its negative inotropic effects through inhibition of β-adrenergic signaling *(61)*.

Like in the acutely infarcted myocardium, these cytokines play an important role in LV remodeling, including myocyte hypertrophy, alterations in fetal gene expression, and progressive myocyte loss through apoptosis. In addition to the above effects, several lines of evidence suggest that TNF may promote LV remodeling through alterations in the extracellular matrix *(56,62)*. Inflammation provokes time-dependent changes in the balance between matrix metalloproteinase (MMP) activity and tissue inhibitors of MMP (TIMP) activity *(63)*. During the early stages of inflammation, there is an increase in the ratio of MMP activity to TIMP levels, which fosters LV dilation. However, with chronic inflammatory signaling, there is a time-dependent increase in TIMP levels, with a resultant decrease in the ratio of MMP activity to TIMP activity and a subsequent increase in myocardial collagen content.

In addition to the effects of inflammatory mediators on cardiac structure and function, there is growing evidence that the concentrations of inflammatory mediators that exist in heart failure are sufficient to contribute to endothelial dysfunction. Pro-inflammatory cytokines such as TNF-α and IL-6 are associated with endothelial dysfunction in patients with CAD or heart failure. When compared with CAD patients and healthy controls, patients with ischemic heart failure and dilated cardiomyopathy exhibited higher levels of pro-inflammatory cytokines *(64)*. Commensurate with increase, patients with ischemic and dilated cardiomyopathy exhibited greater endothelial dysfunction compared to CAD patients ($p < 0.05$) or controls ($p < 0.001$).

Table 3

Biological Effects of Inflammatory Cytokines in Heart Failure

Left ventricular function
  Potent negative inotropes
  Deranged diastolic function
Left ventricular remodeling
  Myocyte hypertrophy
  Alterations in fetal gene expression
  Cardiac myocyte apoptosis
  Alterations in the extracellular matrix
Excitation-contraction uncoupling
Endothelial dysfunction
Decreased catecholamine responsiveness
Pulmonary edema
Decreased skeletal muscle blood flow
Anorexia and cachexia

Growth Factors, Chemokines, and the Failing Heart

The complex pathways involving stimulation of growth factor and chemokine expression remain active in the failing myocardium, but regulatory mechanisms and differential responses serve to modulate these effects, culminating in progressive LV remodeling. Ultimately, the balance of pro- and anti-inflammatory factors as well as factors that stimulate collagen production and degradation dictates the perpetuation or stabilization of myocardial remodeling, respectively *(65)*.

Cardiomyopathy comprises a heterogeneous group of diseases, including the ischemic (ICM) and dilative (DCM) forms. Recent studies in mice show that VEGF is involved in ICM. Whether VEGF played a role in human cardiomyopathy was assessed by examining the mRNA and protein expression of VEGF and its receptors in hearts of patients with end-stage DCM and ICM and in healthy individuals *(66)*. In DCM, mRNA transcript levels of various isoforms of VEGF and the respective protein levels of VEGF and VEGF-R1 were downregulated compared with controls. However, in ICM, mRNA transcript levels of VEGF isoforms and the respective protein levels of VEGF were upregulated. The vascular density was decreased in DCM but increased in ICM compared with controls. Blunted VEGF and VEGF-R1 protein expression and downregulated mRNA of the predominant isoform of VEGF, VEGF-165, provide evidence that the VEGF-165 defect contributes to DCM. Furthermore, other VEGF-independent pathways are also involved in endothelial cell survival *(67)*. The disturbance in the angiogenesis pathways may facilitate the development of a cardiomyopathy *(68)*. Targeting these pathways might be of benefit through upregulating a key component of myocardium, the blood vessels.

Targeting the other component of LV remodeling, the cardiac myocytes, may also contribute to improved LV function in remodeled myocardium. Fibroblast growth factors (FGFs) have diverse effects on the myocardium, but the importance of stimulating angiogenesis vs direct effects of FGFs on cardiac myocytes is unclear. However, the administration of a replication-deficient adenoviral construct overexpressing FGF-5 (AdvFGF-5) to improve flow and function in swine with hibernating myocardium induced profound myocyte cellular hypertrophy and reentry of a small number of myocytes into the mitotic phase of the cell cycle, suggesting that overexpression of

AdvFGF-5 may afford a way to restore function in hibernating myocardium and ameliorate heart failure in chronic ischemic cardiomyopathy (69).

It is postulated that heart failure is related to blood flow and collagen synthesis. HGF, a mesenchyme-derived pleiotropic factor, is known to regulate cell growth, motility, and morphogenesis of various types of cells, but it has also been shown to facilitate the regression of fibrosis in animal injury models of liver and lung. The potent angiogenic and antifibrotic effects of HGF have recently been demonstrated in an animal model of cardiomyopathy. In this model, weekly direct injections of HGF resulted in increased blood flow and capillary density and decreased fibrosis (70).

What these studies emphasize is that remodeled myocardium possesses characteristics that perpetuate dysfunction and preclude the intrinsic myocardial repair mechanisms from stabilizing the decompensation. Consistent with this notion, we have demonstrated that an integral chemokine involved in stem cell homing, SDF-1, is no longer expressed in remodeled myocardium (50). However, the importance of this chemokine to preservation of myocardial function was also demonstrated through recapitulation of its expression profile as well as overexpression in ischemic cardiomyopathy. Although SDF-1 was the first chemokine shown to link the chemokine/stem cell axis in ischemic cardiomyopathy, other factors are becoming elucidated that may facilitate the improvement of LV function through myocardial regeneration.

Apoptosis in the Failing Heart

Apoptosis, a universal mechanism by which organisms clear damaged or unnecessary cells, appears to be an ongoing process in the failing heart that disrupts the contractile infrastructure—the cardiac myocytes. Although heart failure can be the result of a variety of causes, including ischemic, hypertensive, toxic, and inflammatory heart disease, the cellular mechanisms responsible for the progressive deterioration of myocardial function observed in heart failure remain unclear and may result from apoptosis (programmed cell death). Ongoing inflammatory signaling such as that present in the failing myocardium can set into motion the apoptotic pathways and contribute to the loss of cardiomyocytes (71–74) and cardiac stem cells (75). The loss of functionally competent cardiac stem cells in chronic ischemic cardiomyopathy may underlie the progressive functional deterioration and the onset of terminal failure (75). The importance of cardiac apoptosis in the failing heart can be emphasized through studies that have resulted in improved LV function via targeting anti-apoptosis mechanisms through pharmacological, gene, or cell therapy (10,50,76–79).

The regenerative and restorative capacity of stem cell therapy in this patient population may arise, in part, from attenuated apoptosis following an ischemic event, which, ultimately, minimizes LV remodeling, resulting in preserved LV function. The delivery of bone marrow containing endothelial progenitor cells was shown to reduce cardiomyocyte apoptosis and improve myocardial function when delivered early following an MI (10). The benefits of reduced apoptosis have also been demonstrated with enhanced stem cell mobilization in already remodeled myocardium (50). In addition to improved neovascularization with SDF-1-induced stem cell mobilization, a significant reduction in cardiomyocyte apoptosis was observed in a rat model of ischemic cardiomyopathy, supporting the multifaceted mechanisms of benefit of this therapy.

Despite significant achievements in our understanding of the molecular mechanisms responsible for decreased cardiac performance in animals and patients with CHF, numerous hurdles remain before targeting these pathways contributes significantly to treatment of clinical populations with cardiomyopathy.

CLINICAL IMPLICATIONS/CONCLUSIONS

From the discussion above it can be seen that various cytokines, growth factors, and chemokines are produced in significant quantities from the multiple sources following an MI and affect the post-MI milieu through effects on inflammatory cells, myocytes, and the matrix. These agents are also continuously expressed in the failing myocardium, albeit in different proportions. The effects of the response to injury and remodeling are pleiotropic and depend on the balance of other factors, the timing of release, and the cell types involved. In addition, the substantial upregulation of "homing" factors that occurs following an MI may allow for either peripheral or locally infused delivery of stem cells, whereas in the failing myocardium the absence of integral homing factor expression may dictate direct injection of therapies in order to facilitate preservation or regeneration of myocardium.

Although similarities exist between acutely infarcted myocardium and that present in the failing heart, the unique milieu present in each situation may ultimately dictate the optimal therapies. While targeting preservation of as much viable tissue as possible through harnessing and augmenting the natural repair processes may be the goal in the acute MI setting, restoration of the derangements in the myocardial infrastructure through combined cell/gene transfer may be the goal in the heart failure setting. Through a better understanding of the uniqueness of acutely infarcted myocardium and of the myocardium in heart failure, potential novel therapies can be developed that may provide patients with the chance of improved outcomes.

The differences between the acutely infarcted and the failing myocardium suggest that there is a limited therapeutic window early following an MI during which augmentation of the naturally expressed stem cell homing factors and, ultimately, stem cell therapy for the purposes of myocardial regeneration is possible. This pro-regenerative environment can be recapitulated through combined cell therapy and gene transfer in order to awaken the regeneratively quiescent, remodeled myocardium and afford similar benefits of stem cell therapy in the failing myocardium. For example, we demonstrated that the transient expression of a putative homing factor, SDF-1, following an acute MI could be reproduced through transplantation of genetically altered skeletal myoblasts into failing myocardium. This could then be coupled with stem cell mobilization using G-CSF which, ultimately, resulted in improved LV function *(50)*. Because data are compiled with respect to the homing and differentiation capabilities of the different factors expressed in acutely infarcted and failing myocardium, the ability to potentially preserve and regenerate, respectively, myocardium and improve outcomes following an MI will become a reality rather than a dream.

REFERENCES

1. Pfeffer JM, Pfeffer MA, Fletcher PJ, Braunwald E. Progressive ventricular remodeling in rat with myocardial infarction. Am J Physiol 1991;260:H1406–1414.
2. Fuster V, Badimon L, Badimon JJ, Chesebro JH. The pathogenesis of coronary artery disease and the acute coronary syndromes. N Engl J Med 1992;326:242–250.
3. Fletcher PJ, Pfeffer JM, Pfeffer MA, et al. Left ventricular diastolic pressure-volume relations in rats with healed myocardial infarction: effects on systolic function. Circ Res 1981;49:618–626.
4. Eriksson H. Heart failure: a growing public health problem. J Intern Med 1995;237:135–141.

5. Morrow DA, Rifai N, Antman EM, et al. C-reactive protein is a potent predictor of mortality independently and in combination with troponin T in acute coronary syndromes: a TIMI 11A substudy. J Am Coll Cardiol 1998;31:1460–1465.

6. Lindahl B, Toss H, Siegbahn A, Venge P, Wallentin L. Markers of myocardial damage and inflammation in relation to long-term mortality in unstable coronary disease. N Engl J Med 2000;343(16): 1139–1147.

7. Furman MI, Becker RC, Yarzebski J, Savegeau J, Gore JM, Goldberg RJ. Effect of elevated leukocyte count on in-hospital mortality following acute myocardial infarction. Am J Cardiol 1996;78:945–948.

8. Asahara T, Masuda H, Takahashi T, et al. Bone marrow origin of endothelial progenitor cells responsible for postnatal vasculogenesis in physiological and pathological neovascularization. Circ Res 1999;85(3):221–228.

9. Asahara T, Takahashi T, Masuda H, et al. VEGF contributes to postnatal neovascularization by mobilizing bone marrow-derived endothelial progenitor cells. EMBO J 1999;18(14):3964–3972.

10. Kocher AA, Schuster MD, Szabolcs MJ, et al. Neovascularization of ischemic myocardium by human bone-marrow-derived angioblasts prevents cardiomyocyte apoptosis, reduces remodeling and improves cardiac function. Nat Med 2001;7(4):430–436.

11. Shintani S, Murohara T, Ikeda H, et al. Mobilization of endothelial progenitor cells in patients with acute myocardial infarction. Circulation 2001;103(23):2776–2779.

12. Mann DL. Stress-activated cytokines and the heart: from adaptation to maladaptation. Annu Rev Physiol 2003;65:81–101.

13. Deten A, Volz HC, Briest W, Zimmer HG. Cardiac cytokine expression is upregulated in the acute phase after myocardial infarction. Experimental studies in rats. Cardiovasc Res 2002;55(2):329–340.

14. Irwin MW, Mak S, Mann DL, et al. Tissue expression and immunolocalization of tumor necrosis factor-alpha in postinfarction dysfunctional myocardium. Circulation 1999;99(11):1492–1498.

15. White HD, Norris RM, Brown MA, Brandt PW, Whitlock RM, Wild CJ. Left ventricular end-systolic volume as the major determinant of survival after recovery from myocardial infarction. Circulation 1987;76(1):44–51.

16. Kapadia SR, Oral H, Lee J, Nakano M, Taffet GE, Mann DL. Hemodynamic regulation of tumor necrosis factor-alpha gene and protein expression in adult feline myocardium. Circ Res 1997;81(2): 187–195.

17. Ono K, Matsumori A, Shioi T, Furukawa Y, Sasayama S. Cytokine gene expression after myocardial infarction in rat hearts: possible implication in left ventricular remodeling. Circulation 1998;98(2): 149–156.

18. Nakamura K, Fushimi K, Kouchi H, et al. Inhibitory effects of antioxidants on neonatal rat cardiac myocyte hypertrophy induced by tumor necrosis factor-alpha and angiotensin II. Circulation 1998;98(8):794–799.

19. Meldrum DR, Dinarello CA, Cleveland JC, Jr, et al. Hydrogen peroxide induces tumor necrosis factor alpha-mediated cardiac injury by a P38 mitogen-activated protein kinase-dependent mechanism. Surgery 1998;124(2):291–297.

20. Dewald O, Frangogiannis NG, Zoerlein M, et al. Development of murine ischemic cardiomyopathy is associated with a transient inflammatory reaction and depends on reactive oxygen species. Proc Natl Acad Sci USA 2003;100(5):2700–2705.

21. Nakamura H, Umemoto S, Naik G, et al. Induction of left ventricular remodeling and dysfunction in the recipient heart after donor heart myocardial infarction: new insights into the pathologic role of tumor necrosis factor-alpha from a novel heterotopic transplant-coronary ligation rat model. J Am Coll Cardiol 2003;42(1):173–181.

22. Beg AA, Baltimore D. An essential role for NF-kappaB in preventing TNF-alpha-induced cell death. Science 1996;274(5288):782–784.

23. Shiomi T, Tsutsui H, Hayashidani S, et al. Pioglitazone, a peroxisome proliferator-activated receptor-gamma agonist, attenuates left ventricular remodeling and failure after experimental myocardial infarction. Circulation 2002;106(24):3126–3132.

24. Liu HR, Tao L, Gao E, et al. Anti-apoptotic effects of rosiglitazone in hypercholesterolemic rabbits subjected to myocardial ischemia and reperfusion. Cardiovasc Res 2004;62(1):135–144.

25. Deten A, Holzl A, Leicht M, Barth W, Zimmer HG. Changes in extracellular matrix and in transforming growth factor beta isoforms after coronary artery ligation in rats. J Mol Cell Cardiol 2001;33(6): 1191–1207.

26. Deten A, Volz HC, Briest W, Zimmer HG. Differential cytokine expression in myocytes and non-myocytes after myocardial infarction in rats. Mol Cell Biochem 2003;242(1–2):47–55.

27. Hwang MW, Matsumori A, Furukawa Y, et al. Neutralization of interleukin-1beta in the acute phase of myocardial infarction promotes the progression of left ventricular remodeling. J Am Coll Cardiol 2001;38(5):1546–1553.

28. Heba G, Krzeminski T, Porc M, Grzyb J, Dembinska-Kiec A. Relation between expression of TNF alpha, iNOS, VEGF mRNA and development of heart failure after experimental myocardial infarction in rats. J Physiol Pharmacol 2001;52(1):39–52.

29. Orlic D, Kajstura J, Chimenti S, et al. Mobilized bone marrow cells repair the infarcted heart, improving function and survival. Proc Natl Acad Sci USA 2001;98(18):10344–10349.

30. Iwanaga K, Takano H, Ohtsuka M, et al. Effects of G-CSF on cardiac remodeling after acute myocardial infarction in swine. Biochem Biophys Res Commun 2004;325(4):1353–1359.

31. Ince H, Petzsch M, Kleine HD, et al. Final 1-year Results of the Front-Integrated Revascularization and Stem Cell Liberation in Evolving Acute Myocardial Infarction by Granulocyte Colony-Stimulating Factor (FIRSTLINE-AMI) Trial. Circulation 2005;112:I-73–I-80.

32. Ono K, Matsumori A, Shioi T, Furukawa Y, Sasayama S. Enhanced expression of hepatocyte growth factor/c-Met by myocardial ischemia and reperfusion in a rat model. Circulation 1997;95(11): 2552–2558.

33. Kucia M, Dawn B, Hunt G, et al. Cells expressing early cardiac markers reside in the bone marrow and are mobilized into the peripheral blood after myocardial infarction. Circ Res 2004;95(12): 1191–1199.

34. Forte G, Minieri M, Cossa P, et al. Hepatocyte growth factor effects on mesenchymal stem cells: proliferation, migration and differentiation. Stem Cells 2006;24(1):23–33.

35. Lee SH, Wolf PL, Escudero R, Deutsch R, Jamieson SW, Thistlethwaite PA. Early expression of angiogenesis factors in acute myocardial ischemia and infarction. N Engl J Med 2000;342(9): 626–633.

36. Jurgensen JS, Rosenberger C, Wiesener MS, et al. Persistent induction of HIF-1alpha and -2alpha in cardiomyocytes and stromal cells of ischemic myocardium. Faseb J 2004;18(12):1415–1417.

37. Vandervelde S, van Luyn MJ, Tio RA, Harmsen MC. Signaling factors in stem cell-mediated repair of infarcted myocardium. J Mol Cell Cardiol 2005;39(2):363–376.

38. Tang YL, Zhao Q, Zhang YC, et al. Autologous mesenchymal stem cell transplantation induce VEGF and neovascularization in ischemic myocardium. Regul Pept 2004;117(1):3–10.

39. Li F, Chong ZZ, Maiese K. Erythropoietin on a tightrope: balancing neuronal and vascular protection between intrinsic and extrinsic pathways. Neurosignals 2004;13(6):265–289.

40. Genc S, Koroglu TF, Genc K. Erythropoietin and the nervous system. Brain Res 2004;1000(1–2): 19–31.

41. Wright GL, Hanlon P, Amin K, Steenbergen C, Murphy E, Arcasoy MO. Erythropoietin receptor expression in adult rat cardiomyocytes is associated with an acute cardioprotective effect for recombinant erythropoietin during ischemia-reperfusion injury. FASEB J 2004;18(9):1031–1033.

42. van der Meer P, Lipsic E, Henning RH, et al. Erythropoietin improves left ventricular function and coronary flow in an experimental model of ischemia-reperfusion injury. Eur J Heart Fail 2004;6(7):853–859.

43. Bogoyevitch MA. An update on the cardiac effects of erythropoietin cardioprotection by erythropoietin and the lessons learnt from studies in neuroprotection. Cardiovasc Res 2004;63(2):208–216.

44. Calvillo L, Latini R, Kajstura J, et al. Recombinant human erythropoietin protects the myocardium from ischemia-reperfusion injury and promotes beneficial remodeling. Proc Natl Acad Sci USA 2003;100(8):4802–4806.

45. Baxter GF, Mocanu MM, Brar BK, Latchman DS, Yellon DM. Cardioprotective effects of transforming growth factor-beta1 during early reoxygenation or reperfusion are mediated by p42/p44 MAPK. J Cardiovasc Pharmacol 2001;38(6):930–939.

46. Matsumoto-Ida M, Takimoto Y, Aoyama T, Akao M, Takeda T, Kita T. Activation of TGF-β1-TAK1-p38 MAPK pathway in spared cardiomyocytes is involved in left ventricular remodeling after myocardial infarction in rats. Am J Physiol Heart Circ Physiol 2006;290(2):H709–H715.

47. Li TS, Hayashi M, Ito H, et al. Regeneration of infarcted myocardium by intramyocardial implantation of ex vivo transforming growth factor-beta-preprogrammed bone marrow stem cells. Circulation 2005;111(19):2438–2445.

48. Zeineddine D, Papadimou E, Mery A, Menard C, Puceat M. Cardiac commitment of embryonic stem cells for myocardial repair. Methods Mol Med 2005;112:175–182.

49. Li J, Post M, Volk R, et al. PR39, a peptide regulator of angiogenesis. Nat Med 2000;6(1):49–55.

50. Askari AT, Unzek S, Popovic ZB, et al. Effect of stromal-cell-derived factor 1 on stem-cell homing and tissue regeneration in ischaemic cardiomyopathy. Lancet 2003;362(9385):697–703.

51. Zou YR, Kottmann AH, Kuroda M, Taniuchi I, Littman DR. Function of the chemokine receptor CXCR4 in haematopoiesis and in cerebellar development. Nature 1998;393(6685):595–599.

52. Nagasawa T. Role of chemokine SDF-1/PBSF and its receptor CXCR4 in blood vessel development. Ann N Y Acad Sci 2001;947:112–116.

53. Ma J, Ge J, Zhang S, et al. Time course of myocardial stromal cell-derived factor 1 expression and beneficial effects of intravenously administered bone marrow stem cells in rats with experimental myocardial infarction. Basic Res Cardiol 2005;100(3):217–223.

54. Chung ES, Packer M, Lo KH, Fasanmade AA, Willerson JT. Randomized, double-blind, placebo-controlled, pilot trial of infliximab, a chimeric monoclonal antibody to tumor necrosis factor-alpha, in patients with moderate-to-severe heart failure: results of the anti-TNF Therapy Against Congestive Heart Failure (ATTACH) trial. Circulation 2003;107(25):3133–3140.

55. Mann DL, McMurray JJ, Packer M, et al. Targeted anticytokine therapy in patients with chronic heart failure: results of the Randomized Etanercept Worldwide Evaluation (RENEWAL). Circulation 2004;109(13):1594–1602.

56. Pagani FD, Baker LS, Hsi C, Knox M, Fink MP, Visner MS. Left ventricular systolic and diastolic dysfunction after infusion of tumor necrosis factor-alpha in conscious dogs. J Clin Invest 1992;90(2): 389–398.

57. Hosenpud JD, Campbell SM, Mendelson DJ. Interleukin-1-induced myocardial depression in an isolated beating heart preparation. J Heart Transplant 1989;8(6):460–464.

58. Finkel MS, Oddis CV, Jacob TD, Watkins SC, Hattler BG, Simmons RL. Negative inotropic effects of cytokines on the heart mediated by nitric oxide. Science 1992;257(5068):387–389.

59. Rauchhaus M, Doehner W, Francis DP, et al. Plasma cytokine parameters and mortality in patients with chronic heart failure. Circulation 2000;102(25):3060–3067.

60. Panas D, Khadour FH, Szabo C, Schulz R. Proinflammatory cytokines depress cardiac efficiency by a nitric oxide-dependent mechanism. Am J Physiol 1998;275(3 Pt 2):H1016–H1023.

61. Gulick T, Chung MK, Pieper SJ, Lange LG, Schreiner GF. Interleukin 1 and tumor necrosis factor inhibit cardiac myocyte beta-adrenergic responsiveness. Proc Natl Acad Sci USA 1989;86(17): 6753–6757.

62. Li YY, Feng YQ, Kadokami T, et al. Myocardial extracellular matrix remodeling in transgenic mice overexpressing tumor necrosis factor alpha can be modulated by anti-tumor necrosis factor alpha therapy. Proc Natl Acad Sci USA 2000;97(23):12746–12751.

63. Li YY, McTiernan CF, Feldman AM. Interplay of matrix metalloproteinases, tissue inhibitors of metalloproteinases and their regulators in cardiac matrix remodeling. Cardiovasc Res 2000;46(2): 214–224.

64. Tentolouris C, Tousoulis D, Antoniades C, et al. Endothelial function and proinflammatory cytokines in patients with ischemic heart disease and dilated cardiomyopathy. Int J Cardiol 2004;94(2–3): 301–305.

65. Kittleson MM, Minhas KM, Irizarry RA, et al. Gene expression analysis of ischemic and non-ischemic cardiomyopathy: shared and distinct genes in the development of heart failure. Physiol Genomics 2005;21(3):299–307.

66. Abraham D, Hofbauer R, Schafer R, et al. Selective downregulation of VEGF-A(165), VEGF-R(1), and decreased capillary density in patients with dilative but not ischemic cardiomyopathy. Circ Res 2000;87(8):644–647.

67. Schafer R, Abraham D, Paulus P, et al. Impaired VE-cadherin/beta-catenin expression mediates endothelial cell degeneration in dilated cardiomyopathy. Circulation 2003;108(13):1585–1591.

68. Tham E, Wang J, Piehl F, Weber G. Upregulation of VEGF-A without angiogenesis in a mouse model of dilated cardiomyopathy caused by mitochondrial dysfunction. J Histochem Cytochem 2002;50(7): 935–944.

69. Suzuki G, Lee TC, Fallavollita JA, Canty JM, Jr. Adenoviral gene transfer of FGF-5 to hibernating myocardium improves function and stimulates myocytes to hypertrophy and reenter the cell cycle. Circ Res 2005;96(7):767–775.

70. Taniyama Y, Morishita R, Aoki M, et al. Angiogenesis and antifibrotic action by hepatocyte growth factor in cardiomyopathy. Hypertension 2002;40(1):47–53.

71. Narula J, Haider N, Virmani R, et al. Apoptosis in myocytes in end-stage heart failure. N Engl J Med 1996;335(16):1182–1189.

72. Narula J, Pandey P, Arbustini E, et al. Apoptosis in heart failure: release of cytochrome c from mitochondria and activation of caspase-3 in human cardiomyopathy. Proc Natl Acad Sci USA 1999;96(14): 8144–8149.

73. Kubota T, McTiernan CF, Frye CS, et al. Dilated cardiomyopathy in transgenic mice with cardiac-specific overexpression of tumor necrosis factor-alpha. Circ Res 1997;81(4):627–635.

74. Kubota T, Miyagishima M, Frye CS, et al. Overexpression of tumor necrosis factor- alpha activates both anti- and pro-apoptotic pathways in the myocardium. J Mol Cell Cardiol 2001;33(7):1331–1344.

75. Urbanek K, Torella D, Sheikh F, et al. Myocardial regeneration by activation of multipotent cardiac stem cells in ischemic heart failure. Proc Natl Acad Sci USA 2005;102(24):8692–8697.

76. Li Y, Takemura G, Kosai K, et al. Postinfarction treatment with an adenoviral vector expressing hepatocyte growth factor relieves chronic left ventricular remodeling and dysfunction in mice. Circulation 2003;107(19):2499–2506.

77. Schuster MD, Kocher AA, Seki T, et al. Myocardial neovascularization by bone marrow angioblasts results in cardiomyocyte regeneration. Am J Physiol Heart Circ Physiol 2004;287(2):H525–H532.

78. Boyle AJ, Schuster M, Witkowski P, et al. Additive effects of endothelial progenitor cells combined with ACE inhibition and beta-blockade on left ventricular function following acute myocardial infarction. J Renin Angiotensin Aldosterone Syst 2005;6(1):33–37.

79. Perrin C, Ecarnot-Laubriet A, Vergely C, Rochette L. Calpain and caspase-3 inhibitors reduce infarct size and post-ischemic apoptosis in rat heart without modifying contractile recovery. Cell Mol Biol (Noisy-le-grand) 2003;49 Online Pub:OL497–505.

10

Stem Cell Differentiation Toward a Cardiac Myocyte Phenotype

Andrea N. Ladd, PhD

SUMMARY

Understanding cardiac myocyte differentiation during embryonic heart development will provide insight into how to promote cardiac myogenesis in stem cell populations for cell-based therapies. This chapter reviews what is known about the embryonic origin of cardiac myocytes in vertebrates, the signals that induce myocardial cell specification, the factors that regulate transcription during cardiac myocyte differentiation, and the regulatory networks that connect them.

Key Words: Embryonic development; specification; differentiation; lineage establishment; induction; cardiac transcription factors; cardiac myocyte.

All of the tissues of the embryo arise from cells in the inner cell mass of the early blastocyst. These cells are initially totipotent, meaning that a cell from this population can give rise to all the cell types of the body if exposed to the appropriate cues. The developmental potential of these cells is thought to become increasingly more restricted as embryogenesis progresses and the cells terminally differentiate to form the various tissues. Tissues that undergo lifelong regeneration, such as blood and skin, have long been known to maintain populations of stem cells, "embryonic-like" undifferentiated cells that are capable of self-renewal or differentiation, well into adulthood. Findings from studies in the past few years suggest that stem cells are much more widespread in adult tissues than originally anticipated, and both embryonic and adult stem cells may have broad developmental potential. From these findings, the exciting possibility of using stem cells to repair terminally differentiated tissues with little or no regenerative potential has arisen. The idea of stem cell therapy is particularly appealing for regenerating heart muscle tissue because heart disease remains the leading cause of death in the United States.

The promise of stem cell therapy for heart patients depends on the premise that differentiation to a myocardial phenotype can be induced in a stem cell population through purposeful and specific activation of the myocardial program. Understanding myocardial cell development during embryonic heart formation may provide a blueprint for devising a successful stem cell therapy. The purpose of this chapter is to review what is known about the developmental pathways that establish myocardial cell identity in the developing vertebrate embryo.

From: *Contemporary Cardiology: Stem Cells and Myocardial Regeneration*
Edited by: M. S. Penn © Humana Press Inc., Totowa, NJ

EMBRYONIC ORIGIN OF CARDIAC MYOCYTES

The multilayered body plan of the vertebrate organism is established during gastrulation, when embryonic cells are rearranged into three germ layers: inner endoderm, outer ectoderm, and interstitial mesoderm. The endoderm gives rise to the digestive and respiratory tracts, the ectoderm gives rise to skin and nervous tissue, and the mesoderm produces a host of derivatives that form the internal organ systems that lie in between, including the heart. The heart is derived from lateral plate mesoderm, which also forms the blood, blood vessels, linings of the body cavities, and portions of the limbs.

The circulatory system is the first functioning system to form during embryogenesis, and the heart is the first functional organ. Fate maps in fish *(1)*, amphibians *(2)*, birds *(3)*, and mammals *(4)* have revealed considerable conservation in the location and movements of cells that ultimately give rise to cells of heart muscle lineage (Fig. 1). In each case, cells fated to form the heart can be identified in the blastula, scattered broadly throughout the posterior region. The cardiac progenitors progressively localize toward the midline as gastrulation commences and involute early within a broad region of the primitive streak, just caudal to the anterior node *(5)*. As gastrulation proceeds, myocardial precursors migrate out of the streak and form paired heart primordia on either side of the anterior midline. Continued cell migration, along with overall flexion and folding of the embryo during neurulation, brings the bilateral precardiac regions together, where they unite to form a simple tube composed of an outer myocardium surrounding an inner endocardium. Cardiac myocyte differentiation occurs during this process, and by the time fusion is complete the simple heart tube is already a functioning pump. A second population of myocardial progenitors lying anterior and dorsal to the linear heart tube contributes to the forming outflow tract *(6)*. Subsequent looping of the heart tube and remodeling of the endocardium to form the valves and septa gives rise to the familiar four-chambered architecture of the heart.

Although fate-mapping studies provide valuable information concerning the localization of cells that will give rise to the muscle of the heart, they do not address important questions about the developmental state of presumptive myocardial cells. Lineage establishment is a multistep process that includes competence, specification, determination, and, ultimately, differentiation. Competence is the ability of a cell to recognize and respond to external cues that influence cell fate. Specification is the initial assumption of lineage identity by a precursor cell. Operationally, presumptive cells are said to be specified when they are able to differentiate when explanted and cultured in the absence of external inductive factors. Determination occurs when lineage identity becomes set, such that presumptive cells remain committed to their fate even when exposed to external influences that instruct the cells to adopt an alternative fate. The final step, differentiation, is characterized by the activation of genes that define the morphology and function of a cell lineage. In the case of cardiac myocytes, these would include the structural and contractile proteins such as the myosins and troponins.

The timing and position of involution determines the ultimate fate of the mesodermal cell. The regionalization of cell fate within the primitive streak at later stages reflects the spatial relationship of precursors fate-mapped within the epiblast prior to gastrulation, suggesting a role for the streak region in patterning the mesoderm of the embryo. Myocardial specification occurs during gastrulation, as cells fated to form

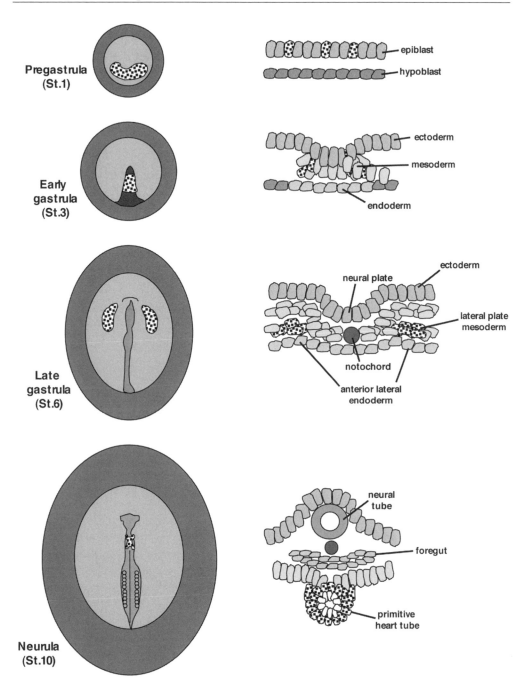

Fig. 1. Origin and movement of precardiac cells. Ventral views (left) and transverse sections (right) of developing chick embryos are shown; cells that form the heart are indicated by black dots. Cells fated to become the heart are broadly distributed throughout the posterior region of the epiblast prior to gastrulation. During gastrulation, cardiac progenitors involute early, and specification of precardiac mesoderm begins while cells are still within the primitive streak. As gastrulation progresses, specified precardiac cells migrate to either side of the anterior midline to form bilateral heart fields. Continued cell migration and overall flexion of the embryo during neurulation bring the heart primordia together, where they fuse to form the primitive heart tube.

heart involute and migrate through the primitive streak. In *Xenopus*, precardiac cells become self-differentiating in culture as soon as cells can be isolated following involution *(7,8)*. Explantation studies in chick and quail have demonstrated that myocardial cell specification has also commenced in avians by early to mid-gastrulation *(9–11)*. Some isolated precardiac cells are already capable of self-differentiating in culture when excised, from within the primitive streak *(11)*.

INDUCTION OF HEART MUSCLE CELL SPECIFICATION

Studies from amphibians, birds, and mammals all suggest that heart muscle cell specification involves inductive signals from two distinct sources (Fig. 2). In amphibians, the organizer region at the dorsal blastopore lip and the deep dorsoanterior endoderm are both important for heart induction *(7,8)*. In birds, the two inductive tissues have been identified as the posterior hypoblast and anterior lateral endoderm. Hypoblast, the avian equivalent of the mammalian trophoblast, has been implicated in axis formation in the posterior region of the pregastrula embryo and may have mesoderm-inducing activity analogous to the amphibian organizer region *(12,13)*. Hypoblast-derived signaling is important prior to gastrulation and may serve to make heart progenitors within the nascent mesoderm competent to respond to inductive signals from the emerging endoderm during gastrulation. Anterior lateral endoderm, which subtends the precardiac mesoderm at late gastrula stages, has heart-inducing capacity and can convert responsive mesoderm, which otherwise would not form heart to a myocardial lineage *(11,14,15)*. In mice, inductive signals are generated by the anterior visceral endoderm, an extraembryonic tissue similar to the avian hypoblast, and the anterior definitive endoderm *(16)*.

Members of the transforming growth factor (TGF)-β superfamily have been implicated in both stages of cardiogenic signaling (Fig. 2). Activin and TGF-β have been detected in the chick pregastrula hypoblast *(17,18)*, and both can promote cardiac myogenesis in avian explant experiments *(19)*. In contrast, the related bone morphogenetic proteins (BMPs) play an early inhibitory role. BMP-2 and BMP-4 are broadly expressed in the chick embryo prior to gastrulation, but their activity is repressed in the posterior region containing the cells fated to form heart by localized expression of chordin and noggin, two BMP antagonists *(20,21)*. Treatment with either BMP-2 or BMP-4 can block the ability of activin or the hypoblast to induce formation of cardiac myocytes in chick precardiac explants *(19)*, and transient inhibition of BMP signaling by noggin can promote cardiac myocyte differentiation in mouse embryonic stem cells *(22)*.

Although BMP signaling inhibits cardiogenic induction prior to gastrulation, it also mediates the positive inductive role of the anterior lateral endoderm during subsequent stages. BMP-2 expression is detectable in anterior lateral endoderm subtending the precardiac mesoderm *(21,23)*. Loss of BMP-2 expression or inhibition of BMP signaling from the endoderm disrupts heart formation and inhibits cardiac differentiation in *Xenopus*, chick, and mouse *(19,23–25)*. Ectopic application of BMP-2 induces expression of cardiac transcription factors in gastrulating chick embryos *(20,23)*, and although treatment with BMP-2 or BMP-4 alone is not sufficient to induce cardiac myocyte differentiation in nonprecardiac mesoderm explants, either will induce full conversion when used in combination with fibroblast growth factor (FGF)-4 *(19,26)*. Combined treatment with FGF-2 and BMP-2 also promotes cardiac myocyte differentiation in mouse embryonic stem cells *(27)*. Members of the FGF family are expressed in precardiac endoderm *(15)*, and ectopic expression of FGF-8 leads to lateral expansion of the

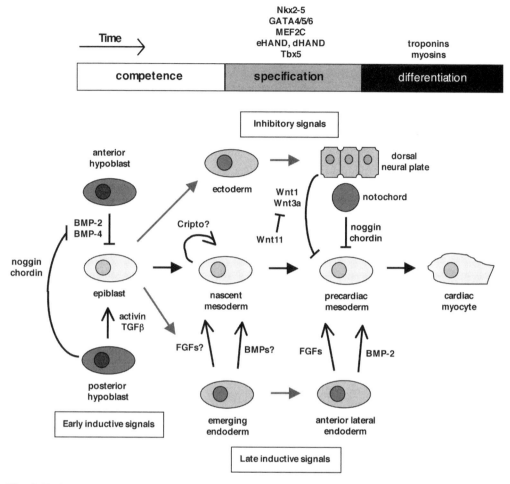

Fig. 2. Early and late signals define the heart fields and commit cells to a myocardial fate. Members of the transforming growth factor (TGF)-β superfamily and fibroblast growth factor (FGF) family mediate signals arising from the hypoblast prior to gastrulation and from the anterior lateral endoderm during gastrulation that are required for induction of cardiac myogenesis. Inhibitory signals involving bone morphogenetic protein (BMP) antagonists and Wnt proteins produced by the axial tissues help restrict the presumptive heart field.

presumptive heart fields *(28)*. These results support a hypothesis that FGFs potentiate the competence of cardiac precursors to respond to BMP signals, although an essential role for FGF signaling in cardiogenic induction has not yet been demonstrated. FGF proteins have also been implicated in the maintenance of cardiac gene expression following specification in chicken and mouse *(28)*.

In addition to members of the TGF-β superfamily and the FGF family, other secreted factors may play a role in myocardial specification. Cripto is a member of the Cripto/FRL/Cryptic family *(29)*, defined by a unique cysteine-rich motif and a divergent epidermal growth factor (EGF)-like motif that fails to bind to the EGF receptor or other known ErgB family receptors *(30)*. Cripto can been detected in prestreak and primitive streak stage mouse embryos in epiblast and forming mesodermal cells, but is later restricted to the developing heart *(31,32)*. Ablation of *Cripto-1 (Cr1)* in mouse embryonic stem cells leads to a specific block in the differentiation of cardiac myocytes in vitro *(33)*, and *Cr1*- null mice exhibit embryonic lethality due to severe deficiency of embryonic mesodermal derivatives, including cardiac muscle *(34,35)*. In these mutants, the anterior–posterior axis does not form, suggesting that the inability of the heart tube to differentiate may be a result of failure to generate the precardiac field within the mesoderm from which the heart would normally develop.

The boundaries of the presumptive heart field are defined not only by the inductive signals produced by cardiogenic tissues, but also by repressive signals emanating from the axial tissues. Juxtaposition of neural tube and notochord blocks BMP-mediated induction of cardiac differentiation in chick precardiac explants *(23)*, effects that are likely mediated in part by noggin and chordin, diffusible BMP antagonists produced by the notochord *(36)*. The dorsal neural plate also expresses two members of the wingless/int (Wnt) family of secreted glycoproteins, Wnt-1 and Wnt-3a, which repress cardiogenesis in culture *(37)*. Wnt antagonists are expressed in the endoderm around the heart fields, and ectopic expression of Wnt antagonists can relieve the repressive effects of the neural plate and activate cardiogenesis in noncardiac mesoderm in frogs and chicks *(37,38)*. Targeted inactivation of β-catenin, which forms a complex in the cytoplasm and enters the nucleus, where it activates transcription of target genes in response to canonical Wnt signaling, results in the formation of ectopic hearts along the anterior–posterior axis in the developing mouse *(39)*. Together, these results support a role for Wnt/β-catenin signaling in limiting cardiac specification to the heart fields. Interestingly, another member of the Wnt family that inhibits the canonical Wnt/β-catenin pathway, Wnt-11, promotes cardiac differentiation *(40,41)*.

The cell surface signaling molecule Notch-1 and its ligand, Serrate, have also been implicated in the refinement of cell fates within the heart field in *Xenopus (42)*. Notch-1 and Serrate are initially expressed throughout the presumptive heart field, but over time Serrate becomes restricted to nonmyogenic cells in the future heart, consistent with a role for activated Notch signaling in the inhibition of myogenesis *(42)*.

TRANSCRIPTIONAL CONTROL OF CARDIAC MYOCYTE DIFFERENTIATION

Specification may be thought of as a state in which a cell has initiated the regulatory program that will in turn activate the genes required for differentiation. Several families of transcription factors have been implicated in the regulation of cardiac myogenesis, including the vertebrate homologs of the *Drosophila* homeobox gene *tinman*, the GATA4/5/6 family, the myocyte enhancer factor 2 (MEF2) proteins, the bHLH transcription factors of the HAND family, and members of the T-box transcription factor (Tbx) family.

The importance of the *tinman* gene in embryonic heart development was first suggested in *Drosophila*, where it was observed that null mutants completely lacked the muscle of the dorsal vessel, the fly equivalent to the vertebrate heart *(43)*. In fish *(44)*, frog *(45)*, chick *(14)*, and mouse *(46,47)*, the vertebrate homolog of *tinman*, the NK-class homeodomain-containing transcription factor *Nkx2-5* (also known as *Csx*), is expressed during gastrulation in the lateral plate mesoderm and currently represents the most commonly used early marker of the presumptive heart field. Several putative downstream target genes for Nkx2-5 have been identified in the cardiac myogenesis pathway, including structural myofibril proteins such as ventricular myosin light chain 2 and other transcriptional regulators, such as eHAND *(48,49)*. Targeted ablation of *Nkx2-5* in mice does not prevent myocardial cell differentiation, although it does lead to disruption of normal cardiac gene expression and morphogenetic defects in the heart tube at later stages *(49,50)*.

The presence of multiple members of the Nkx-2 family in most vertebrate species suggests that some functional redundancy may complicate the interpretation of the Nkx2-5 null phenotype. Injection of dominant inhibitory XNkx-2 constructs that block multiple Nkx-2 family members into *Xenopus* embryos results in the complete elimination of myocardial gene expression and the absence of a morphologically distinguishable heart *(51,52)*. This phenotype is rescuable by coinjection with wild-type homologs *(51,52)*. Although these results suggest that Nkx-2 family members are required for normal cardiac myogenesis, there is no conclusive evidence that Nkx-2 factors initiate the myocardial gene program. The vertebrate *Nkx-2* genes fail to compensate for loss of *tinman* in gene replacement experiments in flies *(53,54)*, suggesting that the vertebrate *tinman* homologs have diverged functionally from their *Drosophila* counterpart and may play a different role in heart development. Overexpression of Nkx2-5 in frog or zebrafish embryos never leads to ectopic heart formation, suggesting that Nkx2-5 is not sufficient for myocardial specification, but overexpression does result in enlargement of the heart, suggesting a possible involvement in defining the heart field *(44,55)*.

The GATA proteins are a family of zinc finger-containing transcription factors. Three GATA family members, *GATA4*, *GATA5*, and *GATA6*, have been detected in the presumptive heart and have been shown to activate numerous myocardial genes *(56)*. Like Nkx2-5, deletion of individual *GATA* genes in the mouse has not revealed determinative roles for these factors in myocardial specification, resulting in part from genetic redundancy *(56–59)*. Interpretation of *GATA* null phenotypes is further confounded by defects caused by developmental roles for the GATA proteins outside of the heart. Early endodermal defects in *GATA4* knockouts and peri-implantation lethality in *GATA6* knockouts hinder our ability to analyze the role of these factors in myocardial differentiation. Nevertheless, a cardiogenic role for these factors has been proposed. $GATA4^{-/-}$ embryonic stem cells have a reduced potential for cardiac differentiation *(60)*, and GATA4 expression in the anterior endoderm and mesoderm may help restrict the mesoderm to a cardiac fate *(28)*. Involvement of GATA factors in the migration of cardiac progenitors during coalescence of the heart tube has also been proposed *(57,58)*. Consistent with this idea, targeted reduction of GATA4 by RNA interference in chick whole embryo cultures and mutation of the *GATA5* gene in zebrafish both result in cardia bifida *(61,62)*.

Members of the Mef2 family of MADS-box transcription factors have been implicated in early steps of both cardiac and skeletal myogenesis *(63)*. MEF2 proteins bind to A/T-rich sequences in the promoters of several cardiac and skeletal muscle-specific genes *(64–67)*. In *Drosophila*, the loss of the single *D-mef2* gene ablates cardiac, visceral, and skeletal muscle *(68)*. In vertebrates, multiple family members are expressed in precardiac mesoderm, and the functional importance of individual MEF2 proteins is not yet fully understood. For example, in mice *Mef2B* and *Mef2C* are expressed in precardiac mesoderm at e7.75, followed by *Mef2A* and *Mef2D* *(63,69)*. Cardiac development is normal in $Mef2B^{-/-}$ mice, while both ventricles are hypoplastic in $Mef2C^{-/-}$ mice *(70)*.

In skeletal muscle, the MyoD family of basic helix-loop-helix (bHLH) proteins is responsible for activation of the skeletal muscle gene program. A different subclass of bHLH proteins may play a similar role in cardiac development. *eHand* (also called *Hand1*) and *dHand* (also called *Hand2*) are bHLH genes expressed in the lateral plate and heart tube, as well as other embryonic tissues *(71,72)*. If antisense oligonucleotides to both of these *Hand* genes are added simultaneously to chick embryos, heart development arrests at the looping stage *(71)*. Heart development also arrests during cardiac looping in both *dHand*[-/-] and *eHand*[-/-] knockout mice *(73,74)*. Thus, early myocardial cell fate decisions can progress without the HAND proteins, but later cardiac morphogenesis requires these factors.

The first indication that T-box transcription factors are important for heart development came in 1997, when mutations in the *Tbx5* gene were identified as being responsible for Holt–Oram syndrome, a human genetic disorder characterized by congenital heart malformations *(75,76)*. Since then, Tbx1, -2, -3, -18, and -20 have also been implicated in cardiac development *(77)*. A differentiated heart tube forms in *Tbx1, -3,* and *-5* null mice, suggesting that loss of a single *Tbx* gene does not impair cardiac lineage specification or differentiation *(78–80)*. Investigations into the function of these factors are still in the early stages, but the Tbx target genes that have been identified to date suggest involvement of cardiac Tbx proteins in regulating chamber-specific gene expression and cardiac myocyte proliferation *(77)*.

Although all of these transcription factor families are expressed in precardiac mesoderm prior to or concurrent with cardiac myocyte differentiation, none are expressed exclusively in the heart, and none are sufficient to drive the differentiation of lateral plate mesoderm into heart by themselves *(81)*. Other transcription factors that may participate in cardiac specification and/or differentiation include the bHLH factors Mesp1 and -2, serum response factor (SRF), the Iroquois homeobox gene family members Irx1-4, Cited1 and -2, the Hairy/Enhancer of Split family proteins Hey1 and -2, Sox6, Pitx2, myocardin, and their homologs *(81–84)*. Some of these, such as the Mesp proteins, may play a more general role in mesoderm development, whereas others, such as myocardin, may play a more specific role in cardiac development, although these roles have not yet been well defined.

INTERACTIONS WITHIN THE REGULATORY NETWORK

It is worth noting that the cardiac transcription factors do not act independently of one another, but rather are integrated in a complex transcriptional network. Investigation of the targets of transcription factor families has revealed numerous physical interactions between factors acting on a variety of target gene promoters. In some cases, transcription factors have been shown to coexist in a stable ternary complex that involves both direct protein–protein interactions and protein–DNA interactions. In many cases, however, it is still not clear whether the transcription factors interact directly with one another or only appear to interact because they bind to elements within the same promoter region.

Nkx2-5, GATA4, and Tbx5 display cooperative binding to DNA, direct protein–protein interactions, and synergistic activation of cardiac transcription *(77)*. Tbx2 and -3 have also been shown to interact with Nkx2-5 when bound to DNA, and Tbx20 interacts with Nkx2-5 and GATA4, although synergistic activation of transcription has not been demonstrated *(77)*. SRF can interact with Nkx2-5 or GATA4 and synergizes with Nkx2-5 and the GATA factors on target promoters *(85)*. GATA4 or -6, but not GATA5, can recruit MEF2 proteins to target promoters that lack MEF2 binding sites, and

GATA4 has been shown to cooperate with MEF2 proteins on a number of cardiac promoters *(86)*.

It is unlikely that all of the possible interactions occur simultaneously on any given promoter. For example, Nkx2-5 can interact with GATA4, Tbx5, Tbx20, and SRF on or near an Nkx2-5 binding site, but it seems improbable that all of these proteins could be physically present on a small stretch of DNA at the same time. The formation of different regulatory complexes may be instrumental for fine-tuning cardiac gene expression. Determining the circumstances in which different combinations arise and their specific consequences for cardiac myogenesis is a major challenge for future investigations.

CHAMBER-SPECIFIC GENE REGULATION IN THE MYOCARDIUM

The muscle cells of the diversified atria and ventricles express distinct subsets of contractile proteins and display different conductive and contractile properties *(87)*. The atrial or ventricular character of cardiac myocytes reflects their position along the anterior/posterior axis, with atrial/ventricular diversification becoming apparent by mid-gastrulation *(87,88)*. This character can be altered prior to differentiation, however, by treatment with retinoic acid, an agent known to influence anterior–posterior identity *(88,89)*. This suggests that final determination occurs concomitantly with terminal differentiation some time following the initial decision to enter the myocardial lineage. Differentiation itself proceeds in an anterior to posterior direction within the cardiogenic mesoderm during neurula stages *(90,91)*.

Few chamber-restricted regulators of cardiac gene expression have been identified to date. eHAND and dHAND develop chamber-restricted expression patterns in the mouse heart, but only after initially being expressed throughout the heart *(73)*. The importance of the HAND proteins for establishment of chamber identity is not clear, as the chamber-restricted expression patterns observed in mouse are not conserved in the chick *(71)*. Irx4 is a homeodomain-containing transcription factor that is expressed only in ventricular myocardium *(92)*. Irx4 is not the only regulator of ventricle-specific gene expression, however, since Irx4-deficient mice display defects in the expression of only a subset of ventricular genes *(92,93)*. Expression of Hey2 (also known as HRT2 or Hesr1) is also restricted to the ventricles *(94)*. The role of Hey2 in ventricular myocyte formation is unknown, but targeted disruption of Hey2 in mice leads to ventricular dysfunction, suggesting a role in the regulation of ventricular gene expression *(95)*. To date, no atrial-specific transcription factors have been identified.

FROM INDUCTIVE SIGNALS TO TRANSCRIPTIONAL CONTROL AND BACK AGAIN

Signaling by the TGF-β superfamily is propagated downstream by the Smad proteins, transcription factors regulated via phosphorylation by TGF-β receptor family members. Smad1, -3, and -5 mediate BMP signaling during cardiac induction and directly activate expression of the early cardiac transcription factors such as *Nkx2-5* *(96,97)*. In addition to the Smad proteins, TGF-β and BMP pathways can activate TAK1, a member of the mitogen-activated protein kinase kinase kinase superfamily, and TAK1 has been implicated in BMP-mediated induction of cardiac transcription programs *(98)*.

Nkx2-5 expression overlaps with the anterior expression domains of the BMPs in the chick embryo and is induced medially in response to ectopic BMP-2 *(20,23)*. Inhibition

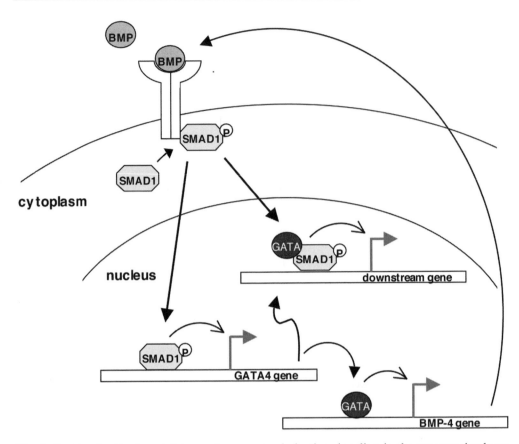

Fig. 3. Positive feedback maintains and propagates inductive signaling in the presumptive heart. Bone morphogenetic protein (BMP) signaling activates expression of cardiac transcription factor genes such as *GATA4*. GATA4 has been shown to activate *Bmp4* gene expression in turn, suggesting that a positive feedback loop maintains BMP expression. GATA4 also interacts with SMAD1, the mediator of BMP signaling, to activate the transcription of BMP target genes.

of BMP signaling by noggin represses *Nkx2-5* expression in cultured precardiac mesendoderm *(23)*. Consistent with the activation of *eHand* by Nkx2-5 *(49)*, in *Xenopus* *eHand* is strongly induced in animal cap assays by ectopic BMP-2 and BMP-4, while induction is blocked by dominant negative BMP receptors *(72)*. *GATA4* expression also overlaps with the expression of BMPs and is induced in response to ectopic BMP-2 in regions medial to its normal domains of expression *(20,23)*.

In addition to the data suggesting that BMP signaling activates expression of the cardiac transcription factors, there is also evidence to suggest that continuation and propagation of BMP signaling in the cardiogenic tissues depends on positive feedback from these same regulatory programs (Fig. 3). BMP-4 has been identified as a direct downstream target of GATA4 and -6 in the mouse *(99)*. Knockdown of GATA6 in *Xenopus* and zebrafish embryos leads to a reduction of BMP-4 in the developing heart despite normal initiation of BMP expression in the early embryo, suggesting a role for GATA factors in maintaining BMP expression during cardiogenesis *(100)*. GATA4, -5, and -6 can physically interact with SMAD-1, the downstream mediator of BMP signaling *(101)*, suggesting the GATA factors not only maintain BMP signaling, but also help mediate its downstream effects.

FUTURE CHALLENGES

Several areas of basic understanding will be helpful for devising and improving successful stem cell therapies to regenerate heart muscle in patients. First, it would be advantageous to maximize the fraction of cells within a stem cell population that commits to a myocardial fate. This will require a more detailed understanding of the signals that induce the cardiac myocyte lineages in the embryo, including the precise order, combination, and dosage of growth factors required for specification, as well as what elements the cells must already possess in order to be competent to respond to these signals. Second, it would be useful to understand what cues promote proliferation of committed progenitor cells, to expand the population, withdraw from the cell cycle when appropriate, and possibly even maintain a subset of self-renewing cells in the repaired heart. Third, it will be important to elucidate how distinct cardiac myocyte lineages (e.g., atrial vs ventricular myocytes) are established in order to fine-tune stem cell differentiation to fit the site of repair. Finally, greater understanding of the regulation of the cardiac gene expression program following differentiation will shed light on how cardiac myocytes mature, a process that must take place if new myocardial cells are to properly integrate into the adult myocardium. A limited capacity for cardiac regeneration has been observed in some species, suggesting that the adult heart maintains an environment conducive for the differentiation and integration of stem cell progenitors into the myocardium. It remains to be seen whether regenerative medicine will be able to tap into that potential.

REFERENCES

1. Stainier DY, Lee RK, Fishman MC. Cardiovascular development in the zebrafish. I. Myocardial fate map and heart tube formation. Development 1993;119(1):31–40.
2. Keller RE. Vital dye mapping of the gastrula and neurula of Xenopus laevis. II. Prospective areas and morphogenetic movements of the deep layer. Dev Biol 1976;51(1):118–137.
3. Hatada Y, Stern CD. A fate map of the epiblast of the early chick embryo. Development 1994;120(10):2879–2889.
4. Parameswaran M, Tam PP. Regionalisation of cell fate and morphogenetic movement of the mesoderm during mouse gastrulation. Dev Genet 1995;17(1):16–28.
5. Garcia-Martinez V, Schoenwolf GC. Primitive-streak origin of the cardiovascular system in avian embryos. Dev Biol 1993;159(2):706–719.
6. Kelly RG, Buckingham ME. The anterior heart-forming field: voyage to the arterial pole of the heart. Trends Genet 2002;18(4):210–216.
7. Sater AK, Jacobson AG. The role of the dorsal lip in the induction of heart mesoderm in Xenopus laevis. Development 1990;108(3):461–470.
8. Nascone N, Mercola M. An inductive role for the endoderm in Xenopus cardiogenesis. Development 1995;121(2):515–523.
9. Antin PB, Taylor RG, Yatskievych T. Precardiac mesoderm is specified during gastrulation in quail. Dev Dyn 1994;200(2):144–154.
10. Montgomery MO, Litvin J, Gonzalez-Sanchez A, Bader D. Staging of commitment and differentiation of avian cardiac myocytes. Dev Biol 1994;164(1):63–71.
11. Yatskievych TA, Ladd AN, Antin PB. Induction of cardiac myogenesis in avian pregastrula epiblast: the role of the hypoblast and activin. Development 1997;124(13):2561–2570.
12. Azar Y, Eyal-Giladi H. Interaction of epiblast and hypoblast in the formation of the primitive streak and the embryonic axis in chick, as revealed by hypoblast-rotation experiments. J Embryol Exp Morphol 1981;61:133–144.
13. Mitrani E, Eyal-Giladi H. Hypoblastic cells can form a disk inducing an embryonic axis in chick epiblast. Nature 1981;289(5800):800–802.
14. Schultheiss TM, Xydas S, Lassar AB. Induction of avian cardiac myogenesis by anterior endoderm. Development 1995;121(12):4203–4214.

15. Sugi Y, Lough J. Activin-A and FGF-2 mimic the inductive effects of anterior endoderm on terminal cardiac myogenesis in vitro. Dev Biol 1995;168(2):567–574.

16. Arai A, Yamamoto K, Toyama J. Murine cardiac progenitor cells require visceral embryonic endoderm and primitive streak for terminal differentiation. Dev Dyn 1997;210(3):344–353.

17. Mitrani E, Ziv T, Thomsen G, Shimoni Y, Melton DA, Bril A. Activin can induce the formation of axial structures and is expressed in the hypoblast of the chick. Cell 1990;63(3):495–501.

18. Sanders E, Hu N, Wride M. Expression of TGFβ1/β3 during early chick embryo development. Anat Res 1994;238:397–406.

19. Ladd AN, Yatskievych TA, Antin PB. Regulation of avian cardiac myogenesis by activin/TGFbeta and bone morphogenetic proteins. Dev Biol 1998;204(2):407–419.

20. Andree B, Duprez D, Vorbusch B, Arnold HH, Brand T. BMP-2 induces ectopic expression of cardiac lineage markers and interferes with somite formation in chicken embryos. Mech Dev 1998;70(1–2):119–131.

21. Streit A, Lee KJ, Woo I, Roberts C, Jessell TM, Stern CD. Chordin regulates primitive streak development and the stability of induced neural cells, but is not sufficient for neural induction in the chick embryo. Development 1998;125(3):507–519.

22. Yuasa S, Itabashi Y, Koshimizu U, et al. Transient inhibition of BMP signaling by Noggin induces cardiomyocyte differentiation of mouse embryonic stem cells. Nat Biotechnol 2005;23(5):607–611.

23. Schultheiss TM, Burch JB, Lassar AB. A role for bone morphogenetic proteins in the induction of cardiac myogenesis. Genes Dev 1997;11(4):451–462.

24. Shi Y, Katsev S, Cai C, Evans S. BMP signaling is required for heart formation in vertebrates. Dev Biol 2000;224(2):226–237.

25. Zhang H, Bradley A. Mice deficient for BMP2 are nonviable and have defects in amnion/chorion and cardiac development. Development 1996;122(10):2977–2986.

26. Lough J, Barron M, Brogley M, Sugi Y, Bolender DL, Zhu X. Combined BMP-2 and FGF-4, but neither factor alone, induces cardiogenesis in non-precardiac embryonic mesoderm. Dev Biol 1996;178(1):198–202.

27. Kawai T, Takahashi T, Esaki M, et al. Efficient cardiomyogenic differentiation of embryonic stem cell by fibroblast growth factor 2 and bone morphogenetic protein 2. Circ J 2004;68(7):691–702.

28. Alsan BH, Schultheiss TM. Regulation of avian cardiogenesis by Fgf8 signaling. Development 2002;129(8):1935–1943.

29. Shen MM, Wang H, Leder P. A differential display strategy identifies Cryptic, a novel EGF-related gene expressed in the axial and lateral mesoderm during mouse gastrulation. Development 1997;124(2): 429–442.

30. Brandt R, Normanno N, Gullick WJ, et al. Identification and biological characterization of an epidermal growth factor-related protein: cripto-1. J Biol Chem 1994;269(25):17,320–17,328.

31. Dono R, Scalera L, Pacifico F, Acampora D, Persico MG, Simeone A. The murine cripto gene: expression during mesoderm induction and early heart morphogenesis. Development 1993;118(4): 1157–1168.

32. Johnson SE, Rothstein JL, Knowles BB. Expression of epidermal growth factor family gene members in early mouse development. Dev Dyn 1994;201(3):216–226.

33. Xu C, Liguori G, Adamson ED, Persico MG. Specific arrest of cardiogenesis in cultured embryonic stem cells lacking Cripto-1. Dev Biol 1998;196(2):237–247.

34. Ding J, Yang L, Yan YT, et al. Cripto is required for correct orientation of the anterior-posterior axis in the mouse embryo. Nature 1998;395(6703):702–707.

35. Xu C, Liguori G, Persico MG, Adamson ED. Abrogation of the Cripto gene in mouse leads to failure of postgastrulation morphogenesis and lack of differentiation of cardiomyocytes. Development 1999;126(3):483–494.

36. Klingensmith J, Ang SL, Bachiller D, Rossant J. Neural induction and patterning in the mouse in the absence of the node and its derivatives. Dev Biol 1999;216(2):535–549.

37. Tzahor E, Lassar AB. Wnt signals from the neural tube block ectopic cardiogenesis. Genes Dev 2001;15(3):255–260.

38. Schneider VA, Mercola M. Wnt antagonism initiates cardiogenesis in Xenopus laevis. Genes Dev 2001;15(3):304–315.

39. Lickert H, Kutsch S, Kanzler B, Tamai Y, Taketo MM, Kemler R. Formation of multiple hearts in mice following deletion of beta-catenin in the embryonic endoderm. Dev Cell 2002;3(2):171–181.

40. Pandur P, Lasche M, Eisenberg LM, Kuhl M. Wnt-11 activation of a non-canonical Wnt signalling pathway is required for cardiogenesis. Nature 2002;418(6898):636–641.

41. Terami H, Hidaka K, Katsumata T, Iio A, Morisaki T. Wnt11 facilitates embryonic stem cell differentiation to Nkx2.5-positive cardiomyocytes. Biochem Biophys Res Commun 2004;325(3):968–975.

42. Rones MS, McLaughlin KA, Raffin M, Mercola M. Serrate and Notch specify cell fates in the heart field by suppressing cardiomyogenesis. Development 2000;127(17):3865–3876.

43. Bodmer R. The gene tinman is required for specification of the heart and visceral muscles in Drosophila. Development 1993;118(3):719–729.

44. Chen JN, Fishman MC. Zebrafish tinman homolog demarcates the heart field and initiates myocardial differentiation. Development 1996;122(12):3809–3816.

45. Tonissen KF, Drysdale TA, Lints TJ, Harvey RP, Krieg PA. XNkx-2.5, a Xenopus gene related to Nkx-2.5 and tinman: evidence for a conserved role in cardiac development. Dev Biol 1994;162(1): 325–328.

46. Komuro I, Izumo S. Csx: a murine homeobox-containing gene specifically expressed in the developing heart. Proc Natl Acad Sci USA 1993;90(17):8145–8149.

47. Lints TJ, Parsons LM, Hartley L, Lyons I, Harvey RP. Nkx-2.5: a novel murine homeobox gene expressed in early heart progenitor cells and their myogenic descendants. Development 1993;119(3):969.

48. O'Brien TX, Lee KJ, Chien KR. Positional specification of ventricular myosin light chain 2 expression in the primitive murine heart tube. Proc Natl Acad Sci USA 1993;90(11):5157–5161.

49. Tanaka M, Chen Z, Bartunkova S, Yamasaki N, Izumo S. The cardiac homeobox gene Csx/Nkx2.5 lies genetically upstream of multiple genes essential for heart development. Development 1999;126(6): 1269–1280.

50. Lyons I, Parsons LM, Hartley L, et al. Myogenic and morphogenetic defects in the heart tubes of murine embryos lacking the homeo box gene Nkx2-5. Genes Dev 1995;9(13):1654–1666.

51. Grow MW, Krieg PA. Tinman function is essential for vertebrate heart development: elimination of cardiac differentiation by dominant inhibitory mutants of the tinman-related genes, XNkx2-3 and XNkx2-5. Dev Biol 1998;204(1):187–196.

52. Fu Y, Yan W, Mohun TJ, Evans SM. Vertebrate tinman homologues XNkx2-3 and XNkx2-5 are required for heart formation in a functionally redundant manner. Development 1998;125(22):4439–4449.

53. Ranganayakulu G, Elliott DA, Harvey RP, Olson EN. Divergent roles for NK-2 class homeobox genes in cardiogenesis in flies and mice. Development 1998;125(16):3037–3048.

54. Park M, Lewis C, Turbay D, et al. Differential rescue of visceral and cardiac defects in Drosophila by vertebrate tinman-related genes. Proc Natl Acad Sci USA 1998;95(16):9366–9371.

55. Cleaver OB, Patterson KD, Krieg PA. Overexpression of the tinman-related genes XNkx-2.5 and XNkx-2.3 in Xenopus embryos results in myocardial hyperplasia. Development 1996;122(11): 3549–3556.

56. Molkentin JD, Tymitz KM, Richardson JA, Olson EN. Abnormalities of the genitourinary tract in female mice lacking GATA5. Mol Cell Biol 2000;20(14):5256–5260.

57. Kuo CT, Morrisey EE, Anandappa R, et al. GATA4 transcription factor is required for ventral morphogenesis and heart tube formation. Genes Dev 1997;11(8):1048–1060.

58. Molkentin JD, Lin Q, Duncan SA, Olson EN. Requirement of the transcription factor GATA4 for heart tube formation and ventral morphogenesis. Genes Dev 1997;11(8):1061–1072.

59. Koutsourakis M, Langeveld A, Patient R, Beddington R, Grosveld F. The transcription factor GATA6 is essential for early extraembryonic development. Development 1999;126(4):723–732.

60. Narita N, Bielinska M, Wilson DB. Cardiomyocyte differentiation by GATA-4-deficient embryonic stem cells. Development 1997;124(19):3755–3764.

61. Reiter JF, Alexander J, Rodaway A, et al. Gata5 is required for the development of the heart and endoderm in zebrafish. Genes Dev 1999;13(22):2983–2995.

62. Zhang H, Toyofuku T, Kamei J, Hori M. GATA-4 regulates cardiac morphogenesis through transactivation of the N-cadherin gene. Biochem Biophys Res Commun 2003;312(4):1033–1038.

63. Edmondson DG, Lyons GE, Martin JF, Olson EN. Mef2 gene expression marks the cardiac and skeletal muscle lineages during mouse embryogenesis. Development 1994;120(5):1251–1263.

64. Iannello RC, Mar JH, Ordahl CP. Characterization of a promoter element required for transcription in myocardial cells. J Biol Chem 1991;266(5):3309–3316.

65. Navankasattusas S, Zhu H, Garcia AV, Evans SM, Chien KR. A ubiquitous factor (HF-1a) and a distinct muscle factor (HF-1b/MEF-2) form an E-box-independent pathway for cardiac muscle gene expression. Mol Cell Biol 1992;12(4):1469–1479.

66. Navankasattusas S, Sawadogo M, van Bilsen M, Dang CV, Chien KR. The basic helix-loop-helix protein upstream stimulating factor regulates the cardiac ventricular myosin light-chain 2 gene via independent cis regulatory elements. Mol Cell Biol 1994;14(11):7331–7339.

67. Zhu H, Nguyen V, Brown A, et al. A novel, tissue restricted zinc finger protein (HR-1b) binds to the cardiac regulatory element (HF-1b/MEF-2) in the rat myosin light chain-2 gene. Mol Cell Biol 1993;13:4432–4444.

68. Lilly B, Zhao B, Ranganayakulu G, Paterson B, Schultz R, Olson EN. Requirement of MADS domain transcription factor D-MEF2 for muscle formation in *Drosophila*. Science 1995;267: 688–693.

69. Molkentin J, Olson E. Combinatorial control of muscle development by basic helix-loop-helix and MADS-box transcription factors. Proc Natl Acad Sci USA 1996;93(18):9366–9373.

70. Lin Q, Schwarz J, Bucana C, Olson EN. Control of mouse cardiac morphogenesis and myogenesis by transcription factor MEF2C. Science 1997;276(5317):1404–1407.

71. Srivastava D, Cserjesi P, Olson EN. A subclass of bHLH proteins required for cardiac morphogenesis. Science 1995;270(5244):1995–1999.

72. Sparrow DB, Kotecha S, Towers N, Mohun TJ. Xenopus eHAND: a marker for the developing cardiovascular system of the embryo that is regulated by bone morphogenetic proteins. Mech Dev 1998;71(1–2):151–163.

73. Srivastava D, Thomas T, Lin Q, Kirby ML, Brown D, Olson EN. Regulation of cardiac mesodermal and neural crest development by the bHLH transcription factor, dHAND. Nat Genet 1997;16(2): 154–160.

74. Firulli AB, McFadden DG, Lin Q, Srivastava D, Olson EN. Heart and extra-embryonic mesodermal defects in mouse embryos lacking the bHLH transcription factor Hand1. Nat Genet 1998;18(3):266–270.

75. Basson CT, Bachinsky DR, Lin RC, et al. Mutations in human TBX5 [corrected] cause limb and cardiac malformation in Holt-Oram syndrome. Nat Genet 1997;15(1):30–35.

76. Li QY, Newbury-Ecob RA, Terrett JA, et al. Holt-Oram syndrome is caused by mutations in TBX5, a member of the Brachyury (T) gene family. Nat Genet 1997;15(1):21–29.

77. Plageman TF, Jr., Yutzey KE. T-box genes and heart development: putting the "T" in heart. Dev Dyn 2005;232(1):11–20.

78. Bruneau BG, Nemer G, Schmitt JP, et al. A murine model of Holt-Oram syndrome defines roles of the T-box transcription factor Tbx5 in cardiogenesis and disease. Cell 2001;106(6):709–721.

79. Jerome LA, Papaioannou VE. DiGeorge syndrome phenotype in mice mutant for the T-box gene, Tbx1. Nat Genet 2001;27(3):286–291.

80. Davenport TG, Jerome-Majewska LA, Papaioannou VE. Mammary gland, limb and yolk sac defects in mice lacking Tbx3, the gene mutated in human ulnar mammary syndrome. Development 2003;130(10):2263–2273.

81. Bruneau BG. Transcriptional regulation of vertebrate cardiac morphogenesis. Circ Res 2002;90(5): 509–519.

82. Cohen-Barak O, Yi Z, Hagiwara N, Monzen K, Komuro I, Brilliant MH. Sox6 regulation of cardiac myocyte development. Nucleic Acids Res 2003;31(20):5941–5948.

83. Satou Y, Imai KS, Satoh N. The ascidian Mesp gene specifies heart precursor cells. Development 2004;131(11):2533–2541.

84. Li J, Zhu X, Chen M, et al. Myocardin-related transcription factor B is required in cardiac neural crest for smooth muscle differentiation and cardiovascular development. Proc Natl Acad Sci USA 2005;102(25):8916–8921.

85. McBride K, Nemer M. Regulation of the ANF and BNP promoters by GATA factors: lessons learned for cardiac transcription. Can J Physiol Pharmacol 2001;79(8):673–681.

86. Morin S, Charron F, Robitaille L, Nemer M. GATA-dependent recruitment of MEF2 proteins to target promoters. EMBO J 2000;19(9):2046–2055.

87. DeHaan R. Morphogenesis of the vertebrate heart. In: DeHaan R, Ursprung H, eds. Organogenesis. Holt, Reinhart, and Winston, New York, 1965, pp. 377–419.

88. Yutzey KE, Rhee JT, Bader D. Expression of the atrial-specific myosin heavy chain AMHC1 and the establishment of anteroposterior polarity in the developing chicken heart. Development 1994;120(4):871–883.

89. Yutzey KE, Bader D. Diversification of cardiomyogenic cell lineages during early heart development. Circ Res 1995;77(2):216–219.

90. Gonzalez-Sanchez A, Bader D. In vitro analysis of cardiac progenitor cell differentiation. Dev Biol 1990;139(1):197–209.

91. Bisaha JG, Bader D. Identification and characterization of a ventricular-specific avian myosin heavy chain, VMHC1: expression in differentiating cardiac and skeletal muscle. Dev Biol 1991;148(1): 355–364.

92. Bao ZZ, Bruneau BG, Seidman JG, Seidman CE, Cepko CL. Regulation of chamber-specific gene expression in the developing heart by Irx4. Science 1999;283(5405):1161–1164.

93. Bruneau BG, Bao ZZ, Fatkin D, et al. Cardiomyopathy in Irx4-deficient mice is preceded by abnormal ventricular gene expression. Mol Cell Biol 2001;21(5):1730–1736.

94. Kokubo H, Lun Y, Johnson RL. Identification and expression of a novel family of bHLH cDNAs related to Drosophila hairy and enhancer of split. Biochem Biophys Res Commun 1999;260(2): 459–465.

95. Kokubo H, Miyagawa-Tomita S, Tomimatsu H, et al. Targeted disruption of hesr2 results in atrioventricular valve anomalies that lead to heart dysfunction. Circ Res 2004;95(5):540–547.

96. Lien CL, McAnally J, Richardson JA, Olson EN. Cardiac-specific activity of an Nkx2-5 enhancer requires an evolutionarily conserved Smad binding site. Dev Biol 2002;244(2):257–266.

97. Liberatore CM, Searcy-Schrick RD, Vincent EB, Yutzey KE. Nkx-2.5 gene induction in mice is mediated by a Smad consensus regulatory region. Dev Biol 2002;244(2):243–256.

98. Monzen K, Hiroi Y, Kudoh S, et al. Smads, TAK1, and their common target ATF-2 play a critical role in cardiomyocyte differentiation. J Cell Biol 2001;153(4):687–698.

99. Nemer G, Nemer M. Transcriptional activation of BMP-4 and regulation of mammalian organogenesis by GATA-4 and -6. Dev Biol 2003;254(1):131–148.

100. Peterkin T, Gibson A, Patient R. GATA-6 maintains BMP-4 and Nkx2 expression during cardiomyocyte precursor maturation. EMBO J 2003;22(16):4260–4273.

101. Brown CO, 3rd, Chi X, Garcia-Gras E, Shirai M, Feng XH, Schwartz RJ. The cardiac determination factor, Nkx2-5, is activated by mutual cofactors GATA-4 and Smad1/4 via a novel upstream enhancer. J Biol Chem 2004;279(11):10,659–10,669.

11

Electrical Coupling and/or Ventricular Tachycardia Risk of Cell Therapy

Dayi Hu, MD and Shuixiang Yang, MD

SUMMARY

Electromechanical coupling is crucial in the process of functional cardiomyocyte regeneration. Experimental and initial clinical studies have showed the high risk of arrhythmia in the animals and patients receiving cell transplantation from pluripotent stem cells. The mechanism underlying these arrhythmogenic properties is still unclear. The communications between the cells via gap junction formed by connexin proteins are essential for activating cardiac tissue, allowing propagation of electrical stimuli and related ionic currents. It has been shown that there is a functional gap junction between cardiomyocytes and most cells used for cell transplantation, such as human embryonic stem cells, human mesenchymal stem cells, bone marrow-derived mononuclear cells, and fibroblasts. Although it is still controversial, a recent study has shown that there are N-cadherin- and connexin-43-mediated junctions between skeletal myoblasts and cardiomyocytes, allowing them to induce synchronous beating. However, it should be emphasized that all of the cells mentioned above have been demonstrated to have pro-arrhythmogenic potentials. These factors must be weighed as we pursue the avenues of cell therapy for failed hearts. Experimental studies and initial clinical experience with cell transplantation has opened new perspectives for treatment of irreversibly injured myocardium. It must be pointed out that further studies, including experimental and clinical studies, are necessary to address the questions regarding the efficacy and long-term safety of cell transplantation.

Key Words: Electromechanical coupling; connexin; gap junction; arrhythmogenic risk.

Cell therapy is emerging as a promising strategy for myocardial repair. This approach is hampered, however, by the absence of direct evidence for functional integration of donor cells into host tissues *(1)*. Electromechanical coupling is a crucial foundation for the strategy of regeneration of cardiomyocyte and revasculization. Electrical coupling is dependent on gap junction formation between original cardiomyocytes (CMs) and stem cell-derived implantation cells. Communications between the cells via gap junctions formed by the connexin proteins are essential for activating the cardiac tissue, allowing propagation of electrical stimuli and related ionic currents. Experimental and initial clinical studies have demonstrated abnormal action potential characteristics and arrhythmogenic properties in CMs derived from pluripotent stem cells *(2)*. Electrical coupling and ventricular tachycardia risk is the focus of scientists paying close attention to experimental and clinical studies and needs further to be addressed and resolved

From: *Contemporary Cardiology: Stem Cells and Myocardial Regeneration*
Edited by: M. S. Penn © Humana Press Inc., Totowa, NJ

in future trials. In this chapter we will discuss these problems and the advances in stem cell implantation therapy.

ELECTRICAL COUPLING AND GAP JUNCTION

Gap Junction

The molecular cloning of connexins and their identification as the protein components of gap junctions heralded a new era. They are in fact channels formed by the oligomerization of connexins: six connexins make a connexon or hemichannel, and two connexons from adjacent cells align in the extracellular space to make a full intercellular gap junction channel that allows direct communication between cells without using the extracellular space to exchange messages (3). With the completion of the human genome sequence, it appears that we have at least 20 connexins. Family members are usually distinguished by their expected molecular weight, so that the best-known connexin (Cx), a protein of 43 kDa, is referred to as Cx43 (4).

Gap junctions are intercellular channels that allow both chemical and electrical signaling between two adjacent cells. Junctions, morphologically represented by intercalated disks, contain adherens and gap junctions for mechanical and electrical coupling, respectively. Adherens junctions are built up from N-cadherin molecules sarcolemma, which allow binding to N-cadherin's neighbor molecules (5). Gap junctions consist mainly of Cx43 transmembrane protein, by which the electrical current can be quickly and freely conducted (6). The presence of intercalated disks represents the ability of CMs to achieve synchronous (gap junction) and effective (adherens junctions, attachment to surrounding tissue) contraction leading to a synchronous contraction of whole left ventricular (LV) cavity. Gap junction intercellular communication has been also implicated in the regulation of various cellular processes, including cell migration, cell proliferation, cell differentiation, and cell apoptosis.

Early-Stage Heart Connexin

Egashira et al.'s (7) research results indicate that Cx45 is an essential connexin for coordinated conduction through early cardiac myocytes. In early-stage heart, the cardiac impulse does not travel through the specialized conduction system but spreads from myocyte to myocyte, because it is the only gap junction protein present in early hearts. Cx45-deficient (Cx45(–/–)) mice die of heart failure, concomitantly displaying other complex defects in the cardiovascular system.

Embryonic Stem Cell Gap Junction

Wong et al. (8), using reverse transcription–polymerase chain reaction and immunocytochemistry, demonstrated that human embryonic stem cells (ESCs) express two gap junction proteins, Cx43 and Cx45. Western blot analysis revealed the presence of three phosphorylated forms (nonphosphorylated [NP], P1, and P2) of Cx43, with NP being prominent. Moreover, scrape loading/dye transfer assay indicates that human ESCs are coupled through functional gap junctions that are inhibited by protein kinase C activation and extracellular signal-regulated kinase inhibition.

hMSC Connexins

Human mesenchymal stem cells (hMSCs) are a multipotent cell population with the potential to be a cellular repair or delivery system provided they communicate with target cells such as cardiac myocytes via gap junctions. hMSC coupling via gap junctions to other cell types provides the basis for considering them as a therapeutic repair or cellular delivery system to syncytia such as the myocardium.

Valiunas et al. *(9)*, using immunostaining, revealed typical punctate staining for Cx43 and Cx40 along regions of intimate cell-to-cell contact between hMSCs. The staining patterns for Cx45 were typified by granular cytoplasmic staining. hMSCs exhibited cell–cell coupling.

The existence of functional gap junctions between hematopoietic progenitor cells (HPCs) and stromal cells of the hematopoietic microenvironment in the human system is a controversial issue. Durig et al.'s *(10)* data indicate that intercellular communication between bone marrow stromal cells and CD34+ hematopoietic progenitor cells is mediated by Cx43-type gap junctions and, thus, may provide an important regulatory pathway in hematopoiesis.

Gap Junction of Bone Marrow-Derived Mononuclear Cells

It is unknown whether or not CMs and bone marrow-derived mononuclear cells (BMCs) can form functioning cell–cell coupling and develop adequate electrophysiological properties. Rastan et al. *(11)* demonstrated that cocultured BMCs have the potential for early expression of muscle specific proteins in about 60% after 14 days and for cardiac gap junction proteins. Synchronous beating indicates an effective electromechanical coupling. From day 7 in coculture, BMCs beat synchronously with neonatal rat CMs. On day 14, 55.9% of BMCs expressed actinin, and 98.3% were positive for gap junction protein Cx43. BMC action potential duration (APD_{90}) was mean 11.1 ms with dV/dt_{max} of 26.8V/s, similar to atrial cardiac type. However, microinjection of Lucifer yellow revealed little dye transfer into adjacent rat CMs.

Fibroblast Gap Junction

Camelliti et al. *(12)* explored the possibility that fibroblasts form functional gap junctions and communicate electrically with other fibroblasts and with CMs in native cardiac tissue (rabbit sinoatrial node). Using confocal laser-scanning microscopy and immunohistochemical techniques to study structure and spread of Lucifer yellow dye to evaluate the functionality of intercellular coupling, they arrived at the following conclusions:

1. Fibroblasts express both Cx40 and Cx45 to form functional gap junctions.
2. Cx40 is found primarily in regions in which fibroblasts are surrounded by other fibroblasts, while Cx45 is expressed mostly where fibroblasts intermingle with myocytes.
3. Gap junctions formed by Cx40 provide fibroblast–fibroblast coupling, while heterogeneous fibroblast–myocyte coupling is provided mostly by the Cx45 isoform.
4. Cx43 is not expressed in nodal tissue from the central region of the sinus node but provides myocyte–myocyte coupling in atrial fibers that protrude into this region. Importantly, the dye-spread studies suggest that fibroblasts can provide conductive pathways between myocytes that are not in direct contact, thus forming bridges for electrical communication.

COUPLING OF SKELETAL MYOBLASTS

Skeletal myoblasts consist of muscle tissue reservoir cells, because they have the ability for self-renewal and differentiation if muscle injury occurs *(13)*. It was shown that after transplantation, myoblasts stay alive for prolonged periods of time *(14)*, form myocyte-like elements, and tend to align parallel to host CMs *(15,16)*. Experimental data and initial clinical studies invariably showed not only engraftment of donor cells, but improvement in global cardiac pump function as well *(15,17–24)*. However, the exact mechanism by which they improve LV function is still debated.

The structure of myocardial and skeletal muscle tissue and their electromechanical properties differ significantly. Skeletal muscle cells are fused together, forming multi-nuclear fibers that are insulated from one another. Although certain data suggest that skeletal myoblasts may acquire few characteristics of CMs *(18)*, it could be assumed that the grafted cells do not transdifferentiate and keep morphological and electrophysiological properties of skeletal muscle. It is speculated that satellite cells are not able to form intercellular junctions characteristic for CMs. This suggests no possibility for electromechanical coupling with the host myocardium, which means that graft cannot be excited by host tissue.

On the other hand, it was shown that the lack of junctions between grafted cells and host tissue does not preclude improvement in LV contractile function *(18)*. This positive effect on contractility seems to last over time and is correlated with the number of implanted cells *(17)*. These results have led to further experiments on electromechanical coupling. Results of the experimental studies performed on myocardial wound strips proved that skeletal myoblast grafts do contract when exogenously stimulated *(15)*. Reinecke and co-workers showed that CMs and skeletal myoblasts, when placed in coculture, forms synchronous beating network *(18)*. On microscopy they even revealed the presence of N-cadherin- and Cx43-mediated junctions between skeletal myoblasts and CMs, allowing them to induce synchronous beating. Although encouraging, it must be emphasized that these results were obtained in cultured myoblasts, which are less differentiated than in vivo graft cells. Cultured myoblasts still express a low level of Cx43, which is undetectable in more matured in vivo cells. It has been suggested that the transplanted cells can contract synchronously even in the absence of connections between cells, because a simple stretch may initiate contraction *(19)*.

Discussing the issue of connections between host and transplanted cells, it must be stated that probably equally valid is the problem of insulation of cells by scar tissue. The scar forms a physical barrier that impedes electromechanical coupling. Therefore, any cell-based therapy that is based on excitation of graft by host tissue must address this problem in future.

Stem Cell Implantation and Ventricular Tachycardia Risk

Experimental and initial clinical studies have demonstrated abnormal action potential characteristics in CMs derived from pluripotent stem cells, which offers experimental evidence confirming that primordial cells may provide the foundation for ultimate repair of the myocardium but, because of their immaturity, may also create an environment conducive to malignant arrhythmias. These factors must be weighed as we pursue avenues of therapy based on the introduction of pluripotent cell lines.

Electrophysiological Properties of Human Stem Cell-Derived Cardiomyocytes

ESCs obviously have the greatest differentiation potential and propagation capacity; on the other hand, the very same advantages give rise to the as yet not fully explored risk of tumor formation. Caspi and Gepstein *(25)* summarized their experience with cardiac myocytes differentiated from human ESCs. Human ESC-derived CMs exhibit nodal, atrial, and ventricular myocyte-like action potentials (AP; most often atrial-like), depolarize and beat spontaneously (~60/min), express a strong sodium current, and interconnect by Cx-positive gap junctions. When co-cultured with neonatal rat CMs, human and rat cells couple electrically and mechanically and beat in synchrony. When embryoid bodies (the cell aggregates embryonic stem CMs are derived from) are injected into the LV of pigs in which the AV had been ablated, ESCs came into contact with the host myocardium and created an "escape pacemaker" that partly took over the endogenous His bundle escape rhythm.

The Arrhythmogenic Properties of Cardiomyocytes Derived From Mouse Embryonic Stem Cells

Zhang et al. *(26)* studied the arrhythmogenic properties of CMs differentiated from mouse pluripotent ESCs in the whole-cell patch-clamp mode and demonstrated that ESCs differentiated into at least three AP phenotypes. CMs showed spontaneous activity, low *dV/dt*, and prolonged AP duration. CMs demonstrated prolonged, spontaneous electrical activity in culture. Frequent triggered activity was observed with and without pharmacological enhancement. Phase 2 or 3 early afterdepolarizations could be induced easily by Bay K8644 plus tetraethylammonium chloride (TEA) or [TEA]o after Cs^+ replacement for $[K^+]i$, respectively. A combination of bradycardic stimulation, hypokalemia, and quinidine resulted in early afterdepolarizations. Delayed afterdepolarizations could be induced easily and reversibly by hypercalcemia or isoproterenol. These findings raise caution about the use of totipotent ESCs in cell transplantation therapy, because they may act as an unanticipated arrhythmogenic source from any of the three classic mechanisms (reentry, automaticity, or triggered activity).

Ion Channels and Currents in hMSCs

The injection transfers undifferentiated cells, which can contain hMSCs, directly into an electrically active environment. Zhang et al. *(27)* demonstrated that hMSCs express a consistent pattern of ion channels and at least three different ion currents. Therefore, the cells have some bioelectrical activity *(28)*. Based on our findings, we cannot judge whether implantation of hMSCs is safe or includes the risk of arrhythmia. However, careful monitoring of patients will be necessary, and will certainly be done, to rule out any pro-arrhythmogenic potential of undifferentiated hMSCs or hMSC-derived CMs.

ARRHYTHMIC POTENTIAL OF STEM CELL-DERIVED CARDIOMYOCYTES

Although it might be related to the intrinsic properties of the infarcted myocardium with LV systolic dysfunction, a major concern with stem cell transplantation is the potential for life-threatening ventricular tachyarrhythmias, especially with skeletal myoblasts *(29)*. Electrical heterogeneity of action potentials exists between the native and transplanted stem cells. Although the exact mechanisms are unknown, there are several proposed hypotheses to explain ventricular tachyarrythmias:

1. Intrinsic arrhythmic potential of transplanted cells
2. Increased nerve sprouting induced by stem cell transplantation
3. Local tissue injury induced by intramyocardial injection

Mesenchymal stem cells also increased cardiac nerve sprouting in both atria and ventricles and increased the magnitude of atrial sympathetic hyperinnervation. However, heterogeneous sympathetic nerve sprouting affects automaticity, triggered activity, refractoriness, and conduction velocity of myocardial cells and, therefore, may represent a substrate for lethal ventricular arrhythmia.

Zhang et al. *(26)* studied the arrhythmogenic properties of CMs differentiated from mouse ESCs. They found that ESCs differentiated into at least four AP phenotypes. CMs showed spontaneous activity, low dV/dt, prolonged AP duration, and easily inducible triggered arrhythmias. These findings raise caution about the use of totipotent ESCs in cell transplantation therapy, because they may act as an unanticipated arrhythmogeic source from any of the three classic mechanisms—reentry, automaticity, or triggered activity.

Arryhthmogenic Risk of Embryonic Stem Cells

Besides the allogenic character and the risk of tumor formation, one potential limitation of the ESC approach is arrhythmogenicity. Dr. Dudley *(26,27)* presented a detailed analysis of ionic currents of ESC-derived CMs from mice. As in humans, these cells come in different electrophysiological flavors—nodal-, atrial-, and ventricular myocyte-like—at different percentages (5, 15, and 80%). The main result was that the ventricular-like, i.e., those one is looking for, exhibit an unusually long action potential (three- to fourfold longer than in adult mouse), a slow propagation velocity, and that classical interventions to induce prolongation of AP duration (low K^+, quinidine, TEA, Bay K 8644) induce early and catecholamines induce late after depolarizations.

Arrhythmogenicity of Skeletal Myoblasts

Menasche et al. *(30–32)* presented the recent state of the art in this field. From animal experiments and the experience in a total of 70 patients treated up to now, the following conclusions can be drawn. The approach is feasible in terms of cell propagation and cell engraftment (survival rate after 2 wk = 5%). Skeletal myoblasts integrate into the host myocardium and survive for a long time, but do not differentiate into CMs and do not electrically couple to them. Animal experiments consistently demonstrate functional improvement. The first data in patients demonstrate an arrhythmogenic potential. The phase 2 trial is therefore conducted with a simultaneous implantation of a cardioverter defibrillator. This will also allow exact quantification of the proarrhythmic potential.

Relative Mechanics of Arrhythmogenic Effect

Based on the published data from clinical studies, we believe that the possible arrhythmogenic effect of myoblast transplantation would be evident only in the initial weeks after the procedure. The possible arrhythmogenic effect of myoblast transplantation is more probably related to its mechanics, including myocardial puncture and the inflammatory response to transplanted cells, some of which die after injection, than to possible problems with electromechanical coupling between newly developed myocytes and CMs. Possible electromechanical coupling problems would result in late arrhythmia as cells differentiate (downregulation of Cx43 and N-cadherin), a situation that has not been observed in clinical trials so far.

FUTURE DIRECTIONS

Initial clinical experience with cell transplantation has opened new perspectives for regeneration of inversibly injured organs, including myocardium. However, future clinical studies are needed to establish the role of cell transplantation in clinical practice and to make cell-delivery techniques more user-friendly and more efficacious. It must also be pointed out that further clinical studies are necessary to address questions regarding efficacy and long-term safety of cell transplantation. Phase 2 and 3 clinical trials must be conducted to prove the clinical efficacy of cellular cardiomyoplasty and to answer many other important questions regarding electric coupling and ventricular tachycardia risk, the need for repeated procedures, and its suitability for myocardial diseases other than post-myocardial infarct dysfunction.

At this stage, with few patients who have undergone autologous stem cell transplantations, it is difficult to predict whether stem cell transplantations are really arrhythmogenic, especially when patients with ischemic LV dysfunction frequently develop ventricular arrhythmia (23,24). Nevertheless, future studies on cell transplantation in patients with postinfarction heart failure will have to focus on the potential arrhythmogenic effect.

ESC-derived CM transplantation approaches are still in their early days, and ESC transplantation still has arrhythmogenic potential. Whether or not this is relevant to the in vivo situation remains to be tested (the former for unresolved safety and efficacy issues, the latter for the problem of ideal cell source). The endothelial progenitor cell and skeletal myoblast strategies, on the other hand, are already under clinical evaluation, but many questions with regard to the efficacy, safety, and mechanism of action appear open and await answers, which will be provided by the ongoing controlled clinical trials and solid experimental research.

REFERENCES

1. Kehat I, Khimovich L, Caspi O, et al. Electromechanical integration of cardiomyocytes derived from human embryonic stem cells. Nat Biotechnol 2004;22(10):1282–1289.
2. Rastan AJ, Walther T, Kostelka M, et al. Morphological, electrophysiological and coupling characteristics of bone marrow-derived mononuclear cells—an in vitro model. Eur J Cardiothorac Surg 2005;27: 104–110.
3. Mummery C, Ward-van Oostwaard D, Doevendans P, et al. Differentiation of human embryonic stem cells to cardiomyocytes. Circulation 2003;107:2733.
4. Valiunas V, Doronin S, Valiuniene L, et al. Human mesenchymal stem cells make cardiac connexins and form functional gap junctions. J Physiol 2004;555(pt 3):617–626. Epub 2004 Feb 6.
5. Volk T, Geiger BA. 135-kD membrane protein of intercellular adherens junctions. EMBO J 1984;3: 2249–2260.
6. Beyer EC, Paul DL, Goodenough DA. Connexin43: a protein form rat heart homologous to a gap junction protein from liver. J Cell Biol 1987;105(pt I):2621–2629.
7. Egashira K, Nishii K, Nakamura K, Kumai M, Morimoto S, Shibata Y. Conduction abnormality in gap junction protein connexin45-deficient embryonic stem cell-derived cardiac myocytes. Anat Rec A Discov Mol Cell Evol Biol 2004;280(2):973–979.
8. Wong RC, Pebay A, Nguyen LT, Koh KL, Pera MF. Presence of functional gap junctions in human embryonic stem cells. Stem Cells 2004;22(6):883–889.
9. Valiunas V, Doronin S, Valiuniene L, et al. Human mesenchymal stem cells make cardiac connexins and form functional gap junctions. J Physiol 2004;555(pt 3):617–626.
10. Durig J, Rosenthal C, Halfmeyer K, et al. Intercellular communication between bone marrow stromal cells and CD34+ haematopoietic progenitor cells is mediated by connexin 43-type gap junctions. Br J Haematol 2000;111(2):416–425.
11. Rastan AJ, Walther T, Kostelka M, et al. Morphological, electrophysiological and coupling characteristics of bone marrow-derived mononuclear cells—an in vitro model. Eur J Cardiothorac Surg 2005;27:104–110.

12. Camelliti P, Borg TK, Kohl P. Structural and functional characterisation of cardiac fibroblasts. Cardiovasc Res 2005;65(1):40–51.
13. Mauro A. Satellite cells of skeletal muscle fibres. J Biophys Biochem Cytol 1961;9:493–497.
14. Koh GY, Klug MG, Soonpaa MH, et al. Differentiation and long-term survival of C2C12 myoblast graft in heart. J Clin Invest 1993;92:1548–1554.
15. Murry CE, Wiseman RW, Schwartz SM, et al. Skeletal myoblast transplantation for repair of myocardial necrosis. J Clin Invest 1996;98:2512–2523.
16. Pagani FD, DerSimonian H, Zawadzka A, et al. Autologous skeletal myoblast transplantation to ischemia-damaged myocardium in humans. Histological analysis of cell survival and differentiation. J Am Coll Cardiol 2003;41:
17. Dorfman J, Duong M, Zibaitis A, et al. Myocardial tissue engineering with autologous myoblast implantation. J Cardiovasc Surg 1998;116:744–751.
18. Taylor DA, Atkins BZ, Hungspreugs P, et al. Regenerating functional myocardium: Improved performance after skeletal myoblast transplantation. Nat Med 1998;4:929–933.
19. Menasché P, Hagege AA, Scorsin M, et al. Myoblast transplantation for heart failure. Lancet 2001;357:279–280.
20. Rajnoch C, Chachques JC, Berrebi A, et al. Cellular therapy reverses myocardial dysfunction. J Thorac Cardiovasc Surg 2001;121:871–878.
21. Kessler PD, Byrne BJ. Myoblast cell grafting into heart muscle: cellular biology and potential applications. Ann Rev Physiol 1999;61:219–242.
22. Atkins BZ, Hueman MT, Meuchel JM, et al. Myogenic cell transplantation improves in vivo regional performance in infarcted rabbit myocardium. J Heart Lung Transplant 1999;18:1173–1180.
23. Ghostine S, Carrion C, Souza LC, et al. Long-term efficacy of myoblast transplantation on regional structure and function after myocardial infarction. Circulation 2002;106:I131–I136.
24. Hagege AA, Carion C, Menasché P, et al. Viability and differentiation of autologous skeletal myoblast grafts in ischaemic cardiomyopathy. Lancet 2003;361:491–492.
25. Caspi O, Gepstein L. Potential applications of human embryonic stem cell-derived cardiomyocytes. Ann NY Acad Sci 2004;1015:285–298.
26. Zhang YM, Hartzell C, Narlow M, Dudley SC, Jr. Stem cell-derived cardiomyocytes demonstrate arrhythmic potential. Circulation 2002;106(10):1294–1299.
27. Zhang YM, Shang L, Hartzell C, Narlow M, Cribbs L, Dudley SC, Jr. Characterization and regulation of T-type Ca2+ channels in embryonic stem cell-derived cardiomyocytes. Am J Physiol Heart Circ Physiol 2003;285(6):H2770–2779.
28. Yanagida E, Shoji S, Hirayama Y. Functional expression of Ca2+ signaling pathways in mouse embryonic stem cells. Cell Calcium 2004;36(2):135–146.
29. Raman SV, Cooke GE, Binkley PF. Stem cell-derived cardiomyocytes demonstrate arrhythmic potential. Circulation 2003;107:e195.
30. Siepe M, Heilmann C, von Samson P, Menasche P, Beyersdorf F. Stem cell research and cell transplantation for myocardial regeneration. Eur J Cardiothorac Surg 2005; [Epub ahead of print].
31. Alfieri O, Livi U, Martinelli L, et al. Myoblast transplantation for heart failure: where are we heading? Ital Heart J 2005;6(4):284–288.
32. Menasche P. Skeletal myoblast for cell therapy. Coron Artery Dis 2005;16(2):105–110.

12   Cell Therapy for Myocardial Damage
Arrhythmia Risk and Mechanisms

William R. Mills, MD
and Kenneth R. Laurita, PhD

SUMMARY

Ischemic heart disease resulting from myocardial infarction (MI) is the leading cause of sudden cardiac death (SCD) in the United States. Recent clinical and basic science investigations have focused on replacing damaged myocardium with skeletal muscle myoblasts (SKMBs) and bone marrow-derived stem cells (BMCs). Such cell therapies for MI have been shown to improve cardiac function; however, it is unknown if electrical viability of damaged myocardium can be restored and, thus, reduce the risk for SCD. Presently, several studies suggest that SKMB therapy for damaged myocardium increases arrhythmia risk, which may be causally related to a lack of SKMB integration into the electrical syncytium of the heart. In contrast, BMCs demonstrate less arrhythmia risk, enhanced electrical viability, and evidence of electrical integration. Other cell types and delivery methods may offer an even greater potential for enhanced electrical viability and reduced arrhythmia risk. Considering that SCD associated with damaged myocardium is primarily caused by arrhythmias, it is clear that an important factor that will determine whether cell therapy will succeed or fail is its electrophysiological consequence.

Key Words: Arrhythmia; myoblasts; stem cells; electrophysiology; myocardial infarction.

INTRODUCTION

Ischemic heart disease resulting from myocardial infarction (MI) is the leading cause of death in the United States. Chronic heart failure and sudden cardiac death (SCD) caused by ventricular arrhythmias are common devastating consequences of MI. MI results in irreversible damage because cardiomyocytes do not have sufficient ability to regenerate cardiac tissue. As a result, recent investigations have focused on replacing injured cardiomyocytes with new, healthy cells such as skeletal muscle myoblasts (SKMBs) and bone marrow-derived stem cells (BMCs). Such cell therapies for MI have been shown to improve cardiac function *(1–6)*, perfusion *(7)*, and symptoms *(8)* and decrease infarct size *(6)*. Given the rapidity in which cell therapy for damaged myocardium has evolved and the fact that cell therapies are already being used in patients, it is critically important to understand the electrophysiological and arrhythmia consequence.

From: *Contemporary Cardiology: Stem Cells and Myocardial Regeneration*
Edited by: M. S. Penn © Humana Press Inc., Totowa, NJ

DOES CELL THERAPY INCREASE ARRHYTHMIA RISK?

Clinical Trials

To date, SKMBs are the most studied cell type used as treatment for damaged myocardium. Several clinical studies have shown that SKMBs can improve hemodynamic function. Early animal studies using SKMBs did not report an incidence of ventricular arrhythmias, but subsequent clinical trials of SKMBs have raised concern. Menasche et al. *(9)* reported a study of SKMB therapy during coronary artery bypass grafting (CABG) in 10 patients with chronic MI and left ventricular (LV) dysfunction (ejection fraction [EF]<35%). Autologous SKMB (>50% SKMB, >70% viable) were injected into areas of scar tissue remote from the revascularized region. They reported a significant improvement in EF, but 4 out of 10 patients had sustained monomorphic ventricular tachycardia (VT) 9–22 days after surgery. Because of the lack of a control group, it was not possible to definitively determine whether SKMB therapy or natural disease progression was directly related to the high incidence of VT. Smits et al. *(10)* reported a small pilot study of five patients with ischemic cardiomyopathy (EF 20–45%) and a history of MI more than 4 weeks old with no previous history of ventricular arrhythmias who received an average of 196 million SKMBs via NOGA-guided transendocardial injection. The authors report that one out of five patients had post-therapy nonsustained VT, but they also report their experience with an additional eight patients and strikingly found that two died suddenly and three had ventricular arrhythmias within 3 months. Consequently, the study was stopped, and all patients enrolled subsequently were mandated to have a pretreatment implantable defibrillator. Recently, Dib et al. *(11)* reported 4-year follow-up data on an American study of SKMB therapy during CABG/LV assist device surgery. They found an 8% increase in EF measured at 24 months postsurgery, improved myocardial viability, and improved ventricular dilatation in patients receiving SKMB therapy, although the lack of a control group made drawing definitive hemodynamic conclusions difficult. Postoperative ventricular arrhythmias were observed in 3 of 24 patients in the CABG group. The authors remark that the incidence of post-SKMB therapy arrhythmias was no different from the 10–15% incidence expected in post-CABG patients with EF below 40% *(10)*. Therefore, despite improvements in cardiac function, clinical trials using SKMBs have not demonstrated a reduction of SCD risk and, importantly, have also raised serious safety concerns.

Several clinical studies have utilized BMCs for treatment of damaged myocardium. The Transplantation of Progenitor Cells and Regeneration Enhancement in Acute Myocardial Infarction (TOPCARE-AMI) trial allocated 20 patients who had MIs and successful percutaneous intervention (PCI) within 5 days to receive either autologous bone marrow cell therapy or peripheral blood progenitor cells via intracoronary catheter delivery *(5)*. Improved EF and myocardial viability (as measured by fluorodeoxyglucose-positron emission tomography) were observed in the cell therapy groups compared with patients receiving PCI and medical treatment. TOPCARE-AMI did not conduct posttreatment arrhythmia monitoring, but by history no patients reported malignant arrhythmias and no deaths occurred. The BOne marrOw transfer to enhance ST-elevation infarct generation (BOOST) trial was the first randomized controlled clinical trial of bone marrow-derived cell therapy *(12)*. After successful PCI for acute MI, 60 patients who had severe post-MI LV dysfunction were randomized to receive either optimal medical therapy or CD34$^+$ bone marrow cell therapy via intracoronary infusion. Patients receiving cell therapy experienced a significant improvement in cardiac function as assessed by cardiac MRI 6 months after MI, whereas non-cell therapy-receiving patients did not. In the follow-up period, 24-hour Holter monitoring at 1 day, 6 weeks, 3 months, and 6 months showed no difference in arrhythmia occurrence between groups. In addition, programmed stimulation 6 months after therapy induced nonsustained VT in one control and one bone marrow cell-receiving patient and induced ventricular fibrillation in one control and zero cell therapy-receiving patients. The authors concluded that bone marrow cell therapy for MI was safe and was associated with improved cardiac function. However, as with SKMB therapy, it is unclear if bone marrow cell therapy can reduce the risk of SCD associated with MI.

Experimental Models

The current understanding of the electrophysiological effects of cell therapy for damaged myocardium has evolved in an unusual manner. Given that early basic studies of cell therapy in animals did not report a significant incidence of posttherapy arrhythmias *(1,13–15)*, the results reported by Menasche *(9)* and Smits *(10)* were surprising. The response has been to re-examine the arrhythmic and electrophysiological effects of cell therapy in experimental models.

As reported by Zhang et al. *(16)*, cardiomyocytes derived from stem cells have demonstrated spontaneous activity, slow upstroke velocity, prolonged action potential duration, and easily inducible triggered arrhythmias. In a recent study by Abraham et al. *(17)*, human SKMBs were co-cultured with rat ventricular myocytes in a monolayer, and optical mapping techniques were used to measure action potential propagation and arrhythmia inducibility. When co-cultures contained more than 30% myoblasts, abnormal impulse propagation and re-entrant excitation were observed. These results suggest a dose dependency of SKMBs on arrhythmia vulnerability; however, it is difficult to extrapolate such results from isolated cells and cell cultures to the whole heart.

Notwithstanding the high rate of ventricular arrhythmias reported in early clinical studies of cell therapy *(9,10)*, few systematic investigations of arrhythmia vulnerability in the whole heart have been reported *(17a)*. Our laboratory has recently developed a rat model of MI specifically designed to determine the electrophysiological and arrhythmic consequences of cell therapy *(18)*. This model of MI shares many of the electrical and hemodynamic characteristics of MI in patients. Compared with normal rats, which have a mean echocardiographic shortening fraction of 50%, our rat model of MI has a mean shortening fraction of approx 10% (*see* Fig. 1). For SKMB therapy, 1–2 million SKMBs were injected from the epicardium into the border zone of the infarct *(19,20)*. For mesenchymal stem cell (MSC) therapy, a similar amount of MSCs was administered intravenously with or without adenoviral myocardial homing factor (SDF-1) overexpression *(19)*. We have shown in this model that both SKMB and MSC therapy typically result in a 50–60% increase in shortening fraction (Fig. 1) *(20)*. These data are comparable to those reported in most clinical trials. Importantly, we have also consistently found that such improvement in cardiac function does not imply a decrease in arrhythmic risk *(20,21)*. Shown in Fig. 2 is arrhythmia inducibility by programmed stimulation 1 month after MI in rats that received SKMB therapy within 24 hours of MI (MI + SKMB 1 month), rats with MI and no cell therapy (control MI), and age-matched normal hearts (normal). Also shown are data from rats 4 months after MI that received homing factor-enhanced (SDF-1) SKMBs 2 months after MI *(21)*. Strikingly, all

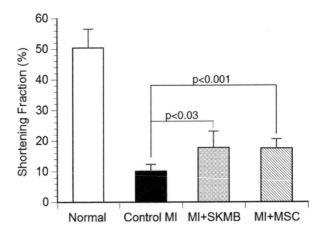

Fig. 1. Shown are shortening fractions measured by echocardiography 1 month after myocardial infarction (MI). Skeletal muscle myoblast (SKMB) and mesenchymal stem cell (MSC) therapy improved cardiac function to a similar extent compared with MI alone (Control MI). *p*-values indicate statistical significance comparing SKMB and MSC therapy groups to control MI.

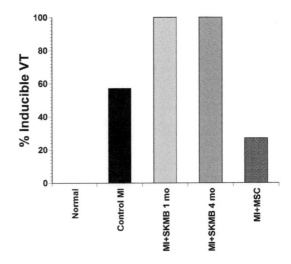

Fig. 2. Arrhythmia vulnerability assessed by percent of preparations inducible during programmed stimulation. Note that skeletal muscle myoblast (SKMB) therapy was associated with increased arrhythmia vulnerability (100% at 1 and 4 months after myocardial infarction [MI]). Note that mesenchymal stem cell (MSC) therapy tended to decrease arrhythmia inducibility compared to control MI. VT; ventricular tachycardia.

SKMB-receiving animals (100%) had inducible VT during programmed stimulation. Also shown in Fig. 2 is arrhythmia inducibility from rats that received intravenous MSCs 24 hours after MI. MI + MSC hearts were significantly less vulnerable to arrhythmias than MI + SKMB hearts and trended toward being less vulnerable than control MIs. The low arrhythmia vulnerability we observed in MI + MSC hearts is also consistent with the low incidence of SCD and ventricular arrhythmias reported in early clinical trials of BMC therapies.

WHY IS CELL THERAPY SOMETIMES ARRHYTHMOGENIC?

Studies in Isolated Cells

Normal myocardium is electrically integrated through intercellular coupling of adjacent myocytes, resulting in a syncytium that promotes rapid and uniform electrical impulse propagation. Electrical coupling occurs through gap junctions that are formed, in part, by connexin proteins. Under conditions of reduced gap junction coupling, cells become electrically uncoupled and can manifest abnormal (e.g., slow, blocked) impulse propagation, a requirement for reentrant arrhythmias. Recent studies suggest that certain cell replacement therapies are unable to form cell-to-cell connections in vivo (e.g., SKMB). Therefore, it is likely that the ability of cells to structurally and electrically couple with neighboring cells is an important determinant of arrhythmia risk associated with cell therapy. In addition, previous studies have also shown that some cell types (i.e., stem cells) express ionic currents that create an inherent arrhythmogenic potential when studied in isolation *(16)*. *See* Chapter 11 for a detailed discussion of the gap junction coupling and cellular electrophysiology.

Studies In Vitro

The cellular electrophysiology of transplanted cells *in situ* and their ability to integrate with host myocardium are important determinants of arrhythmogenesis. In an elegant study, Abraham et al. *(17)* used optical action potential mapping techniques to study impulse propagation in cell monolayers comprised of various ratios of human SKMBs co-plated with neonatal rat ventricular myocytes (NRVMs). The authors demonstrate that neither action potentials nor calcium transients propagated between regions of SKMBs and NRVMs, confirming a lack of electrical integration. The authors also report slow-impulse conduction and prolonged action potential duration in co-cultures, both of which are electrophysiological substrates for arrhythmias. Importantly, all co-cultures with more than 1% SKMBs demonstrated sustained reentry that was terminated by nitrendipine, which also suggests a calcium-dependent mechanism. This study suggests that an important mechanism of arrhythmogenesis associated with SKMB therapy is abnormal impulse propagation directly related to poor electrical integration. At present, there are very few reports of the electrical integration between BMCs and host cardiomyocytes. One such study showed that MSCs can couple with native cardiomyocytes both in vitro and in vivo; however, the percentage of coupling pairs was very low *(22)*.

Studies in the Whole Heart

To determine the mechanisms of arrhythmogenesis associated with cell therapy in the whole heart, we have developed a novel optical action potential mapping system for measuring cellular electrophysiology in a rat MI model. Whole hearts are stained with a fluorescent voltage-sensitive dye (di-4-ANEPPS) using a novel superfusion technique that has been developed and validated previously *(18)*. After dye-superfusion staining, the heart is Langendorff perfused and placed in an imaging chamber (Fig. 3). Excitation light (514 nm) is directed to the surface of the heart, and fluorescence from the heart is focused onto a 256-element photodiode array. Photocurrent, which is linearly related to transmembrane potential, is converted to voltage and digitized at all 256 sites simultaneously. Similar optical action potential mapping techniques have been used to determine the cellular electrophysiological basis of arrhythmias in a variety of heart preparations *(23,24)*.

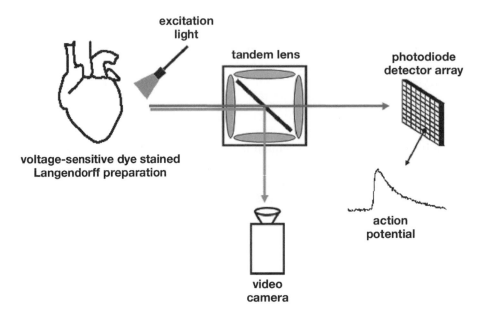

Fig. 3. Optical mapping system for measuring action potential propagation in the intact heart. Excitation light is directed to the heart surface, and resultant fluorescence from membrane-bound di-4-ANEPPS is focused by a tandem lens assembly onto a 256-element photodiode array. Current from each photodiode element is simultaneously converted to an action potential. Reflected light or fluorescence from labeled cells (e.g., DiI or green fluorescent protein) can be redirected by the tandem lens to a change-coupled device video camera.

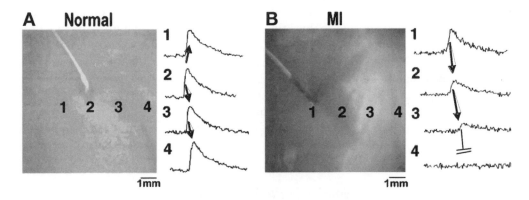

Fig. 4. Myocardial infarction (MI) is associated with conduction block and a lack of significant electrical viability in the infarct border zone as determined by optical mapping. Optically recorded action potentials obtained from normal (**A**) and infarcted rat hearts 1 month after MI. (**B**) The images in each panel show the area mapped in each heart, and the signals beside each image were recorded from the depicted sites, numbered 1–4. *See* text for details. (*See* color insert following p. 114.)

In the rat MI model with cell therapy (SKMB or MSC) or without (control MI), optical action potentials were recorded simultaneously from normal, border zone, and infarcted tissue *(20)*. Shown in Fig. 4 are optically recorded action potentials from a normal heart (Fig. 4A) and a heart with a 1-month-old infarct (Fig. 4B). The image in each panel shows the anterior surface of the heart and the location from which action

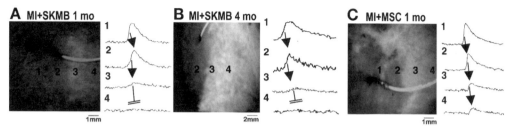

Fig. 5. Mesenchymal stem cell (MSC), but not skeletal muscle myoblast (SKMB), therapy was associated with enhanced electrical viability, including impulse propagation in the infarct border zone. Optically recorded action potentials obtained from myocardial infarct (MI) + SKMB 1 month after MI (**A**), MI + SKMB 4 months after MI (**B**), and MI + MSC 1 month after MI (**C**). The images in each panel show the area mapped in each heart, and the signals beside each photograph were recorded from the depicted sites, numbered 1–4. *See* text for details. (*See* color insert following p. 114.)

potentials were recorded (right) corresponding to normal (site 1), border zone (sites 2 and 3), and infarcted (site 4) tissue. Action potentials recorded from a normal heart demonstrate uniform amplitude and normal action potential morphology. In this example, impulse conduction velocity between sites 1 and 4 is 0.44 m/second. Shown in Fig. 4B are action potentials recorded from a control MI. The action potential recorded from normal tissue (site 1) was similar to those measured from normal hearts, whereas signals recorded from the border zone (sites 2 and 3) demonstrate an abrupt decrease in amplitude and a slower depolarization phase. The decease in optical action potential amplitude likely represents a decrease in the number electrically viable cells. No action potential activity was observed further into the infarct zone (site 4), indicating an absence of electrical viability. On average, conduction velocity from site 1 to site 3 (i.e., in the border zone) was 0.33 ± 0.05 m/second. Shown in Fig. 5 are action potentials recorded from an infarcted heart treated with intramyocardially injected SKMBs (Fig. 5A, 1 month MI; Fig. 5B, 4 months MI) and intravenous infused MSCs (Fig. 5C). For MI + SKMB, action potentials recorded from the normal tissue (site 1) were similar to that measured from normal rats, whereas signals recorded from the border zone (sites 2 and 3) were of low amplitude and had a slower depolarization phase. On average, conduction velocity (0.21 ± 0.05 m/second) was significantly less than that for control MI. No action potential activity was observed at site 4 (similar to control MI), representing failure of impulse propagation (conduction block) and, thus, no change in electrical viability in the infarct zone of SKMB-treated MI. In contrast, action potentials recorded from the border zone of MSC-treated hearts (Fig. 5C, sites 2 and 3) were smaller than normal, but not as small as those recorded from the border zone in control MIs. In addition, unlike control MIs, action potential activity was measured at site 4 (furthest point into the infarct zone), indicating electrical viability including impulse propagation within the infarct zone. Similar results were obtained in four of seven MSC-treated animals. On average, conduction velocity from site 1 to 4 (0.24 ± 0.07) tended to be slower than control MI, but not statistically significant.

Significantly slower conduction velocity compared to control MI and no evidence of electrical viability in the infarct zone associated with SKMB therapy may explain the increase in arrhythmia vulnerability. It has been shown that SKMBs injected into normal or border zone tissue can alter impulse propagation *(25)* and arrhythmia vulnerability *(26)*. Shown in Fig. 6 is abnormal impulse propagation caused by SKMBs injected into normal myocardium *(25)*. In this example, DiI-labeled SKMBs ($\sim 10^8$) were

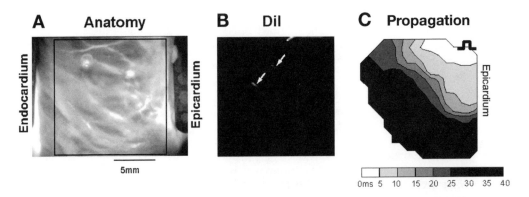

Fig. 6. (A) Image of the transmural surface of the left ventricular wedge preparation under ambient room light. The large box depicts the imaging field from which optical action potentials and DiI fluorescence were measured. **(B)** The same preparation and imaging field during DiI excitation. The illuminated areas depict DiI-labeled cells. **(C)** Pattern of impulse propagation when pacing from the epicardium. The closely spaced isochrone lines of the activation map **(C)** represent a delay in activation, particularly at sites where cells were injected **(B, arrows)**. (*See* color insert following p. 114.)

injected from the epicardium at approx 20–40 sites in the normal canine left ventricle. One month after injections, LV wedge preparations were isolated from each heart and transmural impulse propagation, and the location of SKMB transplanted cells was determined using optical mapping techniques, as described above. Shown in Fig. 6A is the transmural surface of a wedge preparation from a heart that received SKMB injections and the location from which impulse propagation and transplanted cells were imaged (black box). SKMBs were labeled with DiI before transplantation, and the injection sites were clearly visible (arrows, Fig 6B). Interestingly, in this example, impulse propagation (Fig. 6C) was abnormally slow, as indicated by relative crowding of isochrone lines, at the location of SKMB transplantation (arrows). This finding is consistent with recent work by Chang et al., who showed conduction slowing in co-cultures of MSC and cardiomyocytes *(27)*, and Reinecke et al. *(28)*, who showed that SKMBs do not electrically integrate into the myocardium. Moreover, since skeletal myotubes in vivo have not been shown to express connexin-43 *(25)*, SKMB injection sites may impose a significant barrier to impulse conduction.

In contrast to SKMB-treated hearts, evidence of enhanced electrical viability within the infarct zone of MI + MSC hearts may explain the observed reduction in arrhythmia vulnerability. The exact mechanism is not clear, but it is possible that MSC therapy decreased the electrical size of the infarct. Such a decrease would effectively shorten the path length of a reentrant circuit and prevent the induction of VT *(29)*. Electrical coupling between MSCs and native cardiomyocytes may have, at least in part, led to the increase in electrical viability and reduced arrhythmia vulnerability observed. Potapova et al. *(30)* and Valiunas et al. *(22)* have demonstrated low frequency gap junction formation between MSCs and cardiomyocytes.

FUTURE DIRECTIONS

Our present understanding of the electrophysiological substrate and arrhythmia risk associated with cell therapy has been shaped by a small number of clinical and basic studies. In general, these studies have led most investigators to conclude preliminarily that although SKMB therapy can improve hemodynamic function, it may increase arrhythmia vulnerability. This is likely due to the inability of SKMBs to electrically integrate into the myocardium. So far, preliminary studies of bone marrow-derived cell therapies have not demonstrated an increased arrhythmia risk; however, whether or not arrhythmia risk is actually lowered and the underlying mechanisms remain to be determined.

A current limitation of cell therapy is that important proteins that govern ion channel function and cell-to-cell coupling in differentiated cells may not be expressed to the appropriate levels to provide normal electrophysiological function. An advantage of most cell therapy is that while cells are in culture, the expression of such proteins can be genetically engineered. For example, SKMBs have thus far been shown to be incapable of forming gap junctions in vivo *(28)*. However, Abraham et al. *(31)* have shown that overexpression of connexin-43 in SKMB/NRVM co-cultures reduced arrhythmia vulnerability and reentry, suggesting that this technique may increase cell-to-cell coupling of SKMB with host cardiomyocytes. In addition, Reinecke et al. *(32)* and Suzuki et al. *(33)* have shown that overexpression of connexin-43 can improve the formation and function of gap junctions. In addition to overexpressing connexin to improve cell-to-cell coupling, it may also be possible to genetically engineer cells with an ideal action potential phenotype. For example, overexpression of pacemaker current in MSCs *(30)* or potassium channels in fibroblast *(34)* have been shown to restore pacemaker activity and impulse conduction, respectively. Whether or not a similar approach is feasible with damaged myocardium (i.e., MI) has not been tested. Finally, in addition to SKMBs and BMCs, other cells types such as embryonic stems cells *(35–37)* and cardiac stem cells *(38)* are more likely to differentiate into cardiomyocytes with cell-to-cell coupling and ion channel properties that provide a more seamless electrically integration with host myocardial tissue.

The manner by which cells are delivered to the target site (e.g., infarct) may also be an important electrophysiological determinant and, thus, worthy of future investigation. As mentioned above, when cells are directly injected into normal tissue or the infarct border zone, cells have a tendency to cluster at injection sites *(1,26)*, which may form barriers to impulse conduction (*see* Fig. 6). Intracoronary and intravenous delivery of cell therapy has also been shown to improve cardiac function *(5,12,39,40)*. The diffuse delivery of cells using this technique and the resultant absence of cellular clusters or islands may reduce abnormal impulse conduction. In addition, Askari et al. *(19)* showed that overexpression of SDF-1 in transplanted SKMBs increased stem cell engraftment in the infarct zone and was associated with a significant improvement in cardiac function compared with SKMB-null cell therapy.

CONCLUSIONS

Cell therapy may be the first curative treatment for damaged myocardium. This fact makes the field extraordinarily exciting; however, the rapidity with which such a poorly understood therapy has been brought from bench to bedside has raised serious concern. Only after significant arrhythmia risk was recognized did a renewed sense of scientific rigor become apparent. At the present time, clinical and experimental studies strongly suggest that SKMB therapy for damaged myocardium increases arrhythmia risk and, thus, should not be used in humans unless the risks outweigh the benefits, and never without an implantable cardioverter defibrillator. One cannot ignore the experimental data that clearly illustrate the catastrophic flaw of SKMBs: a lack of integration into the electrical syncytium of the heart. Genetically modifying SKMBs to improve intercellular coupling remains a possibility. Other cell types, such as stem cells (e.g., BMCs, embryonic, or cardiac), may offer a greater potential for electrophysiological integration. Further optimization of stem cell therapies may be needed, and many questions remain to be answered (e.g., ideal cell type, delivery method). In conclusion, considering that SCD associated with damaged myocardium is primarily caused by arrhythmias, one of the most important factors that will determine whether cell therapy will succeed or fail is its electrophysiological consequence.

ACKNOWLEDGMENTS

Results reported in this chapter were supported by NIH grants HL68877 (KRL) and HL74400 (MSP), and grants from The Wilson Foundation (MSP), Shalom Foundation (MSP), the Biological Research Technology Transfer Fund of the State of Ohio (MSP and KRL), and Medtronic Inc (KRL). This work was performed during Dr. Mills' tenure as the Michael Bilitch Fellow in Cardiac Pacing and Electrophysiology of the NASPE-Heart Rhythm Society.

REFERENCES

1. Taylor DA, Atkins BZ, Hungspreugs P, et al. Regenerating functional myocardium: improved performance after skeletal myoblast transplantation. Nat Med 1998;4:929–933.
2. Orlic D, Kajstura J, Chimenti S, et al. Bone marrow cells regenerate infarcted myocardium. Nature 2001;410:701–705.
3. Yau TM, Tomita S, Weisel RD, et al. Beneficial effect of autologous cell transplantation on infarcted heart function: comparison between bone marrow stromal cells and heart cells. Ann Thorac Surg 2003;75:169–176.
4. Menasche P, Hagege AA, Scorsin M, et al. Myoblast transplantation for heart failure. Lancet 2001;357:279–280.
5. Assmus B, Schachinger V, Teupe C, et al. Transplantation of Progenitor Cells and Regeneration Enhancement in Acute Myocardial Infarction (TOPCARE-AMI). Circulation 2002;106:3009–3017.
6. Strauer BE, Brehm M, Zeus T, et al. Repair of infarcted myocardium by autologous intracoronary mononuclear bone marrow cell transplantation in humans. Circulation 2002;106:1913–1918.
7. Stamm C, Westphal B, Kleine HD, et al. Autologous bone-marrow stem-cell transplantation for myocardial regeneration. Lancet 2003;361:45–46.
8. Tse HF, Kwong YL, Chan JK, et al. Angiogenesis in ischaemic myocardium by intramyocardial autologous bone marrow mononuclear cell implantation. Lancet 2003;361:47–49.
9. Menasche P, Hagege AA, Vilquin JT, et al. Autologous skeletal myoblast transplantation for severe postinfarction left ventricular dysfunction. J Am Coll Cardiol 2003;41:1078–1083.
10. Smits PC, van Geuns RJ, Poldermans D, et al. Catheter-based intramyocardial injection of autologous skeletal myoblasts as a primary treatment of ischemic heart failure: clinical experience with six-month follow-up. J Am Coll Cardiol 2003;42:2063–2069.
11. Dib N, Michler RE, Pagani FD, et al. Safety and feasibility of autologous myoblast transplantation in patients with ischemic cardiomyopathy: four-year follow-up. Circulation 2005;112:1748–1755.
12. Wollert KC, Meyer GP, Lotz J, et al. Intracoronary autologous bone-marrow cell transfer after myocardial infarction: the BOOST randomised controlled clinical trial. Lancet 2004;364:141–148.
13. Chiu RC, Zibaitis A, Kao RL. Cellular cardiomyoplasty: myocardial regeneration with satellite cell implantation. Ann Thorac Surg 1995;60:12–18.
14. Atkins BZ, Lewis CW, Kraus WE, et al. Intracardiac transplantation of skeletal myoblasts yields two populations of striated cells in situ. Ann Thorac Surg 1999;67:124–129.
15. Murry CE, Wiseman RW, Schwartz SM, et al. Skeletal myoblast transplantation for repair of myocardial necrosis. J Clin Invest 1996;98:2512–2523.
16. Zhang YM, Hartzell C, Narlow M, et al. Stem cell-derived cardiomyocytes demonstrate arrhythmic potential. Circulation 2002;106:1294–1299.

17. Abraham MR, Henrikson CA, Tung L, et al. Antiarrhythmic engineering of skeletal myoblasts for cardiac transplantation. Circ Res 2005;97:159–167.

17a. Fernandes S, Amirault JC, Lande G, et al. Autologous myoblast transplantation after myocardial infarction increases the inducibility of ventricular arrhythmias. Cardiovasc Res 2006;69:348–358.

18. Mills WR, Mal N, Forudi F, Popovic ZB, Penn MS, Laurita KR. Optical mapping of late myocardial infarction in rat. Am J Physiol Heart Circ Physiol 2006;290:H1298–H1306.

19. Askari AT, Unzek S, Popovic ZB, et al. Effect of stromal-cell-derived factor 1 on stem-cell homing and tissue regeneration in ischaemic cardiomyopathy. Lancet 2003;362:697–703.

20. Mills WR, Mal N, Kiedrowski MJ, et al. Stem cell therapy enhances electrical viability in myocardial infarction. Circulation 2005;112:247.

21. Mills WR, Mal N, Kiedrowski MJ, et al. Does transplantation of skeletal myoblasts genetically modified to overexpress stromal-derived Factor 1 restore normal conduction in chronic ischemic heart disease? Heart Rhythm 2005;S141.

22. Valiunas V, Doronin S, Valiuniene L, et al. Human mesenchymal stem cells make cardiac connexins and form functional gap junctions. J Physiol 2004;555:617–626.

23. Laurita KR, Chuck ET, Yang TN, et al. Optical mapping reveals conduction slowing and impulse block in iron-overload cardiomyopathy. J Lab Clin Med 2003;142:83–89.

24. Laurita KR, Rosenbaum DS. Interdependence of modulated dispersion and tissue structure in the mechanism of unidirectional block. Circ Res 2000;87:922–928.

25. Fouts K, Fernandes B, Mal N, Liu J, Laurita KR. Electrophysiological consequence of skeletal myoblast transplantation in normal and infarcted canine myocardium. Heart Rhythm 2006;3:452–461.

26. Krucoff MW, Crater S, Taylor DA, Soliman AM, Morimoto Y. Cell location may be a primary determinant of safety after myoblast transplantation into the infarcted heart. JACC 2004;43.

27. Chang M, Emokpae R, Zhang Y, et al. Co-culture of mesenchymal stem cells and neonatal rat ventricular myocytes produces an arrhythmic substrate. Heart Rhythm 2005;S48.

28. Reinecke H, MacDonald GH, Hauschka SD, et al. Electromechanical coupling between skeletal and cardiac muscle. Implications for infarct repair. J Cell Biol. 2000;149:731–740.

29. Allessie MA. Circus movement in rabbit atrial muscle as a mechanism of tachycardia III. The "leading circle" concept: a new model of circus movement in cardiac tissue without the involvement of an anatomic obstacle. Circ Res 1977;41:9–18.

30. Potapova I, Plotnikov A, Lu Z, et al. Human mesenchymal stem cells as a gene delivery system to create cardiac pacemakers. Circ Res 2004;94:952–959.

31. Abraham R, Lim P, Henrickson CA, et al. Mechanisms and potential pharmacological gene therapy strategies for myoblast transplant-associated ventricular arrhythmias: insights from a unique in vitro model. Circulation 2004;III-1.

32. Reinecke H, Minami E, Virag JI, et al. Gene transfer of connexin43 into skeletal muscle. Hum Gene Ther 2004;15:627–636.

33. Suzuki K, Brand NJ, Allen S, et al. Overexpression of connexin 43 in skeletal myoblasts: relevance to cell transplantation to the heart. J Thorac Cardiovasc Surg 2001;122:759–766.

34. Feld Y, Melamed-Frank M, Kehat Z, et al. Electrophysiological modulation of cardiomyocytic tissue by transfected fibroblasts expressing potassium channels—a novel strategy to manipulate excitability. Circulation 2002;105:522–529.

35. Xue T, Cho HC, Akar FG, et al. Functional integration of electrically active cardiac derivatives from genetically engineered human embryonic stem cells with quiescent recipient ventricular cardiomyocytes: insights into the development of cell-based pacemakers. Circulation 2005;111:11–20.

36. Kehat I, Khimovich L, Caspi O, et al. Electromechanical integration of cardiomyocytes derived from human embryonic stem cells. Nat Biotechnol 2004;22:1282–1289.

37. Singla DK, Hacker TA, Ma L, et al. Transplantation of embryonic stem cells into the infarcted mouse heart: formation of multiple cell types. J Mol Cell Cardiol 2006;40:195–200.

38. Urbanek K, Rota M, Cascapera S, et al. Cardiac stem cells possess growth factor-receptor systems that after activation regenerate the infarcted myocardium, improving ventricular function and long-term survival. Circ Res 2005;97:663–673.

39. Wang JS, Shum-Tim D, Chedrawy E, et al. The coronary delivery of marrow stromal cells for myocardial regeneration: pathophysiologic and therapeutic implications. J Thorac Cardiovasc Surg 2001;122:699–705.

40. Bittira B, Shum-Tim D, Al-Khaldi A, et al. Mobilization and homing of bone marrow stromal cells in myocardial infarction. Eur J Cardiothorac Surg 2003;24:393–398.

III Strategies for Cell Delivery: Advantages/Disadvantages

13 Aspects of Percutaneous Cellular Cardiomyoplasty

Matthew Hook, MD and Patrick Whitlow, MD

SUMMARY

The significant advances achieved over the past decade in the field of percutaneous coronary intervention have significantly increased our ability to use catheter-based techniques to modify cardiac physiology. The ongoing studies demonstrating the significant potential of cell-based therapy for the prevention and treatment of chronic heart failure has led to the development of multiple catheter-based systems for the delivery of cells to the injured myocardium. Advances have also been made in catheter-based systems that exploit electomechanical properties of the heart in order to direct the interventionalist as to the best areas in which to inject cells. In this chapter we will review the different catheter systems currently available or under development as well as discuss how different features of each may be optimal in the different settings of acute myocardial infarction and chronic heart failure.

Key Words: Intracoronary delivery; endocardial injection; electromechanical mapping; ischemic cardiomyopathy.

Percutaneous catheter-directed regenerative cell therapies are being developed for patients with compromised systolic function and prior myocardial infarction (MI), ischemic and nonischemic cardiomyopathy, as well as for patients with acute myocardial injury, presenting for revascularization *(1–3)*. The administration of skeletal myoblasts at the time of acute revascularization for MI is intriguing, as patients may benefit from increased adaptability of the cells in a milieu of intense recruitment of native progenitor cells and better blood supply than those with chronic myocardial scar tissue *(4,5)*.

Some progenitor cells and skeletal myoblasts do not home from the blood stream into the myocardium, and thus, direct delivery of these cells into infarct or peri-infarct beds of myocardium may be required. Although both surgical and percutaneous approaches have been developed and tested in preclinical and clinical studies, a percutaneously based mode of delivery is desirable for several reasons:

1. It helps to avoid an open surgical procedure and the concomitant risks of infection, bleeding, general anesthesia, etc.
2. Surgical/epicardial approaches fail to access the interventricular septum, vital for synchronization of myocardial contraction, while constituting a moderate percentage of ventricular mass.

From: *Contemporary Cardiology: Stem Cells and Myocardial Regeneration*
Edited by: M. S. Penn © Humana Press Inc., Totowa, NJ

3. Percutaneous-based therapies are less invasive in the event of the need for recurrent myocardial injections.
4. If cells need to be delivered at the time of revascularization from an acute MI, it is unlikely that a surgical approach will be readily accessible.

PERCUTANEOUS CELL THERAPY FOR ACUTE MI

If cell delivery is to be undertaken at the time of coronary reperfusion, it implies that an allogeneic cell that is available at the time of patient presentation has been developed. Like a cell that is available at all times, the procedure to deliver them also needs to be available at all times as well. Therefore, the delivery strategy needs to take into account the fact that patients will present at all hours of the day and night. Ideally, patients with an acute MI receiving cell therapy at the time of primary revascularization would do so via a perfusion catheter or an over-the-wire balloon in the infarct-related artery. Concerns regarding this technique relate primarily to ascertaining allogeneic progenitor cells for patients presenting acutely, the adverse effects of cellular embolization in an acutely occluded vessel, as well as a potential for increased rates of in-stent restenosis in target vessels treated with bare-metal stents *(6)*. Delivery via the infarct-related artery would theoretically eliminate the need for electromechanical mapping or other imaging techniques that could prove cumbersome at the time of primary percutaneous coronary intervention (PCI).

Intracoronary injection of cells has recently been proven safe and moderately effective in a small randomized trial of patients with chronic myocardial injury and in the Myoblast Autologous Grafting in Ischemic Cardiomyopathy cell trial, in which patients were randomized only if they presented more than 48 hours after symptom onset and were hemodynamically stable for more than 24 hours prior to randomization *(6,7)*. No trial has yet to address the safety or efficacy of infusing stem cells at the time of revascularization in patients presenting for primary percutaneous revascularization.

CELL THERAPY FOR CHRONIC HEART FAILURE

An ideal route of delivery would be minimally invasive and would send high concentrations of stem cells to a target region of an organ, while avoiding inundating other organs. Direct intramyocardial delivery during surgery and percutaneous delivery via the coronary, arterial-transendocardial, or venous-transendocardial routes is being used or proposed in clinical trials. Intracoronary or intravenous delivery to access a specific region close to the coronary vasculature is effective and is easier to perform than direct injection.

Many have proposed that intramyocardial delivery from the endocardium requires an imaging modality that can discern healthy from injured or dead tissue *(8–10)*. In one study, electromechanical mapping was used to identify viable myocardium for catheter-based transendocardial delivery of mononuclear bone marrow cells in humans using the NOGA system (Cordis) *(11)*. This electromagnetic tracking system used an injection catheter to differentiate and map normal, scarred, and viable myocardial tissue *(8)*. During a standard clinical procedure using the NOGA, three external magnets that emit a low-energy magnetic field are placed at different locations around the patient's chest. The system uses a catheter equipped with three sensing coils and two electrodes on its distal tip that permit measurement of a voltage potential across a short segment of endocardium *(11)*. The coordinates of the catheter tip in three-dimensional space are

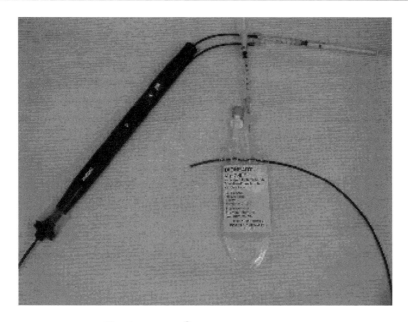

Fig. 1. Myocath® catheter, Bioheart, Inc.

determined by implementing a triangulation algorithm. A three-dimensional, color-coded voltage map reconstruction of the left ventricle that clearly demarcates the area of MI is generated using data collected during these measurements. The system requires X-ray guidance to determine the position of the catheter *(12)* and therefore does not provide an anatomical image of the heart. Thus, the map quality is operator dependent, and the procedure may be lengthy.

CATHETER SYSTEMS

Percutaneous catheters have focused primarily on direct endocardial injection of cells (MyoCath® catheter, Bioheart Inc.; Stiletto® catheter, Boston-Scientific; Myostar®, Cordis/Johnson & Johnson Inc.) or, recently, transvenous, intravascular ultrasound-guided (IVUS) (TransAccess® catheter via the coronary sinus) delivery of cells. Both modes of delivery have demonstrated preclinical and clinical promise. No trials have yet compared these catheters with regard to safety, user-friendliness, transfection efficiency, and myocardial retention of the injectate. Common attributes of these catheters include 7–9 Fr outer lumen diameter, a central injection lumen through which the cellular injectate is instilled, and manually guided, retrograde positioning under fluoroscopic guidance. The TransAccess catheter combines a phased-array IVUS and Nitinol needle. The catheter is placed in the coronary sinus and positioning of the needle confirmed by IVUS and the relationship to the pericardium, atrioventricular artery, and ventricular myocardium. After advancing the Nitinol needle, the injection catheter and cellular injectate is advanced through the needle into the myocardium. Cells are thus introduced into the ventricular myocardium in a circumferential array, in contrast to the perpendicular injection of endocardially based catheters. To optimally use this approach, the operator must be comfortable accessing the coronary sinus and develop expertise with IVUS to ensure proper localization of cellular injectate into the

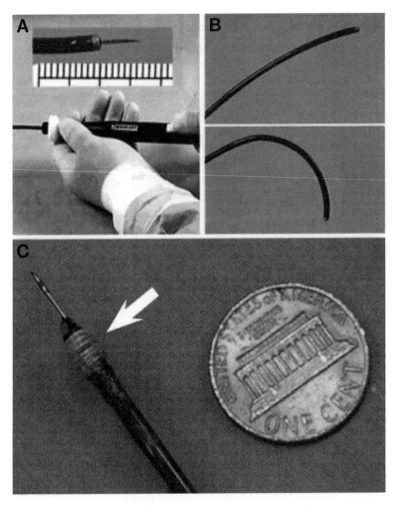

Fig. 2. Magnetic resonance imaging (MRI) steerable modification of Myocath® catheter. (From ref. *13*.)

myocardium and must recognize anatomical landmarks so as not to perforate the coronary sinus or the adjacent atrioventricular artery.

Catheter-mediated injection of endocardial-directed progenitor cells into injured myocardium is a rapidly advancing technology. An extremely thinned myocardial wall is a relative contraindication for this mode of delivery, given the need to inject perpendicularly into the scarred myocardium and the theoretical risk of ventricular perforation. However, cellular injection directly into the endocardium may provide a more durable improvement in ejection fraction given the ability to deliver multiple injections in a target zone of injured ventricular endocardium; this approach has proven safe thus far in phase I/II clinical trials in Europe.

The MyoCath® (Bioheart Inc., Santa Rosa, CA) is a percutaneous microimplant delivery system, utilizing a minimally invasive (8 Fr) steerable catheter, which can be introduced via the venous or arterial system and advanced to the ventricular endocardium. The MyoCath is 115 cm in length, is available in two catheter curvature sizes—medium and large—has an adjustable locking injection needle to allow the

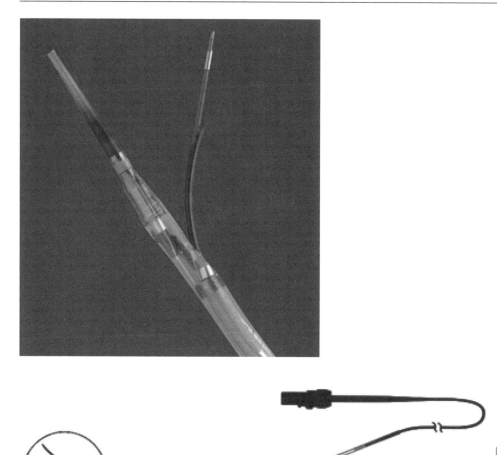

Fig. 3. TransAccess®, intravascular ultrasound (IVUS)-guided catheter, Transvascular/Medtronic Therapeutics, Inc.

operator to change the depth of injection (3–6 mm), and is compatible with standard fluoroscopy. Additionally, the tip of the MyoCath is fairly soft and atraumatic when used properly. Procedurally, after arterial access is obtained, the MyoCath is positioned, under fluoroscopy, with its tip at the desired injection site within the left ventricle and held firmly by the operator. Next, the needle is advanced to its preset length by depressing the needle advance control and the target tissue is penetrated. With the needle extended, the syringe attached to the proximal injection port is used to deliver the injectate (cell-based therapy). After injection, the needle is automatically retracted and the MyoCath can be repositioned to deliver another injection.

The MyoCath is currently being tested in MYOHEART™ (Myogenesis Heart Efficiency and Regeneration Trial), a phase I, open-label, nonrandomized, dose-escalation, multicenter study to assess the safety and cardiovascular effects of autologous skeletal myoblast implantation by a transendocardial catheter-delivery system in chronic heart failure patients post-MI with previous placement of an implantable cardioverter defibrillator (ICD). Patients with ICDs are targeted because of earlier studies demonstrating an increase in ventricular arrythmias after injection of skeletal myoblasts into the epicardium. Patients included will range in age from 30 to 80 years and, in addition to other well-delineated inclusion/exclusion criteria, must have a history of MI and compromised left ventricular function (20% < ejection fraction [EF] < 40%).

The Stiletto® delivery catheter contains a 27-gauge, spring-loaded, retractable needle that advances 3.5 mm. It is manufactured from Nitinol and stainless steel, and the inner lumen contains a proprietary coating, which has been shown to be more biocompatible with adenoviral vectors, resulting in greater transfection efficiency than a similar uncoated Nitinol catheter.

The Myostar® catheter (Cordis, Johnson & Johnson Inc.) is used in conjunction with an electromechanical mapping system (NOGA®, Cordis/Johnson & Johnson), which requires a transmission probe. The 125-cm catheter contains a 27-gauge needle housed in an 8 Fr catheter, which is advanced via the femoral artery, retrograde into the ventricle, and, once in contact with the myocardium, allows measurement of a voltage potential across the myocardium and reconstruction of a color-coded three-dimensional signal map of the endocardial surface. Healthy tissue is differentiated from injured tissue by the difference in voltage potentials across the myocardium, and is reflected in the real-time, color-coded, three-dimensional voltage map *(14,15)*.

Ideally, coincident imaging at the time of cell transfection would provide a measurement of transfection efficiency and injectate retention by the myocardium. Magnetic resonance imaging (MRI) has shown promise in the detection of cellular injectate immediately after cardiomyoplasty and, with proper cellular labeling, may be a modality by which serial studies of myocardial function are compared. Additionally, two MR-guided endomyocardial delivery catheters, one a variation of the Bioheart® catheter the other a variation of the Stiletto® catheter, have been developed and tested in preclinical studies *(13)*. Putatively, these catheters would enable MR-guided precision of endomyocardial injection, simultaneous MR assessment of the efficiency of injectate delivery, and an appraisal of myocardial contractility pre- and posttherapy *(16)*.

REFERENCES

1. Amado LC, Saliaris AP, Schuleri KH, et al. Cardiac repair with intramyocardial injection of allogeneic mesenchymal stem cells after myocardial infarction. Proc Natl Acad Sci USA 2005;102(32): 11,474–11,479.
2. Chachques JC, Salanson-Lajos C, Lajos P, Shafy A, Alshamry, Carpentier A. Cellular cardiomyoplasty for myocardial regeneration. Asian Cardiovasc Thorac Ann 2005;13:287–296.
3. Siminiak T, Fiszer D, Jerzykowska O, et al. Percutaneous trans-coronary-venous transplantation of autologous skeletal myoblasts in the treatment of post-infarction myocardial contractility impairment: the POZNAN trial. Eur Heart J 2005;26:1188–1195.
4. Perin EC, Silva GV. Stem cell therapy for cardiac diseases. Curr Opin Hematol 2004;11:399–403.
5. Orlic D. BM stem cells and cardiac repair: where do we stand in 2004? Cytotherapy 2005;7:3–15.
6. Kang HJ, Kim HS, Zhang SY, et al. Effects of intracoronary infusion of peripheral blood stem-cells mobilised with granulocyte-colony stimulating factor on left ventricular systolic function and restenosis after coronary stenting in myocardial infarction: the MAGIC cell randomised clinical trial. Lancet 2004;363:751–756.
7. Wollert KC, Meyer GP, Lotz J, et al. Intracoronary autologous bone-marrow cell transfer after myocardial infarction: the BOOST randomised controlled clinical trial. Lancet 2004;364:141–148.
8. Perin EC, Dohmann HF, Borojevic R, et al. Transendocardial, autologous bone marrow cell transplantation for severe, chronic ischemic heart failure. Circulation 2003;107(18):2294–2302.
9. Kawamoto A, Tkebuchava T, Yamaguchi J, et al. Intramyocardial transplantation of autologous endothelial progenitor cells for therapeutic neovascularization of myocardial ischemia. Circulation 2003;107:461–468.

10. Losordo DW, Vale PR, Hendel RC, et al. Phase 1/2 placebo-controlled, double-blind, dose-escalating trial of myocardial vascular endothelial growth factor 2 gene transfer by catheter delivery in patients with chronic myocardial ischemia. Circulation 2002;105:2012–2018.
11. Gyongyosi M, Sochor H, Khorsand A, Gepstein L, Glogar D. Online myocardial viability assessment in the catheterization laboratory via NOGA electroanatomic mapping: quantitative comparison with thallium-201 uptake. Circulation 2001;104:1005–1011.
12. Lessick J, Kornowski R, Fuchs S, Ben Haim SA. Assessment of NOGA catheter stability during the entire cardiac cycle by means of a special needle-tipped catheter. Catheter Cardiovasc Interv 2001;52:400–406.
13. Corti R, Badimon J, Mizseif G, et al. Real time magnetic resonance guided endomyocardial local delivery. Heart 2005;91(3):348–353.
14. Gyongyosi M, Khorsand A, Sochor H, et al. Characterization of hibernating myocardium with NOGA electroanatomic endocardial mapping. Am J Cardiol 2005;95:722–728.
15. Gyongyosi M, Khorsand A, Zamini S, et al. NOGA-guided analysis of regional myocardial perfusion abnormalities treated with intramyocardial injections of plasmid encoding vascular endothelial growth factor A-165 in patients with chronic myocardial ischemia: subanalysis of the EUROINJECT-ONE multicenter double-blind randomized study. Circulation 2005;112:I157–I165.
16. Karmarkar PV, Kraitchman DL, Izbudak I, et al. MR-trackable intramyocardial injection catheter. Magn Reson Med 2004;51:1163–1172.

14   Stem Cells and Myocardial Regeneration

Open-Chest/Minimally Invasive Surgical Techniques

Roberto Lorusso, MD, PhD, Josè L. Navia, MD, Cesare Beghi, MD, and Fernando A. Atik, MD

SUMMARY

Chronic heart failure has emerged as a major worldwide epidemic. Recently, a fundamental shift in the underlying etiology of chronic heart failure is becoming evident, in which the most common cause is no longer hypertension or valvular disease, but rather long-term survival after acute myocardial infarction (MI). The costs of this syndrome, both in economic and personal terms, are considerable. American Heart Association statistics indicate that chronic heart failure affects 4.7 million patients in the United States and is responsible for approx 1 million hospitalizations and 300,000 deaths annually.

The societal impact of chronic heart failure is also remarkable. Patients with chronic heart failure often suffer a greatly compromised quality of life. About 30% of diagnosed individuals (i.e.,1.5 million in the United States) experience difficulty breathing with little or no physical exertion and are very restricted in their daily functions. This forced sedentary lifestyle inevitably leads to further physical and mental distress. However, it is evident, running through the different therapeutic strategies of chronic heart failure, that the appropriate treatment of patients with ischemic heart failure is still unknown.

Since 1992, a revolutionary option to treat cardiac disease has come to the scene based on the possibility of using autologous cells, appropriately cultured and expanded, to replace or provide new contractile tissue as well as new sources of blood perfusion. Cell transplantation is currently generating a great deal of interest in that the replacement of akinetic scar tissue by viable myocardium should improve cardiac function, impede progressive left ventricular remodeling, and revascularize the ischemic area. From the original paper of Marelli and colleagues in 1992, presenting for the first time the concept of using autologous skeletal muscle cells to repair a damaged zone of the heart, a procedure termed "cellular cardiomyoplasty," supportive experimental as well as clinical evidence has been published in respect to the potential of cell transplantation for cardiac repair or regeneration. A variety of cell populations have been applied for cardiac repair either experimentally or clinically. Each cell type has its own profile of advantages, limitations, and practicability issues, particularly in the clinical setting. Several options are under evaluation in terms of mode of delivery. In this chapter we will discuss the fundamentals of the direct epicardial approach in cell transplantation using either an open- or closed-chest (endoscopy) technique.

From: *Contemporary Cardiology: Stem Cells and Myocardial Regeneration*
Edited by: M. S. Penn © Humana Press Inc., Totowa, NJ

Key Words: Cardiomyoplasty; thorascopic; robotic control; cell therapy; cell expansion.

Chronic heart failure has emerged as a major worldwide epidemic. Recently, a fundamental shift in the underlying etiology of chronic heart failure is becoming evident, in which the most common cause is no longer hypertension or valvular disease, but rather long-term survival after acute myocardial infarction (MI) *(1,2)*.

The costs of this syndrome, in both economic and personal terms, are considerable *(3)*. American Heart Association statistics indicate that chronic heart failure affects 4.7 million patients in the United States and is responsible for approx 1 million hospitalizations and 300,000 deaths annually. The total annual costs associated with this disorder have been estimated to exceed $22 billion.

The societal impact of chronic heart failure is also remarkable. Patients with chronic heart failure often suffer a greatly compromised quality of life. About 30% of diagnosed individuals (i.e., 1.5 million in the United States) experience difficulty breathing with little or no physical exertion and are very restricted in their daily functions. This forced sedentary lifestyle inevitably leads to further physical and mental distress.

The chronic heart failure problem is growing worse. Chronic heart failure already represents one of our greatest health care problems, and it is expected to become even more severe in the future. By 2010, the number of patients suffering from heart failure will have grown to nearly 7 million—a more than 40% increase.

Coronary artery disease (CAD) is the cause of chronic heart failure in the majority of patients, and chronic heart failure is the only mode of CAD presentation associated with increasing incidence and mortality. However, it is evident, running through the different therapeutical strategies of chronic heart failure, that the appropriate treatment of patients with ischemic heart failure is still unknown *(4,5)*.

Since 1992, a revolutionary option to treat cardiac disease has come to the scene based on the possibility of using autologous cells, appropriately cultured and expanded, to replace or provide new contractile tissue as well as new source of blood perfusio. Cell transplantation is currently generating a great deal of interest in that the replacement of akinetic scar tissue by viable myocardium should improve cardiac function, impede progressive left ventricular (LV) remodeling, and revascularize ischemic area.

The goals of cell therapy are multiple and nonexclusive, leading to the formation of new tissue. One should expect to replace scar tissue with living cells and/or to block or reverse the remodeling process or change its nature and/or to restore the contractility of the cardiac tissue and/or to induce neoangiogenesis that would favor the recruitment of hibernating cardiomyocytes or to enhance transplanted cell engraftment, survival, function, and, ultimately, synergistic interaction with resident cells.

From the original paper of Marelli and colleagues in 1992, presenting for the first time the concept of using autologous skeletal muscle cells to repair a damaged zone of the heart, a procedure termed "cellular cardiomyoplasty" *(5)*, supportive experimental as well as clinical evidence has been published about to the potential of cell transplantation for cardiac repair or regeneration. In 2001, Orlic and collaborators showed that bone marrow-derived cells, already well known in hematology, could be used to engraft an infarcted myocardium, leading to improved heart function, indicating an alternative cell lineage to satellite muscle cells to treat heart damages *(6)*. Many investigators have therefore chosen a pragmatic approach by using unfractionated bone marrow cells (BMCs), which contain different stem and progenitor cell populations, including hematopoietic stem cells (HSCs), endothelial progenitor cells (EPCs), and mesenchymal stem cells (MSCs).

A variety of cell populations have been, therefore, applied for cardiac repair either experimentally or clinically. Each cell type has its own profile of advantages, limitations, and practicability issues, particularly in the clinical setting. Furthermore, besides controversies around the optimal cell to be implanted, several options are under evaluation in terms of mode of delivery. From the initial direct approach consisting of direct cell injection at the epicardial level, other approaches, including endoventricular, intracoronary, and intravenous (either systemic or retrograde through the coronary sinus), have been explored.

In this chapter we will discuss the fundamentals of the direct epicardial approach in cell transplantation using either an open- or closed-chest (endoscopy) technique.

BASIC CONCEPT AND SURGICAL DETAILS OF CELL TRANSPLANT WITH OPEN-CHEST TECHNIQUE

The first open-chest procedure for implanting autologous cells (skeletal myoblasts) in the clinical setting has been performed by Menaschè and co-workers, who have shown the feasibility of transplanting skeletal muscle-derived satellite cells in infarcted regions during a coronary artery bypass graft (CABG) procedure in patients with compromised LV function (7). This pioneering clinical experience opened the route to further clinical series, which encompassed open as well as closed techniques according to the type of cell and mode of delivery (8–22) (Table 1).

The basic concept of open-chest delivery of cell transplantation to the heart, in the clinical setting, is rather straightforward. Indeed, cells are currently taken either from a skeletal muscle biopsy or from progenitors cells, bone-marrow or blood-derived, cultured or processed, and thereafter suspended in phosphate-buffered saline or medium, and then directly injected into the myocardial wall using a small-gauge needle (usually 24 or 26 gauge). Implanted cells are meant not only to repopulate the contractile portion of the cardiac tissue, but also to regenerate vessels, to reperfuse ischemic myocardium, and to promote the formation of a more elastic tissue matrix, which, in turn, may enhance diastolic function and halt ongoing LV dilatation (23).

With different cell lineages and cell selection and expansion protocols, a varying time interval is required between cell tissue extraction, either from a skeletal biopsy or from the stem cell sources (bone marrow or blood in order to allow appropriate cell selection and, in some cases, expansion) and surgical implantation. This interval may vary a great deal, from hours to weeks, according to the cell type or subtype chosen for implantation. Borestein and co-workers have shown in an ovine model that skeletal muscle cells can be injected with successful homing into the myocardium also without culturing and cell expansion after 3 hours from biopsy and start of tissue processing (24). This study, however, assessed cell engraftment in a rather favorable host tissue condition, because no infarct or any other kind of tissue damage was previously induced. Whatever technique is adopted, however, cell transplantation must deal with some inherent shortcomings, which, in turn, may affect early or medium-term results of cell implantation. Injecting cells into the target myocardial region with a needle may indeed either be responsible for a concomitant mechanical effect into the treated cardiac muscle/scar or induce cell damage as a result of the incurring strain linked to the needle passage. Although scar formation is visible at the injection site in mice, in larger animals the needle path is often difficult to identify. The possible angiogenic effect of puncturing the myocardium, giving rise to neo-vessels or to direct new channels through

Table 1
Clinical Open-Chest Series in Cell Transplantation for Cardiac Repair

Ref.	No. of patients	Etiology	Cell	Associated procedure
7	10	ICM	SM	CABG
8	4	ICM	EPC	CABG (3 pts) — CTx (1 pt)
9	8	ICM	BMSC	CABG
10	6	ICM	BMSC	CABG
11	18	ICM	SM	CABG
12	20	ICM	BMSC	OPCAB
13	5	ICM	SM	LVAD
14	10	ICM	SM	CABG
15	17	ICM (13 pts)/DCM (4 pts)	SM	CABG
16	4	ICM	SM	OPCAB
17	5	ICM	SM	CABG
18	10	ICM	EPC	CABG
19	12	ICM	SM	CABG
20	14	ICM	BMSC	CABG
21	5	ICM	BMSC	CABG - TML
22	18	ICM (12 pts)/DCM (6 pts)	SM	CABG (12 pts) — LVAD (6 pts)

ICM, ischemic cardiomyopathy; DCM, idiopathic dilated cardiomyopathy; CTx, isolated cell transplant; SM, skeletal myoblasts; BMSC, bone marrow stem cells; EPC, endothelial progenitor cells; CABG, coronary artery bypass grafting; OPCAB, off-pump coronary artery bypass; LVAD, left ventricular assist device; TML, transmyocardial laser.

which blood may pass and, hence, revascularize the hypoperfused myocardial segments, has been put forward by supporters of transmyocardial laser technology (25). Although the cell transplant tools and syringe are such that relevant blood regurgitation should be unlikely, this event still needs to be elucidated. Neoangiogenesis, however, has also been found in areas not directly located at the needle-puncture site, indicating that a direct angiogenic transdifferentiation or a paracrine effect toward angiogenesis of transplanted cells is likely. On the other hand, the penetration of the needle and the cell culture injection may, by themselves, act as pro-inflammatory stimuli, which may ultimately lead to neoangiogenesis as part of the induced inflammatory process. The latter effect has been also claimed to predispose to cell death following injection, a factor greatly limiting the actual result of direct cell transplantation (26).

An additional element that has been underlined as a major shortcoming is represented by the possible cell loss after needle injection because of backward flow through the needle hole, again markedly limiting cell retention inside the wall thickness and, hence, cell engraftment. For this reason it is recommended to exert a slight compression with the finger for a couple of minutes (27) to avoid cell regurgitation through a channel leakage mechanism. This underestimated but indeed relevant issue has been recently addressed by Chachques and colleagues, who have presented a newly designed surgical catheter (Fig. 1), which was specifically meant to solve several drawbacks of cell delivery through needle techniques (28). This catheter includes some features

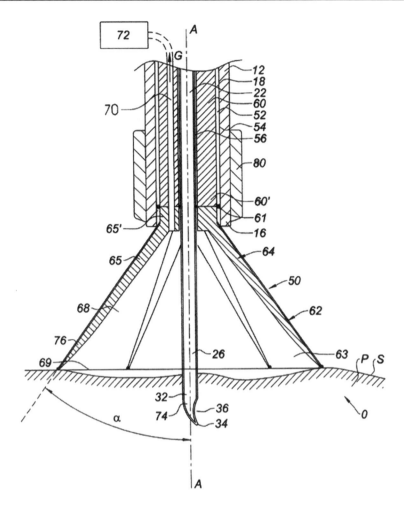

Fig. 1. Patent drawing (USA patent application 20050113760) of the "Cell-Fix" catheter designed for epicardial or endocardial cell transplantation.

drawn by the off-pump coronary artery bypass (OPCAB) and electrophysiology expertise. The catheter ends with a suction cap that should facilitate, particularly if used as endoventricular tool, the myocardial attachment, making the needle/epicardium contact stable and not jeopardized by the heart cyclic movements. Furthermore, the needle, acting as sensing electrode, enhances surface monitoring of the action potential and localized myocardial area with low signal and, hence, true infarcted zones. Finally, the needle design is such that true intrathickness injection should be achieved by means of an angled point and enhanced cell retention into the myocardial tissue. This latter aspect should also be guaranteed by a blunt closure of the induced needle by the maintenance of the catheter on the hole, allowing a spontaneous closure of the epicardial hole and, hence, leaving the majority of the injected cells in the myocardial tissue. This catheter, therefore, might be effective not only in endoventricular delivery, but may also serve as an endoscopic tool thanks to the suction action, which may enhance catheter/myocardial contact even if used through small ports. Apart from a specifically designed catheter, a long needle is advisable because it may avoid the need for multiple injections and, therefore, limit traumatic injury of the myocardium *(27)*.

From the limited clinical series and from the animal experiments, it appears rather definitive that open-chest cell implantation is safe, feasible, and void of peculiar perioperative complications. Besides procedural details directly linked to epicardial puncture, additional factors may be taken into account during an open-chest approach for cell implantation. The implementation of a controlled heart rate, for instance, may enhance cell implantation and reduce premature ventricular beats or malignant ventricular arrhythmia. Controlled heart rate may, therefore, be helpful during open-chest, but intuitively also during closed-chest procedures and, hence, should be advisable in an attempt to further reduce or prevent untoward phenomena, particularly malignant ventricular arrhythmia, during cell delivery.

The use of antiarrhythmic adjutants during cell implantation is certainly useful: lidocaine boluses or infusion or topical application, or amiodarone infusion, together with other drugs meant for heart rate control, are all practical means aimed at preventing or reducing dangerous rhythm disturbances during the epicardial approach. From the published clinical open-chest series, no major intraoperative adverse effects have been reported. Further data and more numerous patient populations are, however, required to conclusively define and predict risks exclusively linked to cell implantation into the myocardium. The use of anti-inflammatory compounds (steroids or nonsteroidal drugs) might have their rationale and role in the light of reducing the local inflammatory reaction, which is considered, as previously mentioned, a potential negative factor for cell engraftment and homing (26), but this issue remains unexplored and certainly deserves further investigation.

CELL TRANSPLANT AS ISOLATED OR ASSOCIATED PROCEDURE WITH OTHER CARDIAC SURGERY?: ISSUES RELATED TO PATIENT SELECTION AND PROCEDURAL INDICATIONS

Despite preliminary experiments with cell implantation in the heart executed in animal models without associated cardiac surgery operations, the first clinical cases, for obvious ethical reasons, have been carried out in combination with traditional revascularization procedures (7). Patients undergoing CABG surgery have undergone cell implantation according to phase I safety studies. Menasché and other authors have, thus, repetitively advised caution in interpreting postoperative data because of the inherent difficulty in extrapolating the actual effects of cell transplants from the effects of concomitant surgical revascularization. Although cell injection was mainly carried out in the myocardial zone void of direct graft reperfusion, any attempt to claim or prove the sole effects of cell engraftment are still difficult to define. Sakakibara and colleagues showed, in an animal model, the effects of cell implantation (fetal cardiomyocytes) in association with LV aneurysmectomy (29). This study showed that, after induced myocardial infarction, surgical remodeling could restore more appropriate LV shape and diameter, but only the adjunct of transplanted cells could substantially improve LV function. This association may have, therefore, its role and indication in the era of the Stitch-or-Restore Trials. If beneficial effects of cell therapy were definitely proved, adjunctive application of cells in the noncontractile segments of the aneurysm left in place might be efficacious and enhance some tissue regeneration and, hence, functional recovery. Although in an extremely preliminary phase, the ongoing research aimed at contractile tissue engineering might represent an additional tool in the cell therapy scenario—the logical prosecution of blind cell injection in the pursuit of designing autologous tissue substitutes for real tissue.

In this light, the application of cell implantation in impaired left ventricle has been advocated and shown in the setting of left ventricular assist device (LVAD) implantation in an attempt to enhance myocardial recovery of function. Pagani and Dib have independently reported about the use of cell implantation in patients undergoing LVAD support *(13,22)*. This application is in its infancy, and many difficulties related to cell type, patient selection, and cell delivery remain unanswered, but preliminary data indicate that cell engraftment occurs, with formation of small vessels. The association of these two procedures may, therefore, have a role, particularly in relation to a durable recovery of function.

Refractory angina, not amenable to catheter or surgical intervention, may represent an increasingly prevalent patient subset to be treated. The induction of neoangiogenesis may indeed represent the sole objective of cell therapy, with recovery of function being a secondary target or not important at all. Recently, Pompilio and colleagues have shown cell delivery in the presence of refractory angina, with or without concomitant CABG *(8)*. They used preoperative stimulation of the bone marrow with hematopoietic growth factor (Lenogastrim) to induce bone marrow production and release: after having collected CD133$^+$ cells by apheresis the day before surgery, they were implanted into the myocardium in an attempt to induce neoangiogenesis or myocyte formation during on- or off-pump surgical revascularization. Interestingly, the authors used two different approaches, including a full sternotomy procedure and a second one characterized by a minimally invasive approach (transdiaphragmatic minilaparotomy approach) at the subxypoid level. This procedure proved to be safe, and cell processing was easy and extremely effective in terms of either cell number or purity, thereby representing an additional option in patients not suitable to CABG or percutaneous transluminal coronary angioplasty, but requiring revascularization for symptom relief.

The ongoing refinements in terms of minimally invasive techniques, as described in this chapter, may also favor the application of cell implant as sole therapy, as opposed as the current mode, which implies a combined procedure.

Patient selection for the open-chest procedure is currently mainly linked to associated surgical revascularization, although a case of isolated cell implantation in which CABG was not indicated has been reported *(8)*. The general advice is to accomplish cell implantation in the area not suitable for conventional CABG procedure and with perfusion defect as assessed by nuclear testing preoperatively. The presence of some persistence of myocardium, despite the occurred infarction, seems advisable *(27)*. The controversy about the injection of autologous cells in a purely scarred myocardial zone remains unsolved. Recent data, either at short or at long term, obtained by surgical remodeling techniques *(3,4)* indicate that the restoration of a more advantageous ventricular shape and volume has effective and durable effects on LV function and patient outcome. It seems reasonable, therefore, to consider that large areas of akinetic, completely scarred, cardiac tissue are unlikely to benefit from cell implantation, whereas a reductive surgical approach may achieve better, or at least, already demonstrated results. In contrast, the presence of a relatively large area of ischemic, partially dead, myocardium (18–30% of the left ventricle) *(27)* may take advantage of cell transplantation, either for contractile restoration or for the angiogenic effects of cell engraftment.

The selection of candidates for cell transplant in the presence of idiopathic dilated cardiomyopathy remains an even more difficult scenario. Despite a few initial experiences of injecting cells at LVAD implantation, it seems unlikely that the implanted cells will play a critical role in the setting of a complete functional recovery in the presence

Table 2

Experimental Studies of Open-Chest Cell Transplantation in Relation to Animal Model, Model of Acute Myocardial Infarction, Timing of Cell Implantation and Postoperative Assessment, Histological and Hemodynamic Findings

Author	Animal model	Cell type	Myocardial Injury model	Time interval AMI-Tx	Cell amount	Number of injections	Cell implantation site	Postop Assessment	Postoperative histology	Cardiac functional effects
Rainoch[32]	ovine	myoblast	snake cardiotoxin injection	3 weeks	2x10^7	undefined	infarct	8 weeks	cell engraftment (only at the peri-infarct zone)	increase in regional function, reduced LVEDD, LVESD, LVESV, and LVEDV, increase in LVEF
Borestein[24]	ovine	myoblasts	no infarct	no AMI	10-20,000,000	10	no infarct	3 weeks	cell engraftment	no functional assessment
Jain[23]	rat	myoblasts	coronary ligation	7 days	10,000,000	6 to 10	infarct and peri-infarct zone	3-6 weeks	cell engraftment	increased contractile function, reduced post-AMI LV dilatation
Thompson[33]	rabbit	myoblast and BMSC	cryoinjury	14 days	100,000,000	3	infarct	4 weeks	cell engraftment, myogenic phenotype from BMSC	improved regional systolic function
Tambara[34]	rat	myoblasts	coronary ligation	4 weeks	5x10^5, 5x10^6, 5x10^7	2	infarct	4 weeks	cell engraftment	LV reverse remodelling, increase in fractional area change, and reduce MI area
Ghostine[35]	ovine	myoblasts	coronary embolization	14 days	100,000	20, 30	infarct and peri-infarct zone	4-12 months	areas of engrafted cells, decreased collagen density	reduced LVEDV and preserved LVEF
Pouzet[26]	rat	myoblasts	coronary ligation	7 days	2-3x10^6	1	undefined	2 months	cell engraftment (no evidence for connection grafted-host cells)	improved contractile LV function (systolic and diastolic)
Taylor[36]	rabbit	myoblasts	cryoinjury	7 days	1x10^7	1	infarct	2-6 weeks	cell engraftment	improved LV function (systolic and diastolic)
Kamihata[37]	rat	BMMC	coronary ligation	60 minutes	1x10^8	25	infarct and peri-infarct zone	3 weeks	neovascularization by angioblasts and angiogenic factors	improved regional blood flow and cardiac function, decreased infarct size
Min[38]	pig	hMSC and fetal CM	coronary ligation	5 minutes	3x10^5	undefined	peri-infarct zone	6 weeks	neocardiomyocytes and angiogenesis	improved contractile LV function
Tomita[39]	pig	BMSC	coronary ligation	4 weeks	100x10^6	5	infarct and peri-infarct zone	4 weeks	neocardiomyocytes and angiogenesis, increased scar thickness	improved contractile LV function, reduced LVEDV
Hamano[40]	dog	BMSC	coronary ligation	30 days	2x10^7	6	infarct and peri-infarct zone	1 month	increased wall thickness, neoangiogenesis	improved contractile LV function
Tomita[41]	rat	BMSC	cryoinjury	3 weeks	1x10^6	1	infarct	8 weeks	neocardiomyocytes and angiogenesis	improved contractile LV function
Min[42]	rat	ESC	coronary ligation	20 minutes	3x10^5	3	infarct and peri-infarct zone	32 weeks	cell engraftment in the infarct, trasdifferentiation in CM, and greater nr. of blood vessels	Improved contractile LV function
Davani[43]	rat	MSC	coronary ligation	7 days	1x10^6	undefined	infarct	1 month	greater vessel density, engrafted cells	Improved contractile LV function
Sakakibara[29]	rat	fetal CM	coronary ligation	4 weeks	undefined	undefined	peri-infarct zone	1 month	cell engraftment	smaller LVEDD, higher LVES elastance

BMSC : Bone marrow stem cells ; BMMC : Bone marrow mononuclear cells ; CM : cardiomyocytes ; ESC : Embrionic stem cells ; AMI : Acute myocardial infarction ; hMSC : human mononuclear stem cells ; LVEDD : Left ventricular end-diastolic diameter ;
LVESD : Left ventricular end-systolic diameter ; LVEF : Left ventricular ejection fraction ; LVEDV : Left ventricular end-diastolic volume

of global impairment of the left ventricle. However, preliminary clinical series appear promising, and the combination of different therapies in this setting may prove beneficial. Ongoing clinical trials will, hopefully, shed some light on the appropriate role of cell transplant in this setting.

DECIDING HOW MANY CELLS TO INJECT

The number of cells injected by an open-chest technique depends on several factors. The first determinant is obviously linked to the amount of cells obtainable from biopsies and, then, from in vitro culture. Usually, the goal is to achieve 500–600 million cells (50–70 million cells/mL). Menasché and colleagues showed that this target is easily achievable, with at least 60% myoblasts obtained within 2–3 weeks of culture *(31)*. In their series an average of 37 injections were administered under cardiac arrest, delivering almost 900 million cells in 6 mL to a mean area of about 30 cm^2. Unfortunately, the appropriate number of cells to be implanted is practically unknown, although it has been documented that the postoperative results are proportionally related to cell number *(26)*. Theoretically, the ultimate goal to repair and regenerate damaged myocardial tissue should be addressed with injections of a huge number of cells because of the evidence that many cells die after implantation. The mechanical damage induced by needle passage, the engraftment into a totally ischemic or relatively hypoperfused tissue, the activation of local inflammatory reaction, and the possible differentiation of transplanted cells into fibroblasts or the occurrence of apoptosis in the implanted cells, are all potential determinants or contributors to limited or unsuccessful cell homing and, hence, functional tissue recovery.

Experimental data do not offer conclusive information, because disparate animal models, cell type, and number of cells injected can be found in the literature *(23,24, 26,29,32–43)*. It seems unrealistic, with the current technology, to predict, given a peculiar tissue condition to be treated, a minimum amount of cells for a certain patient to achieve successful cell implantation and subsequent functional or structural improvement. Table 2 clearly shows that the animal data offer a wide range of cell dose implanted in different animal species as well as tissue conditions. Any attempt to extrapolate conclusive information for cell transplant in the human setting appears extremely difficult. Further studies are obviously warranted to determine a sort of threshold of cell number to be implanted. It is, however, reasonable to foresee that this information may not be available because too many variables and factors linked to cell type, target tissue-related characteristics, and procedural features may confer to any chosen cell quantity the possibility of successfully homing, survival, and effective tissue changes.

DECIDING WHERE TO INJECT CELLS

The controversy surrounding the location of cell implantation appears simple in theory, but encompasses many unsolved issues. The injection of cells, whatever type, into the myocardial scar or deranged cardiac zones, if an infarct is to be treated, appears a logical concept in an attempt to provide new cells in a relatively acellular segment and restore tissue function either by reconstituted contractile tissue or by enhancing neoangiogenesis of the ischemic area. The hypoxic as well as the fibrotic milieau of such a zone may, in contrast, be disadvantageous for cell engraftment for several reasons. The relative hypoperfusion of such a myocardial tissue may markedly limit cell nourishment and, hence, cell survival. Furthermore, the relative lack of viable, contractile resident muscle cells may also limit the positive effect of resident/-transplanted cell interaction. Finally, it was demonstrated that the existence of tissue fibrosis in such an area may direct implanted cell differentiation toward a fibroblast lineage, thereby making the tissue more fibrotic, but certainly not contractile. The latter effect was by some considered not to be a negative result of cell implantation, because a more elastic myocardial scar was also claimed, impeding further tissue thinning and ultimately limiting further ventricular remodeling or preventing ventricular dilatation *(32)*.

Conversely, the injection of cells into the border zone of the infarct area had more supporters among researchers, justified by the fact that a better perfused tissue zone and the presence of still normal cells may influence and positively affect cell homing and functional adaptation. Chachques has recommended injecting approx 70% of transplantable cells at the peri-infarct area, with the remaining 30% into the central portion of the scar *(27)*. This method is meant to induce a centripetal engraftment and repopulation of the necrotic area starting from the healthier and more revascularized myocardial zone. As shown in Table 2, however, experimental experience is not homogeneous in terms of the injection site. The majority of animal models showed concomitant injection of cells into peri-infarct and intrainfarct implantation, but scientific evidence regarding the exact or more appropriate site of implantation is lacking since effective results have been obtained in animal models in which cells were implanted only in the center of the infarcted region. The transplantation of cells in the middle of an infarcted area may still make sense, even if the absence of viable myocardial tissue is confirmed by preoperative investigation, provided that attempts to improve tissue perfusion, by CABG or by alternative methods, are pursued. Bypassing an artery nourishing a dead myocardial area has been considered a futile procedure, but might represent a critical factor in enhancing cell engraftment and survival in cell therapy.

In order to properly localize the infarct and border zones, epicardial echocardiography may be helpful, although transesophageal echocardiography may also be valuable, particularly because it may enhance postoperative comparison to elucidate the cell transplant effect. Additional preoperative examinations may prove valuable in cell transplantation either in terms of injection site identification or as tissue assessment in terms of function or perfusion to be reevaluated after surgery. The preservation of a minimal tissue perfusion, although void of a significant amount of viable cells, might represent a more adequate environment for effective cell engraftment, but these factors remain to be evaluated.

A different perspective may be represented by a diffuse derangement or abnormality of cardiac myocytes, like the situation encountered in idiopathic dilated cardiomyopathy. In this case the target to be addressed by cell repopulation is relatively different from localized necrotic or ischemic area, and the injection of cells should be carried out trying to deliver as many cells as possible in order to provide sufficient new cell population to regenerate or help the resident dysfunctional myocytes. The application of a sufficient number of vital cells in this situation appears unlikely. Myocyte abnormality, myofiber derangement, and diffuse increase in myocardial fibrosis are all common features of idiopathic dilated cardiomyopathy. The application of numerous cell injections, most likely associated with LVAD implantation, may represent a combined technique meant to vigorously assist the failing heart in conjunction with the administration of new and better functional cells. It is, therefore, mandatory to foresee, in addition to the apical area lost for LVAD implantation, how to get a beneficial effect from cell transplant.

DECIDING WHEN TO INJECT CELLS

Current techniques of cell transplant in open-chest clinical procedures imply the presence of chronic CAD and concomitance of CABG procedure, although a case of isolated cell implantation *(8)* has been reported. Stamm and colleagues reported the use of autologous C133[+] bone marrow-derived stem cells injected into the infarct border zone in six patients *(10)*. This limited clinical series showed that global ejection fraction improved in four out of six, and that perfusion defect improved dramatically in five patients. This series was achieved in patients with rather recent acute MI episodes (between 10 days and 3 months) and candidates for CABG in remote areas. It is, therefore, still controversial to define if the surgical candidates for cell transplant are the ones suffering from the sequelae of long-term infarcts and well-established damage without any presence of active inflammatory or ischemic process, or rather soon after an acute MI. Experimental evidence is not helpful in this controversy and offers rather heterogeneous data, showing cell injection from a few hours to weeks from the ischemic or necrotic insult (Table 2). It is, therefore, difficult to define the optimal time for cell implantation after myocardial damage. Many authors discourage the transplantation of cells during or soon after the perfusion of defect-related damage because of the potential negative effects of ongoing ischemia, which predisposes fresh cells to die, or the induced inflammatory pathway that may contribute to implanted cell destruction. Li and associates analyzed the effects of cell implantation in an animal model of myocardial injury where implants were carried out at different times from the induced myocardial damage: interestingly, this experimental model showed that fetal cardiomyocytes had the best outcome if transplanted after the inflammatory reaction subsided. No additional data are available in terms of clinical scenario or with different types of cells—factors that likely play a critical role in cell homing, survival, and long-lasting functional response. Further studies are, therefore, mandatory to fully understand the relationship and proper interval between cell implantation and timing of previous myocardial damage.

INDIRECT OPEN-CHEST CELL TRANSPLANTATION (CYTOKINE-INDUCED CELL MOBILIZATION AND MECHANICALLY ENHANCED MYOCARDIAL HOMING) AND OTHER POTENTIAL MODES OF CELL DELIVERY

Myocardial repopulation by circulating progenitor cells (either endothelial stem cells or mobilized bone marrow-derived stem cells) may be elicited by cytokine-induced cell mobilization or activation. Recently, Actis Dato and co-workers have described a combination of preoperative and intraoperative techniques to enhance bone marrow production and myocardial homing of autologous stem cells *(9)*. Granulocyte–colony-stimulating factor administration for 4 days prior to surgery raises significantly circulating CD34[+] stem cells, and when the cell peak is observed, the patient is scheduled for CABG surgery. This timing ensures the surgical operation is performed with a sufficient stem cell population in the blood circulation. In combination with conventional CABG, several *(50–60)* punctures with a 21 gauge needle are

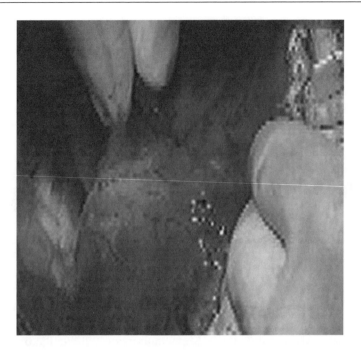

Fig. 2. Intraoperative view of the creation of multiple holes into the ungraftable myocardium to induce diffuse inflammatory reaction. This procedure (Sen procedure) is meant to attract and enhanced engraftment of preoperatively cytokine-mobilized bone marrow stem cells following elective coronary artery bypass graft surgery.

performed at a nonvital area at preoperative diagnostic assessment (Fig. 2) according to an old concept in treating CAD by inducing multiple channels in ischemic regions, the so-called Sen procedure.

This mechanical tissue stress is meant to favor local inflammatory response, which, in turn, should account for and promote capillary leakage and, hence, cell homing and engraftment. A phase II pilot study is ongoing, with 18 patients treated with this technique (unpublished data), with significant improvement of the area treated with needle puncture and without bypass perfusion. Unfortunately, no cell labeling has been possible, and, therefore, no conclusive data can be extrapolated from this experience, although it appears extremely attractive, and might justify bone marrow-derived or resident stem cell activation with an expected neoangiogenetic response in the mechanically treated myocardial zones.

Additional modes of cell injection with an open-chest approach may be achieved by transcatheter delivery of cells through the coronary sinus, particularly in the presence of diffuse and severe CAD, if the percutaneous approach is not feasible or if concomitant surgery should be performed on the heart. Direct injection of processed cells might also be achieved by direct injection inside the coronary artery lumen (arterial or vein puncture) in the presence of a proximal total occlusion and a downstream vessel of poor quality, where vessel grafting may expectedly fail at short term.

ONGOING CLINICAL TRIAL WITH OPEN-CHEST TECHNIQUE

Several clinical studies have been published since the first paper and experience presented by Menaschè and co-workers *(7–22)*. However, limited patient numbers have been reported, with variable results. Ongoing are several multicenter trials, which include different cell types and surgical procedures (the Myoblast Autologous Grafting in Ischemic Cardiomyopathy (MAGIC) Trial includes implantation of automatic defibrillators). These trials should present their clinical data within a few months and will certainly define actual potentials and effects of cell implantation for cardiac repair, but will also enhance further refinement of patient selection, cell type, and mode of delivery. Table 2 presents a summary of the most important clinical series published recently in the literature and demonstrates the limited clinical experience in this setting. Thus far, only one randomized study has been perfomed by Patel and colleagues *(12)*, showing greater improvement of LV function as well as of myocardial perfusion as assessed by single photon emission-computed tomography imaging in patients submitted to OPCAB and stem cell implantation.

MINIMALLY INVASIVE TECHNIQUES

One route for delivering cells in the myocardium is by a direct epicardial injection into predetermined zones of ischemic myocardium or cardiomyocyte loss. This procedure can be achieved at the time of cardiac operation, such as CABG in the setting of ischemic cardiomyopathy or LVAD implant through sternotomy. An alternative approach is the minimally invasive video-assisted and robotic surgery, which offers the main potential advantage of cell injection under vizualization, which allows anatomical identification of the best target area and even distribution of multiple injections through the same surgical approach.

The field of minimally invasive cardiac surgery has grown rapidly in recent years. Over the past 5 years, the surgery has evolved from modified conventional methods to radical changes in micro- and port incision. This rapid technology shift allows the surgeon to use video-assisted and robotic instruments to perform truly endoscopic surgery and reduces surgical trauma 1 *(47)*. The minimally invasive surgical approach to perform cell implantation for cardiac repair can be done in three ways: minithoracotomy, video-assisted thoracoscopic surgery, and robotic surgery.

PATIENT SELECTION FOR A MINIMALLY INVASIVE
SURGICAL APPROACH

Preoperatively, patients need to be assessed by a cardiac anesthesiologist for general anesthesia and single lung ventilation. Intraoperatively, patients are routinely monitored with a 12-lead electrocardiogram and defibrillator pads attached to the skin. Hemodynamics are assessed with invasive arterial pressure, pulmonary artery thermodilution catheter, and transesophageal echocardiography. The status of post-open heart surgery patients must be assessed for feasibility of groin cannulation in an emergency.

General anesthesia is carried out with double lumen endotracheal intubation. At this juncture, the safety of single lung ventilation must be verified.

Indication for a specific surgical approach follows the following general guidelines. Minithoracotomy is selected for two patient populations: those with severely enlarged left ventricles, which are very close to the chest wall, and those who had undergone previous cardiothoracic surgery.

In these patients, total thoracoscopic procedures would be difficult and potentially dangerous, because limited working space restricts safe manipulation of the instruments and they may, inadvertently, trigger life-threatening arrhythmias, ventricular injury, or hemodynamic compromise. Video-assisted thoracoscopic surgery is indicated in patients with adequate anterior–posterior chest diameter, where the thoracoscopic instruments can be freely mobilized inside the chest; reoperations are not a contraindication, but minithoracotomy is preferred in most cases. Robotics is indicated in patients with small cardiothoracic ratio and large anterior–posterior dimension, and left lung downventilation and CO_2 insufflation can cause gentle mediastinal shift, allowing the left ventricle to move toward the right chest, creating an important working space for the robotic arms. Using robotic surgery in reoperation can be challenge as a result of adhesions of the anatomical structures.

SURGICAL TECHNIQUES

Minithoracotomy

A skin incision is made, 3–5 cm long, is made over the fourth or fifth left intercostal spaces just anterior to the mid-axillary line. In a small incision, the use of a self-retaining retractor (Cloward) is helpful because its deep blades allow adequate exposure (Fig. 3).

Single lung ventilation is initiated; if adherent, the left lung is dissected free and retracted posteriorly. The pericardium is tented with forceps and carefully opened anteriorly to the phrenic nerve. Proceeding with extreme caution is advisable for patients who have had previous heart surgery, particularly CABG. Better exposure of the anterior lateral wall of the left ventricle can be obtained by placing stay sutures in the pericardium. The injection of cells is performed through direct vision, similar to the open-chest technique directly injected into the myocardial wall using a small-gauge needle (usually 24 or 26 gauge), or newly designed surgical catheter specifically meant to solve several drawbacks of cell delivery through needle techniques. The catheter ends with a suction cap that should facilitate the myocardial attachment making the needle/epicardium contact stable and not jeopardized by the heart cyclic movements. The needle design is such that true intrathickness injection should be achieved by means of an angled point and enhancing cell retention into the myocardial tissue.

Sometimes the target ventricular wall is not aligned with the incision and makes direct cell implantation difficult. In this case it is helpful to use the a thoracoscopic grasper inserted in a more posterior small incision and redirect the needle to the specific area. This can be used as a draining site.

After adequate hemostasis is obtained, a size 10 Jackson–Pratt drain is placed into the left pleura, double lung ventilation is resumed, and the minithoracotomy incision is closed by layers.

Video-Assisted Thoracic Surgery

The patient is placed in a supine position with the left arm placed slightly below the table level, with a roll along the spine to bring the left chest forward. This maneuver prevents interference with tool manipulation during the procedure. Port position will depend on heart size and position. Usually, a fifth and sixth space anterior and mid-axillary port for working tools and a second or third space mid-anterior clavicular port for the scope is standard (Fig. 4). Sometimes an auxiliary port is placed close to the scope port, allowing better exposure for delivery of the catheter or needle for cell implant. Single lung ventilation is started, and short (10–12 mm) ports will be sufficient for the surgical tools and scope. A valve port allows insufflation of carbon dioxide (CO_2) at pressures of approx 8–10 cmH_2O. A zero-degree telescope is inserted and can immediately see the phrenic nerve line posteriorly. Folding the pericardium somewhere in the middle and holding out

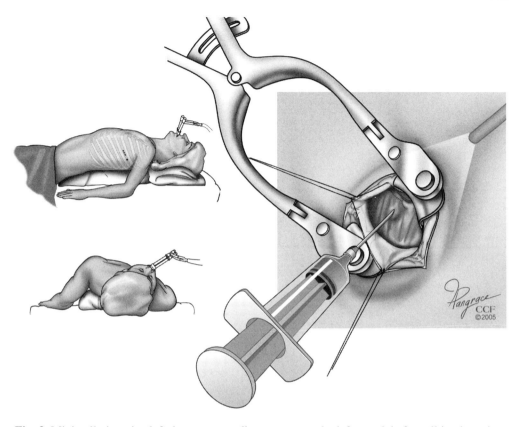

Fig. 3. Minimally invasive left thoracotomy; direct access to the left ventricle for cell implantation.

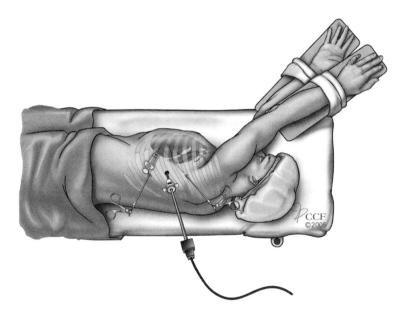

Fig. 4. Video-assisted thoracoscopic surgical approach for cell implantation therapy.

on traction, a small incision is made, which allows some air to get into the pericardial sack and break any capillary traction between the pericardium and the epicardial surface of the left ventricle. Then the pericardium is opened 3 cm above the phrenic nerve in order to expose the antero-lateral wall of the left ventricle, left atrial appendage, and the pulmonary veins, establishing the normal relationship.

If stay sutures are necessary, they can be either brought out through the ports or anchored internally on adjoining chest wall tissue. The goal is to place the needle or catheter in contact with the target area, using grasper tools and sometimes a small suction device, in order to keep the field stabilized, to perform a perfect smooth contact with epicardium and inject the cells deep into the myocardium. If the target area is in the territory of the obtuse marginal artery or adjacent to the anterior aspect of the left atrial appendage, the needle is mounted on the proximal end of the malleable implantation tool and the assembly is inserted in the chest through the most posterior working port to allow direct cell delivery in at right angles to the LV surface. Hemostasis is obtained, the pericardium is closed with interrupted 4-0 polyester (Ticron) sutures, and the port incisions are closed with standard techniques. Double lung ventilation is resumed and a size 10 Jackson–Pratt drain is placed in the left pleural space through the auxiliary port.

Robotically Assisted Surgery

THE DAVINCI SYSTEM

The DaVinci robotic surgical system (Intuitive Surgical Inc., Sunnyvale, CA) is a device composed of a surgeon control console and surgical arm unit that positions and directs the microinstrument. The DaVinci system has three main components: a surgeon console, a computer controller, and specially designed instrument tips attached to the robotic arms (Fig. 5). The surgeon sits at the console and manipulates the instrument handles, and his or her motion is relayed mechanically to the computer controller. These motions are then digitalized and, with specially designed software, filtered and scaled. The surgeon console houses the display system, the surgeon handle, the surgeon user interface, and the electronic controller. The surgeon sits at the control console looking at the image that is displayed in a high-resolution three-dimensional video image, and each movement of the surgeon handles or master is translated in real time into fine movements of the robotic instrument tips at the operative site. This movement can be scaled from 1:1 to 1:3 where the control system is also able to filter out surgeon tremors. The combination of the motion scaling, filter, and image magnification make delicate motion easier to perform than conventional endosopic technique, enhacing surgical dexterity. The excellent three-dimensional system helps compensate for a general lack of force of feedback.

The patient's side cart consists of a fixed base with three passive multilink arms mounted to it. Each arm holds a slave manipulator, two manipulators drive the tools, and one controls the camera.

Each instrument has a mechanical wrist called the Endo-wrist, a key component of the intuitive system that allows the surgeon seven degree of freedom of movement inside the patient (three for translation, three for orientation, and one for grip), compared to what he or she is used to in conventional open surgery. The Endo-wrist is a component that gives the surgeon the ability to reach around, beyond, and behind delicate body structures and is connected to the rest of the system by sophisticated mechanized cable transmission.

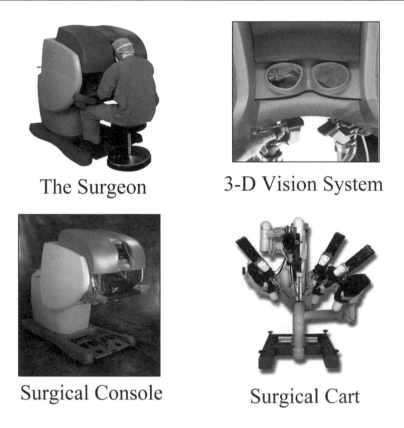

The Surgeon   3-D Vision System

Surgical Console   Surgical Cart

Fig. 5. The daVinci system components.

The term robotic is now used synonymously with computer-assisted surgery, but the major breakthrough of the technology is that for the first time, the surgeon's hand motions are converted to the binary code, allowing enhanced motion to be electronically transferred to a minute instrument inside the chest. All hand and wrist motions are replicated nearly instantaneously to the instrument tips. The three-dimensional vision and Endo-wrist technology allows the surgeon to see and manipulate the instrument as if the surgeon's hands were present inside the chest.

The robotic systems have enabled surgeons around the world to perform different minimally invasive, endoscopic cardiac surgery procedures—the most striking demonstration of the ability of this system to enhance surgical dexterity.

OPERATIVE TECHNIQUE

Anesthesia preparation and monitoring for robotically assisted procedures are the same as described for the previous techniques. The patient should be placed for left ventricle anterior wall surgical approach in a supine position with the left arm placed slightly below the table level, with a roll along the spine to bring the left chest forward, and for obtuse marginal artery target area approach in a full left posterolateral thoracotomy position. The daVinci Robotic Surgical System (Intuitive Surgical Inc., Sunnyvale, CA) is used. Working ports should be placed in the posterior axillary line, adjusted caudad or cephalad, depending on the angle to the left ventricle, to allow placement of the needle or catheter. Flexibility in port positions is important and

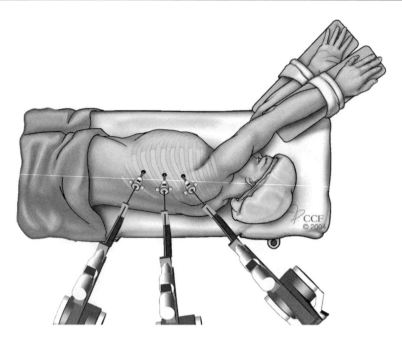

Fig. 6. Ports and arms placed for robotic-assisted surgery.

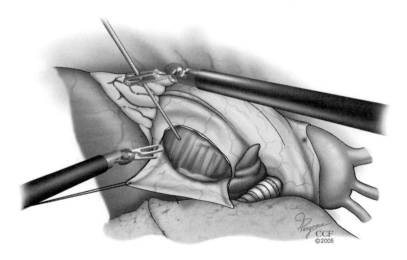

Fig. 7. Robotically assisted left ventricle epicardial injection cell therapy.

should be adjusted based on individual chest wall and cardiac anatomy. Three 1-cm skin port incisions are often made on the third intercostal space for the right instrument, fifth space for the camera, and seventh space for the left instrument, along the left mid-axillary line (Fig. 6), for anterior surgical approach, and on the fifth , seventh, and ninth, along the left posterior axillary line, for the postero-lateral approach. Two lateral robotic arms and a central three-dimensional image camera are placed through the ports into the chest. A carbon dioxide insufflation is used to increase the working space between the heart and the chest wall. A small pericardial incision is made anterior to the phrenic nerve with electrocautery or microsicors in order to reach either target wall of the left ventricle. The needle or catheter is passed through an auxiliary port on the sixth space mid-axillary line, and the cells are injected similarly to the thoracoscopic method, but less space is needed for instrument manipulation (Fig. 7).

The pericardium is closed with interrupted 4-0 polyester (Ticron) suture. The air is evacuated from the pleural space, the left lung is inflated, a Jackson-Pratt N10 drain is placed, and the port incisions are closed as usual. The patient can be extubated in the operating room.

We believe the different minimally invasive surgical alternatives for LV epicardial cell implantation in heart failure patients are viable surgical options and can be helpful in high-risk surgical patients, offering a selection of the best cell implantation sites under direct or indirect visualization with minimal surgical trauma.

SHORTCOMINGS AND COMPLICATIONS OF OPEN-CHEST TECHNIQUE CARDIAC CELL TRANSPLANTATION

As previously mentioned, the first clinical experience was presented by Menaschè and co-workers, who treated 10 patients affected by ischemic cardiomyopathy (LV ejection fraction ≤ 35%). The Paris group showed that at an average follow-up of about 11 mo, New York Heart Association functional class improved from 2.7 to 1.6 ($p < 0.0001$) and that LV ejection fraction increased from 24 to 32% ($p < 0.02$). However, four patients experienced sustained ventricular tachycardia postoperatively, and an automatic implanted cardiac defibrillator (AICD) was implanted. Engrafted skeletal myoblasts seem to possess a pro-arrhythmic electrical activity as a result of increased electrical susceptibility and lack of effective gap junctions with resident myocardial cells. Application of AICDs has been advocated and is currently applied in the clinical series using skeletal muscle-derived cells (MAGIC trial), based on other evidence observed in preliminary clinical experiences *(44)*. Experimental data seem to confirm that skeletal muscle cells might predispose to malignant ventricular arrhythmia, although not constantly. Chachques and colleagues, however, showed that cell irritability might derive not only from the tissue engraftment and cell membrane characteristics, as opposed to cardiomyocyte, but rather from culture technique, with an absence of inducible malignant ventricular rhythm disturbances when cells were cultured in human serum *(45)*.

Stamm reported two cases of marked pericardial effusion after cell transplant, which might be related to the peculiar effects of needle puncture or the elicited inflammatory reaction linked to cell implantation *(10)*. This side effect, however, was not mentioned by the other open chest series, making this postoperative event unlikely related to epicardial cell implantation.

A recent study showed that endoventricular injection may enhance greater retention of injected material inside the ventricular thickness as compare to epicardial implantation *(26)*. A possible explanation for this is that the endoventricular pressure may reduce backward leakage of injected solution, but this effect might be easily achieved with transient external compression or with a dedicated catheter design, as previously mentioned. Incomplete cellular retention, however, seems to happen also with endoventricular cell delivery *(46)*, once again indicating the importance of implantation techniques, modes of delivery, and implantation tools, which are under refinement *(47)*.

In conclusion, open-chest techniques for cell transplantation into the heart have been proved to be feasible, safe, and effective in animal as well as clinical settings in terms of cell engraftment and its related impact on regional or global LV function. Patient-tailored cell type, patient indication, timing of cell implantation, and other issues, however, are far from being fully elucidated for the open-chest approach. Accordingly, several clinical trials and additional experimental studies are eagerly awaited and ongoing and may shed additional light on this promising field. Refinement of catheter design, the use of minimally invasive (thoracoscopy) techniques, and accurate identification of target areas will certainly enhance cell transplantation, as will concomitant techniques to improve cell engraftment and effective grafted cell/resident cell interaction, together with the ingrowth of new blood vessels to treat myocardial ischemia. The current therapy standards and objectives to provide proper amounts of cells to replace or support large areas of dysfunctional myocardium indicate that treatment of large targets, like dilated cardiomyopathy, by this method remains far in the future.

REFERENCES

1. Ansari M, Massie BM. Heart failure: how big is the problem? Who are the patients? What does the future hold? Am Heart J 2003;146:1–4.
2. Berry C, Murdoch DR, McMurray JJ. Economics of chronic heart failure. Eur J Heart Fail 2001;3:283–291.
3. Doenst T, Velazquez EJ, Beyerdorf F, et al. (STITCH Investigators). To STITCH or not to STITCH: we know the answer, but do we understand the question? J Thorac Cardiovasc Surg 2005;129:246–249.
4. Buckberg GD. Early and late results of left ventricular reconstruction in thin-walled chambers: is this our patient population? J Thorac Cardiovasc Surg 2004;128:21–26.
5. Marelli D, Desrosiers C, el-Alfy M, Kao RL, Chiu RC. Cell transplantation for myocardial repair: an experimental approach. Cell Transplant 1992;1:383–390.
6. Orlic D, Kajstura J, Chimenti S, et al. Mobilized bone marrow cells repair the infracted heart, improving function and survival. PNAS 2001;10,344–10,349.
7. Menaschè P, Hagege AA, Scorsin M, et al. Myoblast transplantation for heart failure. Lancet 2001;357:279–280.
8. Pompilio G, Cannata A, Peccatori F, et al. Autologous peripheral blood stem cell transplantation for myocardial regeneration: a novel strategy for cell collection and surgical. Ann Thorac Surg 2004;78:1808–1813.
9. Actis Dato G, Tarella C, Calafiore AM. Stem cell mobilization and auto-implantation by Sen procedure in post-ischemic chronic heart failure: results of a pilot phase II study. Int J Cardiol 2004; 95(suppl 1):S61.
10. Stamm C, Westphal B, Klein HD, et al. Autologous bone marrow stem-cell transplantation for myocardial regeneration. Lancet 2003;361:45–46.
11. Chachques JC, Duarte F, Herreros J, et al. Cellular myogenic and angiogenic therapy for patients with cardiac or limb ischemia. Bas Appl Myol 2003;13:29–37.
12. Patel AN, Vina RE, Geffner L, Kormos R Urschel HC, Benetti F. Surgicakl treatment for congestive heart failure using autologous adult stem cell transplantation: a prospective randomized study. Proceedings of the 84th Annual Meeting of the AATS, Toronto, 2004, p. 50.
13. Pagani F, DerSimonian H, Zawadzka A, et al. Autologous skeletal myoblasts transplanted to ischemia-damaged myocardium in humans. J Am Coll Cardiol 2003;41:879–888.
14. Siminiak T, Kalawski R, Fiszer D, et al. Autologous skeletal myoblast transplantation for the treatment of postinfarction myocardial injury: phase I clinical study with 12 months of follow up. Am Heart J 2004;148:531–537.
15. Akhmedov SD, Babokin VE, Suslova TE, et al. Clinical experience using autologous mononuclear bone marrow cells in patients undergoing cardiac surgery procedures. Int J Cardiol 2004;95(suppl 1):S63.
16. Schluter M, Sambuceti G, Limbruno U, et al. Scintigraphic evaluation of bone marrow cell implantation in patients with previous myocardial infarction and dominance scar. Int J Cardiol 2004;95 (suppl 1):S63.

17. Trainini J. Autologous myoblast cardiac implant in ventricular dysfunction. Int J Cardiol 2004; 95(suppl 1):S62.

18. Trainini J, Lago N, Klein G, et al. Autologous bone marrow cell transplantation in patients with myocardial infarction. Int J Cardiol 2004;95(suppl 1):S62.

19. Herreros J, Prosper F, Perrez A, et al. Autologous intramyocardial injection of cultured skeletal muscle-derived stem cells in patients with non-acute myocardial infarction. Eur Heart J 2003;24:2012–2020.

20. Galinanes M, Loubani M, Davies J, Chin D, Pasi J, Bell P. Safety and efficacy of transplantation of autologous bone marrow into scarred myocardium for the enhancement of cardiac function in man. Circulation 2002;106(suppl 2):463.

21. Ghodsizad A, Klein HM, Borowski A, et al. Intraoperative isolation and processing of BM-derived stem cells. Cytotherapy 2004;5:523–526.

22. Dib N McCarthy P, Campbell A, et al. Two-year follow-up of the safety and feasibility of autologous myoblast transplantation in patients with ischemic cardiomyopathy: results from the United States experience. Circulation 2003;108(suppl IV):623.

23. Jain M, DerSimonian H, Brenner DA, et al. Cell therapy attenuates deleterious ventricular remodelling and improves cardiac performance after myocardial infarction. Circulation 2001;103:1920–1927.

24. Borestein N, Bruneval P, Hekmati M, et al. Noncultured, autologous, skeletal muscle cells can successfully engraft into ovine myocardium. Circulation 2003;107:3088–3092.

25. Chu VF, Giaid A, Kuang JQ, et al. Angiogenesis in transmyocardial revascularization : comparison of laser versus mechanical punctures. Ann Thorac Surg 1999;68:301–308.

26. Pouzet B, Vilquin JT, Hagège AA, et al. Factors affecting functional outcome after autologous skeletal myoblast transplantation. Ann Thorac Surg 2001;71:844–851.

27. Chachques JC, Acar C, Herreros J, et al. Cellular cardiomyoplasty: clinical application. Ann Thorac Surg 2004;77:1121–1130.

28. Chachques JC, Herreros J, Lorusso R. New "Cell-Fix" catheter for infarct detection and cell delivery. Int J Cardiol 2004;95(suppl 1):S66.

29. Sakikabara Y, Tambara K, Lu F, et al. Combined procedure of surgical repair and cell transplantation for left ventricular aneurysm: an experimental study. Circualtion 2002;106(suppl I):193–197.

30. Dor V. Left ventricular reconstruction: the aim and the reality after twenty years. J Thorac Cardiovasc Surg 2004;128:17–20.

31. Menasché P, Hagege AA, Vilquin JT, et al. Autologus skeletal myoblast trasplantation for severe postinfarction LV dysfunction. J Am Coll Cardiol 2003;41:1078–1083.

32. Rainoch C, Chachques JC, Berrebi A, Bruneval P, Benoit MO, Carpentier A. Cellular therapy reverses myocardial dysfunction. J Thorac Cardiovasc Surg 2001;121:871–878.

33. Thompson RB, Emani SM, Davis BH, et al. Comparison of intracardiac cell transplantation: autologous skeletal myoblasts versus bone marrow cells. Circulation 2003;108(suppl II)264–271.

34. Tambara K, Sakakibara Y, Sakaguchi G, et al. Transplanted skeletal myoblasts can fully replace the infacrted myocardium when they survive in the host in large numbers. Circulation 2003; 108(suppl II):259–263.

35. Ghostine S, Carrion C, Souza LCG, et al. Long-term efficacy of myoblast transplantation on regional structure and function after myocardial infarction. Circulation 2002;106(suppl I):131–136.

36. Taylor DA, Atkins ZB, Hungspreugs P, et al. Regenerating functional myocardium: improved performance after skeletal myoblast transplantation. Nat Med 1998;4:929–933.

37. Kamihata H, Matsubara H, Nishiue T, et al. Implantation of bone marrow mononuclear cells into ischemic myocardium enhances collateral perfusion and regional function via side supply of angioblasts, angiogenic ligands, and cytokines. Circulation 2001;104:1046–1052.

38. Min JY, Sullivan MF, Yang Y, et al. Significant improvement of heart function by cotransplantation of human mesenchymal stem cells and fetal cardiomyocytes in postinfarcted pigs. Ann Thorac Surg 2002;74:1568–1575.

39. Tomita S, Mickle DAG, Weisel RD, et al. Improved heart function with myogenesis and angiogenesis after autologous porcine bone marrow stromal cell transplantation. J Thorac Cardiovasc Surg 2002;123:1132–1140.

40. Hamano K, Li TS, Kobayashi T, et al. Therapeutic angiogenesis induced by local autologous bone marrow cell transplantation. Ann Thorac Surg 2002;73:1210–1215.

41. Tomita S, Li RK, Weisel RD, et al. Autologous transplantation of bone marrow cells improves damaged heart function. Circulation 1999;100(suppl II):247–256.

42. Min JY, Yang Y, Sullivan MF, et al. Long-term improvement of cardiac function in rats after infarction by transplantation of embryonic stem cells. J Thorac Cardiovasc Surg 2003;125:361–369.

43. Davani S, Marandin A, Mersin N, et al. Mesenchymal progenitor cells differentiate into an endothelial phenotype, enhance vascular density, and improve heart function in a rat cellular cardiomyoplasty model. Circulation 2003;108(suppl II):253–258.

44. Smits PC, van Geuns RJ, Poldermans D, et al. Catheter-based intramyocardial injection of autologous skeletal myoblasts as a primary treatment of ischemic heart failuire: clinical experience with six-month follow-up. J Am Coll Cardiol 2003;42:2070–2072.

45. Chachques JC, Herreros J, Trainini JC, et al. Autologous human serum for cell culture avoids the implantation of cardioverter-defibrillators in cellular cardiomyoplasty. Int J Cardiol 2004;95(Suppl1): S29–S33.

46. Grossman PM, Han Z, Palasis M, Barry JJ, Lederman RJ. Incomplete retention after direct myocardial injection. Cathet Cardiovasc Intervent 2002;55:392–397.

47. Navia JL, Atik F. Minimally invasive surgical alternatives for left ventricle epicardial lead implantation in heart failure patients. Ann Thorac Surg 2005;80(2):751–754.

IV STEM CELL-BASED CLINICAL TRIALS FOR CARDIAC DYSFUNCTION

15

Measures of Effective Cell-Based Therapy

Wael A. Jaber, MD
and Manuel D. Cerqueira, MD

SUMMARY

Ischemic heart disease remains a leading cause of morbidity and mortality despite advances in medical therapy and revascularization techniques. Born out of this burden of ischemic heart disease is a burgeoning body of literature in both the preclinical and clinical settings that demonstrates the benefits of cell therapy. Central to the acceptance of cell therapy as a viable treatment strategy is determining the fate of the cells employed, the overall effect on ventricular function, and, ultimately, clinical outcomes. Although these assessments are readily attainable through invasive hemodynamic studies and histological analysis in the preclinical setting, the use of clinical parameters and noninvasive imaging modalities have been employed in the clinical setting. In addition to establishing the safety of cell therapy by focusing on "hard endpoints," such as death, myocardial infarctiion, arrhythmias, the efficacy of cell therapy in achieving the outcome of myocardial regeneration may be feasible through advances in magnetic resonance and nuclear imaging as well as echocardiography. This chapter will discuss potential strategies that have been employed and those strategies that should continue to be utilized in the assessment of the cardiac response to cell therapy.

Key Words: Stress testing; nuclear imaging; strain imaging; echocardiography.

The American Heart Association reports that nearly 800,000 patients (60% of all deaths in the United States) die of heart disease each year. In this setting, and despite important advances in reperfusion therapies, cardiomyocyte death (an irreversible process) often remains a final common pathway for functional deterioration and death. The clinical manifestation of the failure to overcome this hurdle manifests itself in a rising epidemic of heart failure.

In the past two decades several developments have provided new promise for treatment of once thought irreversible myocardial cell death.

1. Skeletal myoblasts: Satellite cells residing in a dormant state in the basal membrane of the skeletal muscle fiber. These myogenic precursor cells are mobilized to proliferate and replace damaged muscle tissue after injury. These cells have the capability of rapidly proliferating in culture media without the danger of tumor formation associated with fetal and adult stem cells *(1–5)*. However, these skeletal myoblasts are capable

From: *Contemporary Cardiology: Stem Cells and Myocardial Regeneration*
Edited by: M. S. Penn © Humana Press Inc., Totowa, NJ

only of forming myocytes and not other supporting tissues needed for true myocardial regeneration. They are capable of functioning under lower oxygen saturation conditions than normally required by myocytes. This makes them good candidates for transplantation into poorly revascularized areas of the myocardium.

2. Bone marrow-derived cells (adult stem cells): Mononuclear cells derived from the bone marrow were initially known to differentiate into mesenchymal lineage (6) and recently into ectodermal and endodermal lineages (7). The potential therapeutic applications of these "adult stem cells" may alleviate some of the ethical and immunological concerns associated with fetal stem cells.

3. Fetal stem cells: In 1981 mouse embryonic stem cells were isolated for the first time (8). Almost two decades later in 1998, human embryonic stem cells were isolated (9). The pluripotent nature and plasticity of this type of cells created another opportunity for cell-based therapies.

These opportunities, coupled with advances in techniques of cell isolation and harvesting, culture media, and cell transfer to scarred myocardium, paved the way to a long list of preclinical and clinical trials over the past decade to explore the potentials for "true" cardiac restoration therapies. The direct target of all these efforts is to transform the heart from being a postmitotic organ to a continuously or "on-demand" regenerating organ. The simplistic view of cell-based therapy is that heart failure is a mechanical manifestation of permanent myocyte net loss/dysfunction and that replacing the damaged myocytes with new cells that can be integrated as a functional unit in the damaged heart can ameliorate the heart failure symptoms. In addition, cell-based transplantation may contribute to enhanced neovasculerization and improve perfusion to areas of myocardium that cannot be revascularized or salvage myocardium at the time of acute ischemic injury or revascularization procedures.

PRECLINICAL TRIALS

The initial experience by Chiu et al. (10) demonstrated in two separate canine models the survival of the transplanted skeletal myoblasts in cryoinjured scarred myocardial tissue. Furthermore, the transplanted over time showed histological evidence of intercalated discs and centrally located nuclei, similar to those seen in functioning cardiac muscle fibers. Since this landmark study, other investigators have implemented multiple different cell types in preclinical animal studies to determine their potential efficacy in the treatment of left ventricular (LV) dysfunction in acute myocardial infarction (MI) or heart failure. These preclinical studies used invasive hemodynamics and/or echocardiography to quantify the effects of cell therapy. A clear advantage that preclinical studies have over clinical studies is the ability to perform histological analyses in a controlled fashion, as well as to used tagged cells, so that they can be identified later. Although important clinical histological data is slowly being developed from explanted hearts from patients who later undergo cardiac transplantation and patients who die at some time after cell therapy, we will obviously never have the ability to obtain histological data in clinical populations. The goal of this chapter is to review potential clinical strategies for quantification of cardiac responses to cell therapy.

CLINICAL MEASURES OF EFFECTIVE CELL THERAPY

It is important during the process of developing new therapies to have measurement techniques and clearly defined endpoints to evaluate the successes and failures of each therapeutic intervention as well as to establish a mechanistic explanation for the expected effects.

When considering cell-based therapies, not only are the therapies changing rapidly, but the target population for the therapies is heterogeneous. In this respect both the weapons and the targets are in motion and ever-changing. Fortunately, many of the lessons learned from pharmaceutical and mechanical interventional devices for treating myocardial disease can be applied in the era of cell-based therapies.

The primary aim of any therapeutic intervention should always be to improve survival or to ameliorate symptoms. Keeping these endpoints in mind, a researcher should always try to design a clinical trial that uses overall mortality comparisons as a primary endpoint. However, in the early to intermediate phases of developing cell-based therapies, it is usually difficult to do mortality comparisons for various reasons:

1. Small sample size of the trial.
2. Short follow-up period.
3. The population enrolled in phase 1 and 2 clinical trials inherently at high risk/high mortality.
4. The absence of a true control cohort.
5. The concomitant use of other effective procedures and therapies (coronary artery bypass graft [CABG], percutaneous coronary intervention [PCI], medications) makes the cause and effect relationship hard to trace.
6. The complicated processes of harvesting the cells, growing them, purifying and delivering the cells to the target (scarred myocardium) creates many opportunities for failure.

In order to work within these limitations, several intermediate surrogate endpoints have been used in the absence of mortality data. The collection of these surrogate endpoints relies heavily on the dramatic advances in the in vivo noninvasive assessment of cardiac perfusion, metabolism, and function. Cardiac magnetic resonance imaging (MRI), X-ray-based computed tomography (CT), single photon emission computed tomography (SPECT), positron emission tomography (PET), and ultrasound-based techniques (echocardiography) are the most widely available and clinically useful tools to collect intermediate endpoints in the early stages of clinical trials. In addition to these imaging endpoints, simple but practical measurements such as quality of life, functional class, exercise duration, and time to chest pain are very relevant measurements that can be quantified and reproducibly measured.

Cardiac Magnetic Resonance Imaging

This noninvasive tool uses the signal produced by the hydrogen nuclei in a strong magnetic field to create an image of the water composition of the heart. The advantage of MRI is that no ionizing radiation is used in the process and it has very high spatial resolution. Furthermore, MRI can image the heart in any plane without regard to acoustic windows, a common problem with echocardiography. The three-dimensional nature of the images allows accurate and reproducible volumetric measurements and evaluation. These capabilities were described in 1985 by Longmore et al. *(11)*. Many contributions since then have confirmed these findings in various patient populations. One such early contribution was made by Gaudio et al. *(12)*, who compared left ventricular ejection fraction (LVEF) measurements by MRI to equilibrium radionuclide ventriculography in 32 patients with idiopathic dilated cardiomyopathy and found an excellent correlation ($r = 0.91$). In addition to these excellent global characteristics,

MRI was also proven to be a powerful tool in assessing regional segmental myocardial function throughout the cardiac cycle. In addition to the qualitative visual assessment available with other techniques (echocardiography), utilizing the quantitative tools available in MRI (strain rate, myocardial tagging, and systolic/diastolic deformation of myocardial segments) is an accurate and sensitive strategy to detect the very small changes in myocardial performance seen with cell-based therapies. These changes may be missed by qualitative methods or techniques with poor spatial resolution and be interpreted as a lack of efficacy for the therapeutic strategy being tested.

These clear advantages of MRI will become even more important once scanning parameter adjustments become interactive and instantaneous. Also, real-time display will enhance the standing of MRI as a tool in stress testing. A major obstacle for MRI is the growing use of implanted intracardiac defibrillators in compliance with new guidelines. Such devices pose a danger to patients due to inactivation of the pacemaker function in the magnetic field and local heating at the lead insertion site. The issue of defibrillators and cardiac resynchronization is even more complicated because many if not all the patients considered for cell-based myocardial restoration therapy are candidates for implantable cardioverter defibrillator (ICD) insertion. Serial follow-up is not possible when an ICD is inserted at the time of treatment.

Computed Tomography

CT has not been used in clinical trials of cell-based therapy but has the potential to measure function and perfusion and to define coronary anatomy using the fast multislice detector systems.

Echocardiography

This modality is one of the safest, relatively inexpensive, and widely available diagnostic tests used in cardiology. It has been the main benchmark used in many heart failure, LV remodeling, and sudden death prevention trials. To date, the echocardiogram-derived ejection fraction, LV end-systolic, and end-diastolic dimensions remain very robust tools to predict symptom improvement, prognosis, and mortality. Building on these semiquantitative measures of global cardiac performance, recent techniques (tissue Doppler imaging, strain and torsion, three-dimansional echo, Doppler assessment of filling parameters, contrast echo) have been introduced in day-to-day clinical practice. As a result, echocardiography-derived endpoints were used in many phase 1 and 2 trials of cell-based myocardial restoration therapy. In the current era, most of the intermediate endpoints needed to evaluate the efficacy of cell-based therapies can be derived from echocardiography. These include the following:

1. Global LVEF: this important marker for severity of disease and potential impact of therapy is easily estimated/calculated by echocardiography.
2. LV dimensions/volumes are also readily available from standard echocardiographic studies.
3. Regional/segmental wall motion abnormalities are at least qualitatively assessed by standard echocardiography and more recently quantitatively via tissue Doppler and strain/strain rate measurements.
4. Echocardiography is the gold standard for evaluation of valvular function. In this instance, evaluation of the competency of the mitral valve and regression of mitral regurgitation post-cell-based therapy can be easily assessed serially by echocardiography.
5. Diastolic function and cardiac filling pressures are easily evaluated by echocardiography. These filling pressures and diastolic function are considered a better reflection

of clinical symptomatology than LV systolic function and size. In addition, echocardiographically derived filling pressures correlate well with measurements collected invasively *(13–17)*.

Technical limitations resulting from poor acoustic windows still pose a problem when obtaining cardiac images, especially serial measurements, by echocardiography. This is frequently encountered in obese patients, patients with lung disease, and postop patients. Despite these limitations, our group was recently involved in a phase 1 clinical trial that used echocardiography to successfully monitor the impact of myoblast transplantation (GenVec Inc., in press).

Nuclear Cardiology Imaging

Radionuclide approaches for patient selection and monitoring the effects of cell-based restoration therapy include SPECT and PET. Both techniques can be used in clinical trials to show changes in blood flow, function, and metabolism. The techniques are accurate and highly reproducible. SPECT offers advantages in terms of availability and cost, but is limited by poor resolution and ability to look at metabolism or other mechanistic processes. Equilibrium radionuclide angiography, or multiple uptake gated acquisition (MUGA) scans, can provide reliable information on global and regional systolic and diastolic ventricular function, but echocardiography is capable of providing so much more clinically useful information that it is the preferred method for assessment. All the radionuclide methods expose patients to low levels of radiation, but the risks to the patient or the transplanted cells are minimal. The integration of CT with SPECT and PET into a single unit allows a comprehensive examination of the heart that includes measures such as calcium scoring, assessment of function, infarct sizing, and the ability to perform coronary angiography using 16-, 31-, 40-, or 64-slice detector systems capable of achieving adequate temporal resolution to freeze coronary motion. To date, these hybrid systems have not been used in human studies of cell-based therapy.

SPECT

This is the most widely utilized method to measure myocardial blood flow and is generally performed as the first test to identify areas of ischemic myocardium that may benefit from revascularization with an improvement in function and relief of anginal symptoms. Such methods should be attempted before considering cell-based restoration therapy. SPECT has also been used to measure changes in perfusion, global, and regional function and myocardial mass. Despite the very small sample size in the majority of these studies, SPECT imaging has documented improved perfusion. The advantages of SPECT are the relatively small number of technical limitations to getting good quality studies in nearly all patients, established prognostic data on short- and long-term outcomes, and the ability to perform accurate and reproducible quantitative and semi-quantitative baseline and serial measurements. The disadvantages of SPECT are the poor spatial resolution in comparison to MRI, echocardiography, and PET, limitations imposed by radiation attenuation and scatter, and the inability to adequately measure metabolism with currently available radiotracers.

PET

This technique offers a superior spatial resolution of 4–5 mm compared with 15–16 mm for SPECT, highly accurate attenuation correction, and is the standard for assessment of myocardial viability using F-18 fluorodeoxyglucose and absolute myocardial blood flow using N-13 ammonia. The ability to make and image C-14 and

O-15 allows radiolabeling of biologically important molecules that can be used to understand basic biological processes occurring after transplantation. The disadvantages of PET imaging is the relatively small number of imaging systems available, an even fewer number of onsite cyclotrons for production of non F-18 radiopharmaceuticals, and a greater cost for studies. When CT is used in conjunction PET, there is the additional radiation exposure as a result of the CT component.

IMPLEMENTATION IN CLINICAL TRIALS

Skeletal Myoblasts

The earliest published report of human transplant of myoblasts came from the group lead by Menasché et al. in France *(18)*. In this single patient report, a 72-year-old male in New York Heart Association (NYHA) Class III heart failure undergoing CABG was injected with an autologous myoblast cell suspension. The cells were injected into the border zone between the postinfarct myocardium and the uninjured myocardium. At 5 months, the group reported an improvement in heart failure symptoms by one NYHA class, an increase in regional inferior wall segmental function and contractility, as well as an overall improvement in LV function from 21 to 30%. One could speculate that in this single case the improvements noted could be related to the unblinded nature of the protocol or a result of the revascularization process alone. However, assessment of viability using PET showed an increase in tracer uptake indicating *de novo* metabolic activity in a previously proven nonviable and scarred myocardium. Almost simultaneously, a Polish group led by Siminiak and colleagues *(19)* in a case report described a single case experience of autologous myoblast transplant in a 55-year-old female. The patient suffered a transmural anterior wall MI with scarring as demonstrated by dobutamine echocardiography. A solution containing 1.2 million autologous myoblasts was injected in a non-revascularized and scarred area of the left ventricle during routine CABG. The authors reported that at 1 month there was improvement in LV segmental contractility in the previously scarred segments that were injected with myoblasts.

The cautious optimism from these two single case experiments paved the way for these two groups from Paris and Posnañ to independently carry out two phase 1 clinical trials on autologous skeletal muscle myoblast transplantation in patients undergoing CABG *(20,21)*. The French protocol by Menasche et al. *(20)* reported on 10 patients (EF < 35%) who received autologous skeletal myoblasts injection directly into akinetic segments of the myocardium at the time of coronary artery bypass surgery. A total of 37 akinetic segments were injected with a mean of 874 million cells. One patient died shortly after the procedure from noncardiac causes. On the clinical side, after 11 months of follow-up, the NYHA mean functional class improved from 2.7 before the procedure to 1.6 after the procedure. The average EF improved from 24 to 32%. A blinded echocardiographic analysis showed that 63% of the cell-implanted scars demonstrated improved systolic thickening. On the negative side, four patients showed delayed episodes of sustained ventricular tachycardia and required an internal defibrillator. It was postulated by the investigators that this serious side effect might be related to reentry circuits established by the myoblast engraftment. One additional death occurred at 17.5 months from noncardiac causes.

The Polish investigators also enrolled 10 patients with a mean EF of 35.2% with myocardial scarring identified by dobutamine stress echocardiograms *(21)*. The selected akinetic/dyskinetic segments were injected with an average of 20 million myoblasts at the time of coronary artery bypass surgery. One patient died 7 days postop from an infarct in another part of the ventricle not involved in the myoblast transplant. In the surviving patients and up to 12 months after the procedure, the EF was 42%. Segmental contractility in the scarred but transplanted segments showed improvement. In 9 dyskinetic segments, 5 became akinetic, and in 10 akinetic segments, 4 became hypokinetic. However, the potential hazard from ventricular arrhythmia was also present in this group of patients. Sustained ventricular arrhythmia occurred early (2–4 hours) in 2 patients and late in another 2 patients (2 weeks). Based on these observations, the protocol was amended, and all patients received amiodarone-suppressive therapy with no subsequent significant arrhythmias. The encouraging results of these phase 1 clinical trials gave the researchers many positive leads, but left them with several challenges.

- Is the improvement in LVEF and regional contractility related to the myoblast injection, or is it a result simply of coronary revascularization? The promising limited data from these two trials is that areas that are deemed scarred and historically do not improve with revascularization are responding to myoblast transplantation and showing improvement in contractility.
- What is the optimal number of cells one should inject per akinetic segment to be able to detect improvement in regional contractility? In an animal model Tambara et al. *(22,23)* demonstrated that the improvement in LV dimensions and function were related directly to the number of cells injected. Furthermore, a large number of transplanted myocytes could survive and proliferate to replace the full thickness of the myocardium. Testing of this observation in human clinical trials is underway *(24)*.
- Is there dissociation between the myoblasts injected and the surrounding myocardium that can lead to electrical instability? Or is it that transplanted myoblasts retain a different action potential compared to that of the adjacent myocardium *(25)*. Pagani et al. *(26)* in a small experiment reported histological observations in which skeletal muscle cells survived and differentiated into mature myofibers. Theis data were obtained in three out of four explanted hearts were examined after cardiac transplantation. However, the question remains as to whether new "colonizers" can electrically couple with the rest of the myocardium and act as a syncytium.
- Is the electrical instability a result of the mechanical trauma (injection site, edema)? Given that most ventricular arrhythmia occurred very early in the postinjection period, local irritation (injection, or inflammatory) was postulated as an etiology for early arrhythmia. Furthermore, the population studied (EF < 35%) is known to be at high risk for cardiac arrhythmia irrespective of instrumentation and treatment protocols. On the other hand, and following the recent results of the Multicenter Automatic Defibrillator Implantation (MADIT)-II Trial *(27,28)*, the patient population targeted for myoblasts transplant will qualify and likely get an ICD.
- Are there any better tools that are less invasive that can deliver the cells to the affected myocardium? A percutaneous delivery system was used as a stand-alone therapy by Smits et al. *(29)* to transplant myoblast cells in the infarct zone of five patients with symptomatic heart failure. There were no procedural events. Compared with baseline, the LV ejection fraction increased from 36 to 41% at 3 months and 45% at 6 months. Regional wall thickening in the targeted but infarcted area improved on subsequent MRI exams.

More recently, Herreros et al. *(30)* reported their experience with 12 patients who had old MIs. The sites of infarcts were injected with autologous skeletal muscle cells at the time of CABG. In this study there was a remarkable improvement in LV regional and global contractility from 35% at baseline to 54% at 12 weeks. This was in conjunction with improvement in fluorodeoxyglucose (FDG) uptake in the scarred segments indicating restoration of viability. In this study, there was no excess arrhythmia reported during the 3 months of follow-up.

However, the limited availability of autologous myoblasts and the need to have a "waiting period" to generate enough myoblasts in vivo led some scientists to explore the possibility of transplanting allogenic myoblasts. Law and collaborators *(31)* reported early success with transplanting two patients with chronic heart failure with allogenic myoblasts. This experiment could remove many of the supply barriers limiting autologous transplants and providing "on-demand" myoblasts in the future.

The results of these promising experiments ushered in the era of larger clinical trials. These industry-sponsored trials were done almost simultaneously in Europe and the United States. The American experience was lead by Nabil Dib at the Arizona Heart Institute in collaboration with GenVec Inc. (formerly Diacrin). The initial report by Pagani et al. was from five patients who, at the time of implanting a LV assist device, received transepicardial autologous skeletal myoblasts *(26)*. Histological examination of the explanted hearts at the time of cardiac transplant revealed evidence of engrafted skeletal myoblasts in the previously scarred segments. The second phase 1 study (22 patients) conducted by the same company used an escalating dose of 10 (3 patients), 30 (3 patients), 100 (3 patients), and 300 (13 patients) million myoblasts injected transepicardially at the time of bypass surgery. The total experience from this work was reported earlier *(35)* and recently at the American College of Cardiology annual meeting in 2005 with a 3-year follow-up on patients who received 10– 300 million cells (mean 214 million). In this 24-patient report, postprocedural monitoring included PET and MRI. The safety of the procedure remains excellent, with no perioperative complications. PET and MRI studies show evidence of new skeletal myoblast formation at the site of injection mostly in patients who received 300 million cells, LVEF increased from 27 to 36%, and an improvement in NYHA function class from 2.1 to 1.7. There was one death at 3 years and two strokes. Importantly, there were seven documented ventricular arrhythmia episodes. In five patients there were documented arrhythmias before the procedure. An ICD shock was delivered in another patient, and one patient had a nonsustained ventricular tachycardia not requiring shock. This group now is working on a new delivery device (NOGA) to deliver the myoblasts to the scarred myocardium percutaneously. Recently, Bioheart, Inc. announced a phase 1, open-label, nonrandomized, dose-escalation, multicenter study to assess the safety and cardiovascular effects of autologous skeletal myoblast implantation by a transendocardial catheter (MyoCath™) delivery system in chronic heart failure patients post MI with previous placement of an ICD. The study is expected to enroll 15 patients and report the results in late 2006. A similar study by the same company is currently under consideration for patients who are having bypass surgery.

Dr. Tomasz Siminiak presented the Percutaneous Transvenous Transplantation of Autologous Myoblasts in the Treatment of Postinfarction Heart Failure (POZNAN) trial at the American College of Cardiology in 2004, and the results were published recently *(32)*. POZNAN was a phase 1 trial designed to evaluate the safety and feasibility of this approach in 10 patients with postinfarction heart failure, no viable myocardium, and good coronary flow resulting from revascularization or collateral vessels. Nine patients were receiving prophylactic amiodarone, and one patient had an ICD. Skeletal myoblast transplantation was performed using a catheter system enabling intramyocardial injections from the lumen of cardiac veins under intravascular ultrasound guidance.

The ICD patient had an episode of ventricular tachycardia. The other nine patients had no arrhythmic events. NYHA heart failure class improved in all nine patients. A modest increase in EF was seen in four patients. Bioheart is currently sponsoring two phase 1/2 safety studies in Europe using different catheters to deliver the MyoCell™ product. One of these studies is near completion with active enrollment at sites in The Netherlands and Germany. A pilot phase 2 study (SEISMIC trial) has been finalized and will be initiated shortly after the safety study is complete. This study will be a randomized, multicenter, blinded study.

The European (Myoblast Autologous Grafting in Ischemic Cardiomyopathy [MAGIC] trial) lead by Menasché in Paris and sponsored by MG Biotherapeutics, LLC, a Medtronic-Genzyme joint venture, currently includes centers in Belgium, France, Germany, Italy, Switzerland, and the United Kingdom, with partial funding from Assistance Publique–Hôpitaux de Paris in France. This study is planned to enroll up to 300 patients. This multicenter phase 2 clinical trial is designed to assess the safety and efficacy of two doses of autologous skeletal myoblasts (400 vs 800 million cells, as compared to placebo) in the treatment of ischemic heart failure. Patients met the following three inclusion criteria: (1) a severe LV dysfunction reflected by an echocardiographically measured EF ≤ 35%), (2) a postinfarction discrete akinetic and nonviable scar, as assessed by dobutamine echocardiography, and (3) an indication for coronary artery bypass surgery in remote ischemic areas, i.e., areas different from those in which the cells (or placebo) are injected *(33,34)*. All patients in the MAGIC trial will get an ICD. The primary endpoint of this trial is the improvement in contractility in the myoblast-grafted segments as assessed by a blinded echocardiography core laboratory. The expectation is to complete enrollment in the MAGIC phase 2 trial by the end of calendar year 2006. If this trial is successful, the companies anticipate conducting a phase 3 clinical trial, which will involve the use of catheter delivery. This trial would begin in early 2008. In the first blinded assessment of the safety of this trial, 5 out 44 arrhythmic events were detected by ICDs, and only 2 required ICD therapy *(34)*.

In the summer of 2005, Dib et al. reported the findings from 24 patients who had autologous skeletal myoblast transplantation concurrent with CABG or LV assist device *(35)*. No acute or long-term (2 yr) complications were noted. The average EF improved from 28 to 36% at 2 yr. New viability in the infarcted area was demonstrated on PET-FDG scans. Furthermore, histopathology of the explanted hearts demonstrated successful homing and survival of the transplanted myoblasts.

It is obvious from the wealth of clinical data collected over the past 2–3 yr (*see* Table 1) that:

1. Myoblast in vivo growth and transplant is feasible both epicardially during bypass and percutaneously (arterial and venous).
2. It has been reported earlier that over 90% of grafted cells die within 24–48 h after transplantation *(36,37)*. Using human allograft serum-supplement myoblast culture medium has been proposed to reduce immunogenicity of the cells *(38)*. Also, the dose of myocardial cells required will most likely be in the high range (>300 million) to ensure clinically detectable engrafting.
3. Irrespective of the delivery method, the procedure of cell transplant to the scarred tissue is safe.
4. The incidence of peri-procedural arrhythmia is not as high as reported earlier. We also learned that injecting in the middle of the infarcted zone leads to a lower incidence of arrhythmia then injecting in the border zones at the interface of normal tissue and

Table 1
Clinical Reports of Stem Cell Therapy for Heart Disease

Cell type	Cell delivery	Result (Reference)
Skeletal myoblasts	im at CABG, transepicardial	Improved symptoms and function (4)
Skeletal myoblasts	im at CABG, transepicardial	Improved symptoms and function (5)
Skeletal myoblasts	im with NOGA®ᵃ transendocardial	Improved function and regional wall motion (29)
Skeletal myoblasts and BMC	im, transvenous	Feasibility studies (19,21)
Skeletal myoblasts	im at CABG, transepicardial	Improved function and regional wall motion (30)
Skeletal myoblasts	im at LVAD transepicardial	Confirmed myoblast engraftment (26)
Mononuclear BMC	ic at PCI	Improved function and regional wall motion (39)
AC133+BMC	im at CABG, transepicardial	Improved function and perfusion (41)
Mononuclear BMC	im with NOGA, transendocardial	Improved symptoms and function (42)
Mononuclear BMC	im with NOGA, transendocardial	Improved symptoms and perfusion (43)
Mononuclear BMC	im with NOGA, transendocardial	Improved symptoms and function (44)
BMC and circulating progenitor cells	ic at PCI	Improved function (52)
BMC	ic	Trend toward improved function (53)
Mononuclear BMC	im at CABG, transepicardial	Improved symptoms and function (47)
Mobilized BMC	ic at PCI	Improved exercise capacity, perfusion, and function (48)
BMC	ic at PCI	Improved wall velocity, LVEF, and reduction and perfusion defects (51)
BMC	ic at PCI	Improved function (49)
Skeletal myoblast	CABG, LVAD	Improved EF and viability by PET (24,35)
BMC	ic	Slight increase in EF, increase perfusion, increased metabolism (54)
GCSF	Trauma	One case, increase EF after G-CSF-treated BMC injection (53)
GCSF	CHF	4 patients, indeterminate results, probably safe (56)
GCSF	AMI	Increased EF, increased segmental wall motion, increased perfusion (57)

ᵃNOGA is a cardiac navigator system from Cordis Corp.

im, intramuscular; CABG, coronary artery bypass graft; LVAD, left ventricular assist device; BMC, bone marrow cell; ic, intracoronary; PCI, percutaneous coronary intervention; LVEF, left ventricular ejection fraction; EF, ejection fraction; PET, positron emisson tomography; G-CSF, granulocyte–colony-stimulating factor.

214

infarcted tissue. Most, not all patients (EF < 35%) who will derive benefit from myoblast transplant therapy will be "protected" by an ICD. However, the use of ICDs in this population makes monitoring the process of LV remodeling/function and improvement in wall thickness by the currently accepted gold standard (MRI) challenging in clinical trials.

5. Mechanistically, the clinical detection of benefit form myoblast transplant was clear despite the small sample size in all these trials. There was always an improvement in functional class as well as LV functional parameters. Furthermore, new myocardial cells could be detected clinically by MRI and PET.

Reproduction of these observations awaits the results of the phase 2 trials now underway. It remains to be seen whether these results can be seen in stand-alone myoblast transplant procedures independent of surgical or percutaneous revascularization.

Bone Marrow-Derived Cells (Adult Stem Cells)

The first published report of clinical use of autologous bone marrow-derived stem cells (BMSCs) came from Strauer et al. in 2002 (39). They analyzed 10 patients as part of a phase 1 trial who were treated by infarct-related artery intracoronary transplantation of autologous, mononuclear BMSCs in addition to standard therapy after MI. These patients were compared to another set of 10 patients who received standard care. The BMSC recipients had a smaller infarct zone, a better regional contractility, stroke volume index, and regional perfusion at 3 months. Decisive conclusions from this limited data set were hard to make given the nonrandomized nature of the study. The feasibility of the combination of BMSC transplantation in conjunction with bypass was studied by Stamm et al. and reported in the *Lancet (40)*. An improvement in EF from 39 to 48% was seen in their experience from 12 patients with MIs who had scarred myocardium and were referred for bypass (41). Nuclear perfusion imaging on these patients revealed local improvement in tracer uptake in the scarred segments that were treated with BMSCs. More interestingly, there were no arrhythmias or neoplasia reported in these 12 subjects. The results of this trial were again encouraging. However, absence of a control arm and the bypass surgery confounded the validity of these results.

Improvement in patients' symptoms corresponding to the improvement in LVEF with BMSC transplant was reported by Tse et al. (42). Autologous mononuclear BMSCs were implanted into the ischemic myocardium of eight patients with severe ischemic heart disease (EF > 30%) as guided by electromechanical mapping with a percutaneous catheter procedure. After 3 mo of follow-up, there was improvement in symptoms (less angina and use of nitroglycerin), myocardial perfusion, and function of the ischemic region on MRI. No tachyarrhythmias were reported. This study also lacked a control group. Almost simultaneously, a report by Fuchs et al. (43) on 10 patients, who received transendocardial catheter-based transplantation of BMSCs for severe symptomatic chronic myocardial ischemia not amenable to conventional revascularization, revealed an improvement in Canadian anginal class from 3.1 to 2 and a reduction in the amount of myocardial ischemia as detected by nuclear stress testing. No ventricular arrhythmias were reported in this study. Perin et al. (44) published a similar experience in 21 patients (7 served as controls) who were treated also with transendocardial catheter-based transplantation of BMSCs. In this report, at 4 mo there was an increase in EF from 20 to 29% and a reduction in the areas of stress-induced ischemia by SPECT imaging.

Two reports from the cardiology departments at J.W. Goethe-University and University of Frankfurt helped us understand some of the mechanistic (homing and migratory) properties that determine successful engrafting of BMSCs *(45,46)*. In 28 patients who were assigned to receive intracoronary circulating blood or BMSCs, at 4 mo there was an increase in EF from 44 to 49% and a reduction in the infarct size from 46 to 37 mL in the BMSC arm as detected by MRI. These two reports also showed that BMSC homing is increased with larger infarct size and predominantly to the infarct border zone.

Galinanes et al. reported a clinically noticeable improvement in cardiac function with bone marrow cell transplant in 2004 *(47)*. In this study, 14 patients received unmanipulated autologous bone marrow cell injections directly into scarred myocardium at the time of coronary bypass surgery. Only the scarred segments that were revascularized and received the bone marrow cells showed improvement is segmental contractility on echocardiography 6 weeks and 10 months later. There were no mortalities or procedural complications in this report. Importantly, the bone marrow cells were harvested from the patient's sternum at the time of the surgery and were injected immediately into the myocardium without any further processing.

The MAGIC cell trial conducted in Korea planned to randomize 27 patients to receive intracoronary bone marrow cell infusion ($n = 10$), granulocyte–colony-stimulating factor (G-CSF) alone ($n = 10$), and a control group ($n = 7$) at the time of target vessel stenting. In the first results from this trial, the G-CSF arm was stopped as a result of high and unacceptable rates of in-stent restenosis. However, the patients who received the bone marrow cells had an exercise capacity of 450 seconds at baseline vs 578 seconds at 6-month follow-up, a smaller myocardial perfusion (perfusion defect 11.6% vs 5.3%), and a better systolic function (LVEF 48.7% vs 55.1%) *(48)*.

One of the largest completed clinical trials on autologous bone marrow cell transplant was done in Germany *(49)*. In this study, 60 patients were randomized to receive either optimal medical management after percutaneous intervention for acute ST-elevation MI or intracoronary transfer of autologous bone-marrow cells 4.8 days after PCI. Changes in LVEF from baseline to 6 months were used as the primary endpoint of this trial. After 6 months, mean global EF had increased by 0.7 % in the control group and 6.7 % in the bone marrow-cell group ($p = 0.0026$). The regional improvement in contractility was seen most in the peri-infarct zone. Cell transfer did not increase the risk of adverse clinical events, in-stent restenosis, or proarrhythmic effects. However, this study enrolled patients with relatively good EF (mean 50%), who received "immediate" and "complete" revascularization. It remains to be seen whether these results will be reproducible in patients with chronically poor LV function who have poor targets for revascularization. These questions are important given that in a situation of progressive chronic LV dysfunction there is, in addition to myocardial cell loss, continuous loss of matrix tissue and architectural deformation *(50)*.

The results of another trial by Chen et al. reported on the outcomes of 78 patients randomized to receive either bone marrow cells/percutaneous intervention ($n = 34$) or percutaneous intervention in the remaining patients *(51)*. The LVEF improved in cell-transplanted patients together with a reduction in the size of perfusion defects as detected by PET. These improvements occurred early at 3 mo and were maintained at the end of the 6-month follow-up period.

BMSC mobilization and homing to the scarred myocardium using growth factors and cytokines is currently being evaluated in preclinical studies, but no clinical trials were available as of 2006.

FUTURE DIRECTIONS

It is clear that cardiac regenerative cell therapy using various cellular sources is a therapy that will be attracting scientific and public attention for years to come. Evaluating the efficacy and safety of this therapeutic option is currently in the hands of few centers around the globe. The methodology of conducting the validation studies varies greatly among the centers. To ensure a proper scrutiny of cellular therapy, we think that the research should be conducted in an environment that will yield the benefits desired without compromising safety. Therefore, at least in the initial period, several issues should be addressed:

1. Patients participating in these trials should be in advanced heart failure (classes III, VI).
2. Patients with the lowest EF (<35%) and with advanced diastolic dysfunction should be the subjects of these trials.
3. All patients should be on maximal recommended medical therapy at time of cell transplantation.
4. All patients should have implantable defibrillators as recommended by the recent guidelines. This will ensure continuous electric monitoring and patient safety.
5. Delivery methods and cell quantity should be as uniform as possible across the trials.
6. More clinically relevant endpoints should be used for the upcoming large clinical trials: death, recurrent heart failure, functional class, 6-minute walk test, $V_{O2\,max}$, and others.
7. Mechanistic intermediate endpoints should not be ignored as we move to larger trials. More precise measurements of EF, diastolic dysfunction, and volumes can be achieved using echocardiographic and nuclear techniques. Also, assessment of new myocardial viability by SPECT, PET, and potentially CT will be conducted in future.
8. A framework must be offered to prove that cellular-based therapies will provide an incremental benefit over surgical and pharmacological therapies available now.

REFERENCES

1. Mauro A. Satellite cell of skeletal muscle fibers. J Biophys Biochem Cytol 1961;9:493–495.
2. Menasche P. Myoblast-based cell transplantation. Heart Fail Rev 2003;8(3):221–227.
3. Menasche P. (Cell therapy for heart failure). Bull Mem Acad R Med Belg 2003;158(10–12): 409–423.
4. Menasche P. Skeletal muscle satellite cell transplantation. Cardiovasc Res 2003;58(2):351–357.
5. Hagege AA, et al. Viability and differentiation of autologous skeletal myoblast grafts in ischaemic cardiomyopathy. Lancet 2003;361(9356):491–492.
6. Caplan AI. Mesenchymal stem cells. J Orthop Res 1991;9(5):641–650.
7. McKay R. Stem cells in the central nervous system. Science 1997;276(5309):66–71.
8. Evans MJ, Kaufman MH. Establishment in culture of pluripotential cells from mouse embryos. Nature 1981;292(5819):154–156.
9. Thomson JA, et al. Embryonic stem cell lines derived from human blastocysts. Science 1998;282(5391): 1145–1147.
10. Chiu RC, Zibaitis A, Kao RL. Cellular cardiomyoplasty: myocardial regeneration with satellite cell implantation. Ann Thorac Surg 1995;60(1):12–18.
11. Longmore DB, et al. Dimensional accuracy of magnetic resonance in studies of the heart. Lancet 1985;1(8442):1360–1362.
12. Gaudio C, et al. Comparison of left ventricular ejection fraction by magnetic resonance imaging and radionuclide ventriculography in idiopathic dilated cardiomyopathy. Am J Cardiol 1991;67(5): 411–415.
13. Garcia MJ, Thomas JD. Tissue Doppler to assess diastolic left ventricular function. Echocardiography 1999;16(5):501–508.

14. Garcia MJ, et al. Estimation of left ventricular operating stiffness from Doppler early filling deceleration time in humans. Am J Physiol Heart Circ Physiol 2001;280(2):H554–H561.

15. Garcia MJ. A step closer in the quest for reliable quantification in echocardiography. Eur J Echocardiogr 2003;4(1):1–2.

16. Garcia MJ. Echocardiographic assessment in cell transplantation. Int J Cardiol 2004;95 (suppl 1): S50–S52.

17. Pasquet A, Garcia MJ, Thomas JD. New approaches to the Doppler echocardiographic assessment of diastolic function: from research laboratory to clinical practice. Prog Pediatr Cardiol 1999;10(2): 105–112.

18. Menasche P, et al. Myoblast transplantation for heart failure. Lancet 2001;357(9252):279–280.

19. Siminiak T, Kalawski R, Kurpisz M. Myoblast transplantation in the treatment of post infarction myocardial contractility impairment—a case report. Kardiol Pol 2002;53:131–136.

20. Menasche P, et al. Autologous skeletal myoblast transplantation for severe postinfarction left ventricular dysfunction. J Am Coll Cardiol 2003;41(7):1078–1083.

21. Siminiak T, et al. Autologous skeletal myoblast transplantation for the treatment of postinfarction myocardial injury: phase I clinical study with 12 months of follow-up. Am Heart J 2004;148(3): 531–537.

22. Tambara K, et al. Transplanted skeletal myoblasts can fully replace the infarcted myocardium when they survive in the host in large numbers. Circulation 2003;108 (suppl 1):II259–II263.

23. Tambara K, Tabata Y, Komeda M. Factors related to the efficacy of skeletal muscle cell transplantation and future approaches with control-released cell growth factors and minimally invasive surgery. Int J Cardiol 2004;95 (suppl 1):S13–S15.

24. Dib N, et al. Feasibility and safety of autologous myoblast transplantation in patients with ischemic cardiomyopathy. Cell Transplant 2005;14(1):11–19.

25. Makkar RR, Lill M, Chen PS. Stem cell therapy for myocardial repair: is it arrhythmogenic? J Am Coll Cardiol 2003;42(12):2070–2072.

26. Pagani FD, et al. Autologous skeletal myoblasts transplanted to ischemia-damaged myocardium in humans. Histological analysis of cell survival and differentiation. J Am Coll Cardiol 2003;41(5): 879–888.

27. Moss AJ, et al. Prophylactic implantation of a defibrillator in patients with myocardial infarction and reduced ejection fraction. N Engl J Med 2002;346(12):877–883.

28. Moss AJ. MADIT-II and implications for noninvasive electrophysiologic testing. Ann Noninvasive Electrocardiol 2002;7(3):179–180.

29. Smits PC, et al. Catheter-based intramyocardial injection of autologous skeletal myoblasts as a primary treatment of ischemic heart failure: clinical experience with six-month follow-up. J Am Coll Cardiol 2003;42(12):2063–2069.

30. Herreros J, et al. Autologous intramyocardial injection of cultured skeletal muscle-derived stem cells in patients with non-acute myocardial infarction. Eur Heart J 2003;24(22):2012–2020.

31. Law P. First human heart myoblast allograft. J Am Coll Cardiol 2004;43:39A.

32. Siminiak T, et al. Percutaneous trans-coronary-venous transplantation of autologous skeletal myoblasts in the treatment of post-infarction myocardial contractility impairment: the POZNAN trial. Eur Heart J 2005;26(12):1188–1195.

33. Menasche P, Hagege AA, Desnos M. (Myoblast transplantation for heart failure: where are we heading?). Arch Mal Coeur Vaiss 2005;98(6):649–654.

34. Alfieri O, et al. Myoblast transplantation for heart failure: where are we heading? Ital Heart J 2005;6(4):284–288.

35. Dib N, et al. Safety and feasibility of autologous myoblast transplantation in patients with ischemic cardiomyopathy: four-year follow-up. Circulation 2005;112(12):1748–1755.

36. Irintchev A, Zweyer M, Wernig A. Cellular and molecular reactions in mouse muscles after myoblast implantation. J Neurocytol 1995;24(4):319–331.

37. Pouzet B, et al. Intramyocardial transplantation of autologous myoblasts: can tissue processing be optimized? Circulation 2000;102(19 suppl 3):III210–III215.

38. Chachques JC, et al. Treatment of heart failure with autologous skeletal myoblasts. Herz 2002;27(7):570–578.

39. Strauer BE, et al. Repair of infarcted myocardium by autologous intracoronary mononuclear bone marrow cell transplantation in humans. Circulation 2002;106(15):1913–1918.

40. Stamm C, et al. Autologous bone-marrow stem-cell transplantation for myocardial regeneration. Lancet 2003;361(9351):45–46.

41. Stamm C, et al. CABG and bone marrow stem cell transplantation after myocardial infarction. Thorac Cardiovasc Surg 2004;52(3):152–158.

42. Tse HF, et al. Angiogenesis in ischaemic myocardium by intramyocardial autologous bone marrow mononuclear cell implantation. Lancet 2003;361(9351):47–49.

43. Fuchs S, et al. Catheter-based autologous bone marrow myocardial injection in no-option patients with advanced coronary artery disease: a feasibility study. J Am Coll Cardiol 2003;41(10):1721–1724.

44. Perin EC, et al. Transendocardial, autologous bone marrow cell transplantation for severe, chronic ischemic heart failure. Circulation 2003;107(18):2294–2302.

45. Britten MB, et al. Infarct remodeling after intracoronary progenitor cell treatment in patients with acute myocardial infarction (TOPCARE-AMI): mechanistic insights from serial contrast-enhanced magnetic resonance imaging. Circulation 2003;108(18):2212–2218.

46. Aicher A, et al. Assessment of the tissue distribution of transplanted human endothelial progenitor cells by radioactive labeling. Circulation 2003;107(16):2134–2139.

47. Galinanes M, et al. Autotransplantation of unmanipulated bone marrow into scarred myocardium is safe and enhances cardiac function in humans. Cell Transplant 2004;13(1):7–13.

48. Kang HJ, et al. Effects of intracoronary infusion of peripheral blood stem-cells mobilised with granulocyte-colony stimulating factor on left ventricular systolic function and restenosis after coronary stenting in myocardial infarction: the MAGIC cell randomised clinical trial. Lancet 2004;363(9411):751–756.

49. Wollert KC, et al. Intracoronary autologous bone-marrow cell transfer after myocardial infarction: the BOOST randomised controlled clinical trial. Lancet 2004;364(9429):141–148.

50. Fedak PW, et al. Matrix remodeling in experimental and human heart failure: a possible regulatory role for TIMP-3. Am J Physiol Heart Circ Physiol 2003;284(2):H626–H634.

51. Chen SL, et al. Effect on left ventricular function of intracoronary transplantation of autologous bone marrow mesenchymal stem cell in patients with acute myocardial infarction. Am J Cardiol 2004;94(1):92–95.

52. Assmus B, et al. Transplantation of progenitor cells and regeneration enhancement in acute myocardial infarction (TOPCARE-AMI). Circulation 2002;106(24):3009–3017.

53. Aviles FF, et al. Intracoronary stem cell transplantation in acute myocardial infarction. Rev Esp Cardiol 2004;57(3):201–208.

54. Dobert N, et al. Transplantation of progenitor cells after reperfused acute myocardial infarction: evaluation of perfusion and myocardial viability with FDG-PET and thallium SPECT. Eur J Nucl Med Mol Imaging 2004;31(8):1146–1151.

55. Grines C, et al. Angiogenic gene therapy with adenovirus 5 fibroblast growth factor-4(Ad5FGF-4): a new option for the treatment of coronary artery disease. Am J Cardiol 2003;92(9B):29N–31N.

56. Belenkov Iu N, et al. Moblization of bone marrow stem cells in the management of patients with heart failure. Protocol and first results of ROT FRONT trial. Kardiologiia 2003;43(3):7–12.

57. Kuethe F, et al. Lack of regeneration of myocardium by autologous intracoronary mononuclear bone marrow cell transplantation in humans with large anterior myocardial infarctions. Int J Cardiol 2004;97(1):123–127.

A

Chronic Heart Failure

16

Whole Bone Marrow Transplantation

Emerson C. Perin, MD, PhD
and Guilherme V. Silva, MD

SUMMARY

Treating ischemic heart failure remains one of the most challenging tasks in current cardiology practice. Despite recent technological advances, many heart failure patients are not ideal candidates for percutaneous or surgical revascularization. This so-called "no-option" patient group usually comprises those individuals who have undergone multiple revascularization procedures and have significant residual myocardial ischemia. The hallmark of the so-called no-option group of patients is that the current treatment approach yields unsatisfactory results once they continue to have unmanageable symptoms of refractory angina or heart failure.

For treatment of no-option patients, clinical cardiology researchers have pursued different strategies, including percutaneous and surgical laser therapy and angiogenesis via delivery of growth factors, but limited and conflicting clinical results have been discouraging and led to the development of further therapies. As a result, stem cell therapy has emerged as an alternative for patients with end-stage heart disease. New insights into the mechanisms of cardiac repair have provided evidence that the heart can undergo a repair process in adulthood. Currently, several types of stem cells are under investigation for use in cardiac stem cell therapy. Bone marrow-derived stem cells were among the first to be studied in clinical trials. The present chapter will address current understanding of bone marrow-derived cardiac stem cell therapy for the treatment of ischemic heart failure and will discuss experimental and clinical evidence supporting its utilization.

Key Words: Regenerative medicine; cardiac myocytes; progenitor cells; chronic heart failure; electro-mechanical mapping; endocardial injection.

Treating ischemic heart failure remains one of the most challenging tasks in current cardiology practice. Despite recent technological advances, many heart failure patients are not ideal candidates for percutaneous or surgical revascularization *(1)*. This so-called no-option patient group usually comprises those individuals who have undergone multiple revascularization procedures and have significant residual myocardial ischemia *(2)*. The hallmark of the no-option group of patients is that the current treatment approach yields unsatisfactory results once they continue to have unmanageable symptoms of refractory angina or heart failure *(3)*.

For treatment of no-option patients, clinical cardiology researchers have pursued different strategies, including percutaneous and surgical laser therapy and angiogenesis

From: *Contemporary Cardiology: Stem Cells and Myocardial Regeneration*
Edited by: M. S. Penn © Humana Press Inc., Totowa, NJ

via delivery of growth factors *(4,5)*, but limited and conflicting clinical results have been discouraging and led to the development of further therapies. As a result, stem cell therapy has emerged as an alternative for patients with end-stage heart disease. Until recently, cardiologists believed that myocardial damage followed by ventricular remodeling was irreversible and that the heart was incapable of self-renewal. However, new insights into the mechanisms of cardiac repair have provided evidence that the heart can undergo a repair process in adulthood *(6)*. Because ischemic heart failure is a result of myocardial cell loss and/or untreated myocardial ischemia, cardiac stem cell therapy is promising because stem cells may be capable of myocardial regeneration or neovascularization.

Currently, several types of stem cells are under investigation for use in cardiac stem cell therapy *(6)*. Bone marrow-derived stem cells were among the first to be studied in clinical trials. The present chapter will address current understanding of bone marrow-derived cardiac stem cell therapy for the treatment of ischemic heart failure and discuss experimental and clinical evidence supporting its utilization.

ADULT BONE MARROW STEM CELLS: WHAT ARE THEY?

Adult stem cells are tissue-specific cells found in the adult organism. Hematologists have long studied adult bone marrow stem cells, given their widespread utilization for bone marrow transplantation. This involves the intravenous infusion of hematopoietic progenitor cells to reestablish marrow function in patients with damaged or defective bone marrow, which has been successfully performed for more than 40 years.

Currently, adult bone marrow-derived stem cells are the most widely used cell source for cardiac cell therapy. Bone marrow stem cells are collected by taking an aspirate from the iliac crest of the patient with the aid of local anesthesia. Alternatively, for direct surgical injections, bone marrow is isolated from the sternal marrow when surgeons gain direct access to the mediastinum. The mononuclear subfraction is isolated by Ficoll density centrifugation and filtered through 100-μm nylon mesh to remove cell aggregates or bone spicules. Cells are washed several times in phosphate-buffered saline and can then be utilized for therapy or expanded in an endothelial cell-specific culture medium.

The bone marrow is a complex organ with specific geometric organization and intricate cell-to-cell interaction and signaling. Bone marrow is composed of hematopoietic progenitors, osteocytes and osteoblasts, and supporting mesenchymal cells (stromal cells) (Fig. 1). The bone marrow mononuclear cell subset contains mesenchymal stem cells (MSCs), hematopoietic progenitor cells (HPCs), endothelial progenitor cells (EPCs), and more committed cell lineages such as natural killer lymphocytes, T-lymphocytes, B-lymphocytes, and others *(6)*.

The mononuclear cell subset is the most extensively studied of the adult stem cells, such as MSCs and EPCs. Because MSCs and EPCs have been described in previous chapters, only a brief description of those cell subtypes and any newly described bone marrow mononuclear cell (BMMNC) subtypes with therapeutic potential will follow.

Mesenchymal Stem Cells

MSCs are defined as any selected cell from adult tissue that can be expanded in a culture and that has the capacity for self-renewal and differentiation into several specific mesenchymal cell lineages. MSCs are present in different niches throughout the body, such as bone marrow and adipose tissue. Initially, bone marrow MSCs were most

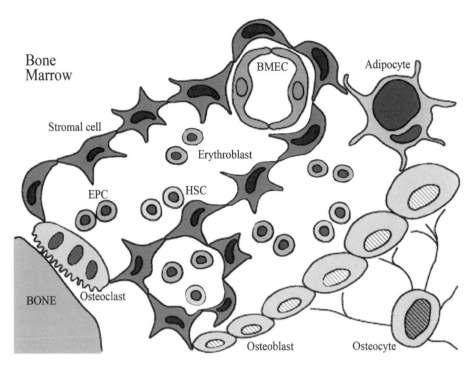

Fig. 1. Bone and bone marrow constitute a single organ, in which marrow cells reside in close vicinity to bone cells. Within the marrow, hematopoietic stem cells (HSC) produce the angiogenic factor (VEGF), and erythroblasts are a source of both VEGF and its homolog, PlGF, placental growth factor; BMEC, bone marrow endothelial cell.

studied because researchers realized that bone marrow stroma was essential for providing an adequate microenvironment for hematopoiesis; further studies revealed MSCs' high degree of plasticity. Both in vitro and in vivo, MSCs can develop into terminally differentiated mesenchymal phenotypes, including bone *(7,8)*, cartilage *(9)*, tendon *(10,11)*, muscle *(12,13)*, adipose tissue *(14)*, and hematopoietic-supporting stroma *(15)*. MSCs differentiate not only into tissues of the mesenchymal lineage, but also into cells derived from other embryonic layers, including neurons *(16)* and epithelia in the skin, lung, liver, intestines, kidney, and spleen *(17–19)*. The high degree of MSC plasticity has led to increasing interest in this cell subtype for use in cardiac regeneration.

Plating studies indicate that MSCs are a rare population of cells in the bone marrow, representing perhaps less than 0.01% of the nucleated cells in bone marrow. They are 10-fold less abundant than HSCs and are identified as CD45 and CD34. The gold standard for identifying MSCs in culture is the colony-forming unit-fibroblast assay, which identifies adherent, spindle-shaped cells that proliferate to form colonies *(20)*. By using different culture techniques, slightly different adherent fibroblast-like cells from the bone marrow can be obtained with different cell surface markers as well *(21,22)*. Bone marrow likely has different subpopulations of MSCs that vary from early tissue-committed cells to more "primitive" cells.

Endothelial Progenitor Cells

EPCs are isolated from the mononuclear fraction of the bone marrow or the peripheral blood, and they also can be isolated from fetal liver or umbilical cord blood

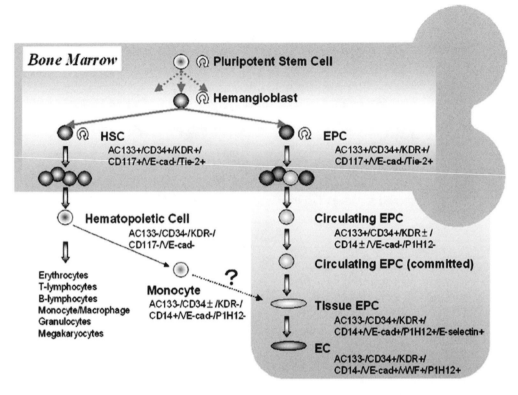

Fig. 2. Putative cascade and expressional profiles of human bone-marrow-derived endothelial progenitor cell differentiation. +, positive; –, negative; EC, endothelial cell; EPC, endothelial progenitor cells; HSC, hematopoietic stem cell. (From ref. *23*.)

(23–26). In animal models of ischemia, heterologous, homologous, and autologous EPCs were shown to incorporate into sites of active neovascularization in different biological scenarios *(26).*

Either in vitro or in vivo, EPCs can differentiate into endothelial cells, smooth muscle cells, or cardiomyocytes *(26).* EPCs have been identified by different research groups using different methodologies *(26).* The classical isolation methods include the use of adherence culture of total peripheral blood mononuclear cells (PBMCs) or the use of magnetic microbeads coated with anti-CD133 or anti-CD34 antibodies. After isolation, the cells are cultured in medium with specific growth factors (e.g., vascular endothelial growth factor [VEGF] and epidermal growth factor) that facilitate the growth of endothelial-like cells. In vitro, EPC proliferation and differentiation are probably influenced by incubation with growth factors and adhesion to specific substrates (such as fibronectin). In vivo, EPC proliferation and differentiation may be influenced by contact with different cell phenotypes (e.g., mature endothelial cells) and extracellular matrix. After initial adhesion in vitro, EPCs begin to lose their progenitor characteristics and within 3–4 wk start to differentiate and form monolayers with an endothelial appearance *(27,28).* EPCs also incorporate acetylated low-density lipoprotein and bind endothelial-specific lectin when cultured with CD34⁻ cells *(29).*

"Immature" or "primitive" EPCs have a similar profile to that of HSCs, and both are thought to be generated from a common precursor, the hemangioblast (Fig. 2). Within the bone marrow, "immature" EPCs and HSCs share common cell surface markers:

CD34, CD133, and VEGFR2 (KDR). Similarly, in the peripheral circulation, the more "primitive" cell population, which has the capacity of differentiation into EPCs, also expresses CD34, VEGFR2, and CD133. In the peripheral circulation, the more committed EPCs "lose" CD133 but retain CD34 and VEGFR2 expression.

Intriguingly, however, EPCs isolated from PBMCs have been demonstrated to express CD14, MAC-1, and CD11-c, which are monocyte/macrophage markers, suggesting a possible monocyte/macrophage origin *(30)*. Harraz et al. *(31)* describe CD34⁻ cells within mononuclear peripheral cells that are CD14⁺ and that also differentiate into cells of the endothelial lineage. Taken together, these findings may represent plasticity of the so-called EPCs (CD34, VEGFR2, and CD133⁺), different stages of development of a common precursor progenitor cell, or distinguished cell subtypes that could be further differentiated by surface markers yet to be discovered.

Other Bone Marrow Cells

It is clear at this time that bone marrow harbors a reservoir of cells with a regenerative capacity extending beyond the hematopoietic lineage. Using cell surface markers for stem cell identification has limitations that may delay the discovery of additional tissue-specific stem cell subtypes. Regardless, the stem cell field is rapidly advancing. Kucia et al. *(32)* report that postnatal bone marrow harbors a nonhematopoietic population of cells that express markers for cardiac differentiation, corroborating the early work of Deb et al. *(33)* reporting the presence of Y chromosome-positive cardiac myocytes in female recipients of male bone marrow transplants. The percentage of cardiomyocytes harboring the Y chromosome was quite small (0.23%), but there was no evidence of either pseudonuclei or cell fusion. The newly described bone marrow cardiac precursors are identified as bone marrow mononuclear cells (BMMNCs) expressing cardiac markers within a population of nonhematopoietic CXCR4⁺/Sca-1⁺/lin⁻/CD45⁻ BMMNCs in mice and within a population of nonhematopoietic CXCR4⁺/CD34⁺/AC133⁺/CD45⁻ BMMNCs in humans. Those nonhematopoietic BMMNCs expressing cardiac precursors are mobilized into the peripheral blood after myocardial infarction (MI) and are chemoattracted to the infarcted myocardium in an SDF-1-CXCR4-, HGF-c-Met-, and LIF-LIF-R-dependent manner *(32)*.

Summary

The BMMNC fraction is a very heterogeneous subgroup of stem cells. BMMNCs retain a high degree of plasticity, and there is evidence they transdifferentiate into several cell lines. The complexity of bone marrow as a stem cell reservoir is far from being fully elucidated, in part because of our limited capacity to differentiate cell subtypes using surface markers. A "functional approach" of cell sorting, such as enzymatic expression or identification of transcriptional factors, would be desirable. Such a method would allow for better understanding of the cell product administered clinically and further refinement of clinical strategies.

Experimental Evidence

As outlined above, there is abundant evidence that bone marrow stem cells can transdifferentiate into cardiomyocytes and endothelial and smooth muscle cells. In experimental studies, bone marrow-derived cells have been shown to regenerate areas of infarcted myocardium and the coronary capillaries, thus limiting functional impairment after an MI.

Table 1
Regional Myocardial Perfusion in Ischemic Animals

	Baseline	Follow-up	p-value
Rest			
ABM (%)	83 ± 12	98 ± 14	0.001
Control (%)	89 ± 9	92 ±10	0.49
Adenosine			
ABM (%)	78 ± 12	89 ± 18	0.025
Control (%)	77 ± 5	78 ± 11	0.75

ABM, autologous bone marrow.
From ref. *36.*

Despite these initial encouraging results in the acute infarct experimental model, chronic reversible myocardial ischemia has an utterly different pathophysiology when compared to that of acute MI. Therefore, to study how bone marrow stem cell therapy affects chronic myocardial ischemia, experimental studies were performed utilizing the ameroid constrictor model. Ameroid constrictors are implanted in large animals through a left thoracotomy. The ameroid itself is a C-shaped device with an outer metallic ring and an inner ring of a hygroscopic material *(34).* Over time, this inner material will swell, creating progressive occlusion of the targeted epicardial coronary artery and ischemia in the distal vascular bed. Usually, the targeted coronary artery will be totally occluded 3–4 weeks after ameroid implantation. In general, ameroids are placed in the left anterior descending artery in dogs and in the left circumflex artery in pigs. It is important to consider the animal's anatomy so as to produce a sizable amount of myocardial ischemia (i.e., proximal implant of the ameroid). One drawback of this chronic ischemia model is the intra/interanimal variability of the amount of subendo-cardial scar generated by ameroid placement.

Advances in cell-based therapies for chronic myocardial ischemia can be attributed in part to previous experience from angiogenesis preclinical studies. Therapeutic angio-genesis via injection of growth factors has been proposed as an alternative treatment for patients with refractory angina and for no-option patients in whom further revascular-ization procedures are not feasible. Experimental angiogenesis trials have focused on the chronic ischemia model (using ameroid constrictors) and have validated the safety of the transendocardial delivery route *(35).* Using the groundwork set during angiogen-esis preclinical work, Fuchs et al. *(36)* report the first experience of transendocardial delivery of whole autologous bone marrow (ABM) (including neutrophils and erythro-cytes) into ischemic myocardial zones in a pig ameroid chronic ischemia model. The most important finding of that study was a significant improvement in myocardial per-fusion at rest and during adenosine infusion in the ABM cell-treated group, along with improvement in regional myocardial contractility both at rest and during stress (Table 1). In addition, results of in vitro studies performed by the same investigators demon-strated the remarkable secretory capacity of ABM cells—specifically regarding VEGF. Histopathological quantification of vascularity, however, did not reveal increased vessel numbers in the ABM-treated animals. Therefore, the marked functional improvement in the ABM-treated animals could be attributed to decreased myocardial flow resistance in collateral vessels not detected by conventional angiography or histopathological examination *(36).*

Further experimental studies compare the anti-ischemic effects of mononuclear ABM stem cells (BMMNCs) obtained via bone marrow aspirate with those of peripherally harvested mononuclear stem cells (peripheral bone marrow-mononuclear cells [PBMNCs]). Both cell types were implanted into ischemic myocardial areas generated by placement of an ameroid constrictor around the left circumflex artery in swine *(37)*. BMMNC and PBMNC injections were targeted and exclusively injected into ischemic areas as assessed by electromechanical mapping (EMM) (preserved unipolar voltage and impaired linear local shortening [contractility]). BMMNC transendocardial injections were associated with increased perfusion at endocardial and epicardial regions as opposed to the PBMNC injections, which resulted in improved endocardial perfusion alone. However, injection of either cell type resulted in significant functional improvement as assessed by echocardiography and EMM parameters *(37)*.

Other bone marrow cell subtypes were also utilized in experimental models of chronic myocardial ischemia. Kawamoto et al. *(38)* studied peripheral circulating bone marrow endothelial progenitor cells. Four weeks after ameroid placement, CD31[+] mononuclear cells were harvested from the peripheral blood of swine and cultured overnight. The nonadhesive cells were then separated and injected transendocardially into ischemic myocardial areas. Histological, functional, and angiographic evidence of neovascularization was obtained 4 weeks after cell transplantation *(38)*.

The above preclinical studies show that functional improvement occurs after bone marrow stem cell treatment of hearts with chronic myocardial ischemia. Moreover, in accordance with the previously described angiogenesis experience, transendocardial delivery of stem cells appeared safe.

CLINICAL APPLICATION OF MONONUCLEAR BONE MARROW-DERIVED STEM CELLS

Targeted Cell Delivery in Ischemic Heart Failure

Stem cells have been delivered through coronary arteries and veins or by means of peripheral vein infusion. Alternatively, direct intramyocardial injections have been performed using a surgical, transendocardial, or transvenous approach. Another delivery strategy may involve mobilization of stem cells from the bone marrow using cytokine therapy, with or without peripheral harvesting.

The main objective of any cell-delivery mode is to achieve the ideal concentration of stem cells needed for repairing the myocardial region of interest. Therefore, cell-delivery strategies must take into account different clinical settings and local milieus, because it is believed that stem cells perform differently according to local signaling. Notwithstanding the importance of signaling, the cardiac environment may help determine the amount of cell retention; the cardiac microenvironment may ultimately determine the fate and therapeutic effects of injected stem cells.

Acute MI is followed by massive release of cytokines and inflammatory mediators, with a consequent systemic increase in serum concentration of growth factor and possible recruitment of bone marrow-derived stem cells into the peripheral blood *(39)*. In theory, stem cell homing signaling is more intense in the AMI setting. Interestingly, in a proof-of-concept study, Saito et al. *(40)* performed intravenous injections of MSCs transduced with a *LacZ* reporter gene. When infused into healthy rats, the MSCs preferentially engrafted within the bone marrow. When infused into

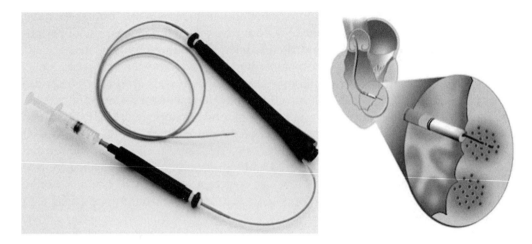

Fig. 3. (Left) Myostar catheter with attached syringe. **(Right)** Artist's illustration showing the catheter traversing the aortic valve and transendocardial extension of the needle with cell delivery **(inset)**. (From ref. *47*.)

rats subjected to ischemia/reperfusion cycles, however, the MSCs engrafted in the infarcted regions of the heart, were positive for cardiomyocyte-specific proteins, and participated in angiogenesis. When injected 10 days after a myocardial injury, MSCs were found preferentially in the bone marrow, suggesting that, in the first days after such an injury, a specific cell signal causes these cells to home in on the affected myocardial areas.

In contrast to acute MI, chronic myocardial ischemia is associated with a paucity of bone marrow cell recruitment signaling. Therefore, human trials of stem cell therapy have relied on the transendocardial-delivery approach, which enhances cell retention and assures accurate delivery into the needed environment.

Transendocardial injection is performed by means of a percutaneous femoral approach. After an injection needle catheter has been advanced in a retrograde fashion across the aortic valve and positioned against the endocardial surface, cells can be injected directly into any area of the left ventricular (LV) wall. The Myostar (Fig. 3) is an injection catheter that takes advantage of nonfluoroscopic magnetic guidance. Injections take place inside a three-dimensional LV "shell," or NOGA-EMM representing the endocardial surface of the left ventricle. The shell is constructed by acquiring a series of points at multiple locations on the endocardial surface, which are then gated to a surface electrocardiogram *(41)*. The technique uses ultra-low magnetic fields (10– to 10^{-6} tesla) that are generated by a triangular magnetic pad positioned beneath the patient. The magnetic fields intersect with a location sensor just proximal to the deflectable tip of a 7 Fr mapping catheter, which helps determine the real-time location and orientation of the catheter tip inside the left ventricle. The NOGA system uses an algorithm to calculate and analyze the movement of the catheter tip or the location of an endocardial point throughout systole and diastole. That movement is then compared with the movement of neighboring points in an area of interest. The resulting value, called linear local shortening (LLS), is expressed as a percentage that represents the degree of mechanical function of the LV region at that endocardial point. Data are obtained only when the catheter tip is in stable contact with the endocardium. This contact is determined automatically.

The mapping catheter also incorporates electrodes that measure endocardial electrical signals (unipolar or bipolar voltage). Voltage values are assigned to each point acquired during LV mapping, and an electrical map is constructed concurrently with the mechanical map. Each data point has an LLS value and a voltage value. When the map is complete, all the data points are integrated by the NOGA workstation. The points are presented in a three-dimensional color-coded reconstruction of the endocardial surface, as well as 9- and 12-segment bull's-eye views that show average values for the LLS and voltage data in each myocardial segment. These maps can be spatially manipulated in real time on a Silicon Graphics workstation (Mountain View, CA). The three-dimensional representations acquired during the cardiac cycle can also be used to LV volumes and ejection fraction.

The EMM thus provides a three-dimensional platform in which the catheter can navigate the left ventricle and provide orientation for transendocardial injections as well as a diagnostic platform that can distinguish ischemic areas (which have low LLS and preserved UniV) from areas of infarct (which have low LLS and low UniV). Moreover, the Myostar catheter allows assessment of myocardial viability at each specific injection site where the catheter touches the endocardial surface (42). The operator thus has the ability to target therapy to viable tissue, which is desirable in situations of chronic ischemia where neoangiogenesis may play an important role, and to avoid nonviable tissue. Because of the patchy nature of myocardial involvement in human ischemic heart disease, the ability to distinguish underlying tissue characteristics is important when performing cell delivery.

The argument in favor of targeted stem cell delivery gains strength because accumulating evidence from preclinical and basic science studies points toward an enhanced angiogenic effect associated with stem cell therapy. Angiogenesis has been studied in depth over the past years and is known to involve a series of complex, well-orchestrated events. The angiogenic process entails proliferation of endothelial cells, breakdown of extracellular matrix, attraction and attachment of pericytes, and migration and proliferation of smooth muscle cells (43), all of which result in the formation of new vessels. Therefore, an area of nonscarred, viable myocardium is needed to support the process of required cell signaling and proliferation.

The ineffectiveness of injecting BMMNCs into scar tissue has become increasingly evident. Agbulut et al. (44) found that injection of bone marrow-derived CD133[+] cells into scarred myocardium was associated with less engraftment (and therefore less efficacy) than was injection of skeletal myoblasts.

The need for targeted cell delivery, the fact that patients may require injections into areas not limited to those supplied by patent coronary arteries (thus hindering the utilization of the intracoronary route), and the findings from current clinical experience all demonstrate that the transendocardial route is likely the first choice for cell delivery in patients with chronic myocardial ischemia.

Clinical Evidence

Autologous bone marrow stem cell therapy has been used for the treatment of chronic myocardial ischemia, including ischemic heart failure with or without systolic functional compromise and in patients who are not candidates for myocardial revascularization (Table 2). Very preliminary clinical evidence supports the efficacy of this new therapy, and, at this point, all the evidence appears to substantiate its safety.

Table 2

Cell Therapy Trials in Patients With Myocardial Ischemia and No Revascularization Option

Study (ref.)	Number	LVEF	Cell type	Dose	Delivery	Outcomes	
						Subjective	Objective
Tse et al. (45)	8 treated	58 ± 11%	BMMNC	From 40 mL BM	Transendocardial (guided by EMM)	Angina ↓[†]	Perfusion ↑[†]; regional wall motion ↑[†]
Fuchs et al. (44)	10 treated	47 ± 10%	NC	$7.8 \pm 6.6 \times 10^7$	Transendocardial (guided by EMM)	Angina ↓[†]	Perfusion ↑[†]
Perin et al. (47,48)	14 treated 7 controls*	30 ± 6%	BMMNC	$3.0 \pm 0.4 \times 10^7$	Transendocardial (guided by EMM)	Angina ↓; NYHA class ↓	Perfusion regional wall motion ↑[†]; global LVEF ↑
Hamano et al. (49)	5 treated		BMMNC	$0.3 - 2.2 \times 10^9$	Transepicardial (during CABG)		Perfusion ↑[†]

BM, bone marrow; CABG, coronary artery bypass grafting; EMM, electromechanical mapping; LVEF, left ventricular ejection fraction; BMMNC, bone marrow–derived mononuclear cells; NC, bone marrow–derived nucleated cells; NYHA, New York Heart Association.
*Nonrandomized control group; [†]effects reported only within cell therapy groups. Values are mean ± standard deviation.

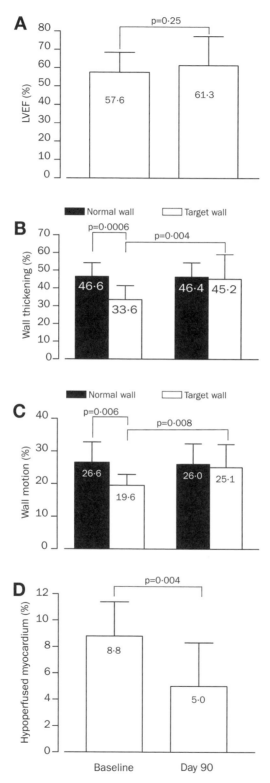

Fig. 4. (A) Left ventricular ejection fraction, **(B)** regional wall thickening, and **(C)** regional wall motion of the normal and target wall; **(D)** percent of hypoperfused myocardium at baseline and 90 d after implantation of bone marrow cells. LVEF; left ventricular ejection fraction. Data are mean SD. (From ref. *45.*)

Tse et al. *(45)* report transendocardial injection of autologous BMMNCs in eight patients with severe ischemic heart disease and preserved LV function (preserved LV ejection fraction [LVEF]). After 3 months of follow-up, there was improvement in symptomatology and myocardial perfusion. Cardiac magnetic resonance imaging showed improved regional perfusion and contractility at the ischemic region (Fig. 4).

Fuchs et al. *(46)* conducted a feasibility clinical study of transendocardial delivery of filtered unfractionated ABM (not mononuclear) cells in 10 patients with severe, symptomatic, chronic myocardial ischemia not amenable to conventional revascularization. Twelve targeted injections (0.2 mL each) were administered into ischemic, noninfarcted myocardium that was preidentified by single-photon emission computed tomography (SPECT) perfusion imaging. Notably, no serious adverse effects occurred (i.e., arrhythmia, infection, myocardial inflammation, or increased scar formation). Treadmill exercise duration results (available for nine patients) did not change significantly (391 ± 155 vs 485 ± 198; $p = 0.11$), but there was improvement in Canadian Cardiovascular Society angina scores (3.1 ± 0.3 vs 2.0 ± 0.94; $p = 0.001$) and in stress scores in segments within the injected regions (2.1 ± 0.8 vs 1.6 ± 0.8; $p < 0.001$).

Our group performed the first clinical trial designed to use transendocardial injection of autologous BMMCs to treat heart failure patients *(47)*. We published the results of 2- and 4-month noninvasive and invasive follow-up *(47)* and of 6- and 12-month follow-up evaluation *(48)*. This study, performed in collaboration with physicians and scientists at the Hospital Pro-Cardiaco in Rio de Janeiro, Brazil, used EMM-guided transendocardial delivery of stem cells.

Twenty-one patients were enrolled (treatment group, first 14 patients; control group, last 7 patients). Baseline evaluations included complete clinical and laboratory tests, exercise stress (ramp treadmill) studies, two-dimensional Doppler echocardiography, SPECT perfusion scanning, and 24-hour Holter monitoring. BMMNCs were harvested, isolated, washed, and resuspended in saline for injection by the NOGA catheter (15 injections of 0.2 cc, totaling 30×10^6 cells per patient). Electromechanical mapping was used to identify viable myocardium (unipolar voltage ≥ 6.9 mV) for treatment. All patients underwent noninvasive follow-up tests at 2 months, and the treatment group also underwent invasive studies at 4 mo, using standard protocols and the same procedures as at baseline. The demographic and exercise test variables did not differ significantly between the treatment and control groups. There were no procedural complications. At 2 months there was a significant reduction in the total reversible defect in the treatment group and between the treatment and control groups ($p = 0.02$) on quantitative SPECT analysis. At 4 months the LVEF improved from a baseline of 20 to 29% ($p = 0.003$), and the end-systolic volume was reduced ($p = 0.03$) in the treated patients. Electromechanical mapping revealed significant mechanical improvement of the injected segments ($p < 0.0005$). We concluded that transendocardial injection of BMMNCs was safe and that additional investigation of this therapy was warranted to further evaluate efficacy endpoints. This was the first time that objective data suggesting perfusion and functional improvement had been seen in a group of severely impaired patients solely on the basis of cell therapy. The significant improvement seen at 2 and 4 months was maintained at 6 and 12 months, as exercise capacity improved slightly in the treatment group (Table 3). Monocyte, B-cell, HPC, and early HPC subpopulations correlated with improvement in reversible perfusion defects at 6 months (Table 4).

Table 3
Comparison of Clinical Values for the Treatment and Control Groups at Baseline, 2 Months, 6 Months, and 12 Months

Variable	Baseline		2 Months		6 Months		12 Months		p-Value[a]
	Rx	Control	Rx	Control	Rx	Control	Rx	Control	
SPECT									
Total reversible defect, %	14.8–14.5	20–25.4	4.45–11.5	37–38.4	8.8–9	32.7–37	11.3–12.8	34.3–30.8	0.01
Total fixed defect (50%), %	42.6–10.3	38–12	39.8–6.9	39.1–11.2	38–6.7	36.4–12	38.2–8.5	35.2–9.3	0.3
Ramp Treadmill Test									
VO_2 max, mL/kg/min	17.3–8	17.5–6.7	23.2–8	18.3–9.6	24.2–7	17.3–6	25.1–8.7	18.2–6.7	0.03
METS	5.0–2.3	5.0–1.91	6.6–2.3	5.2–2.7	7.2–2.4	4.9–1.7	7.2–2.5	5.1–1.9	0.02
LVEF	30–6	37–14	37–6	27–6	30–10	28–4	35.1–6.9	34–3	0.9
Functional Class									
NYHA	2.2–0.9	2.7–0.8	1.5–0.5	2.4–1.0	1.3–0.6	2.4–0.5	1.4–0.7	2.7–0.5	0.01
CCSAS	2.6–0.8	2.9–1.0	1.8–0.6	2.5–0.8	1.4–0.5	2–0.1	1.2–0.4	2.7–0.5	0.002
PVCs, n	2507–6243	672–1085	901–1236	2034–4528	3902–8267	1041–1971	—	—	0.4
dQRS, ms	136–15	145–61	145.9–25	130–27	144.8–25	140–61	—	—	0.62
LAS 40, ms	50–24	70–76	54–33	48–20	25–25	66–79	—	—	0.47
RMS 40, mV	22.2–22	23.3–23	23.3–19	24.6–28	25–25	30–27	—	—	0.7

[a]p-value for comparisons between the treatment and control groups, as assessed by ANOVA, relating to treatment over time. CCSAS, Canadian Cardiovascular Society Angina Score; dQRS, filtered QRS duration; LAS 40, duration of terminal low-amplitude signal less than 40 mV; LEVF, left ventricular ejection fraction; METS, metabolic equivalents; NYHA, New York Heart Association; PVCs, premature ventricular contractions; RMS 40, root mean square voltage in the terminal 40 ms of the QRS complex; Rx, treatment; SPECT, single-photon emission computed tomography; VO_2 max, maximal rate of oxygen consumption. (Reprinted from ref. 48 with permission.)

Table 4
Correlation of Bone Marrow Mononuclear Cell Subpopulations
and Reduction in Total Reversible Perfusion Defects

Cell population and phenotype	r	p
Hematopoietic progenitor cells (CD45^{lo}CD34$^+$)	0.6	0.04
Early hematopoietic progenitor cells (CD45^{lo}CD34$^+$HLA-DR$^-$)	0.6	0.04
CD4$^+$ T cells (CD45$^+$CD3$^+$CD4$^+$)	0.5	0.1
CD8$^+$ T cells (CD45$^+$CD3$^+$CD8$^+$)	0.5	0.07
B cells (CD45$^+$CD19$^+$)	0.7	0.02
Monocytes (CD45$^+$CD14$^+$)	0.8	0.03
NK cells (CD45$^+$CD56$^+$)	0.1	0.9
B-cell progenitors (CD34$^+$CD19$^+$)	0.5	0.3
CRU-F	0.7	0.06

r indicates Pearson correlation coefficient; CFU-F, fibroblast colony-forming unit; NK, natural killer.

MECHANISTIC ASPECTS OF AUTOLOGOUS BMMNC-INDUCED FUNCTIONAL IMPROVEMENT IN CHRONIC MYOCARDIAL ISCHEMIA

Preclinical Evidence

Preclinical experiments have provided solid evidence supporting the efficacy of cardiac autologous BMMNC therapy; however, further investigation is needed at the molecular level to elucidate the mechanistic aspects of stem cell therapy—an area where researchers have more questions than answers.

Numerous research groups, using various detection methods in diverse experimental settings, have proposed different mechanisms for the apparent transformation of stem cells into cells of a variety of tissues (6). Some investigators attribute the transformation to the transdifferentiation potential of stem cells (58–60), while others have demonstrated that the transformation is a result of cell fusion (61).

Initial evidence indicated that BMMNCs transdifferentiate into endothelial cells and cardiac myocytes. Recent studies in mice, however, have challenged this belief, thereby generating enormous controversy (61). In a recent study by Murry et al. (61), researchers failed to detect BMMNC transdifferentiation into a cardiomyocyte phenotype, despite the use of sophisticated genetic techniques to follow cell fate and engraftment. In experimental models, BMMNCs have been shown to depend on external signals that trigger secretory properties and differentiation (62). The local environment of viable myocardial cells may provide the milieu necessary for inducing BMMNC myocyte differentiation (63). In recent studies of occlusion-induced MI in rats, few (if any) BMMNCs might be expected to differentiate and express specific cardiac myocyte proteins, depending on the injection site. To further clarify the issue of transdifferentiation vs fusion, Zhang et al. (64) performed an elegant study involving flow cytometry analysis of heart cell isolates from mice that had received human CD34$^+$ cells. Human leukocyte antigen (HLA)-ABC and cardiac troponin T or Nkx2.5 were used as markers for cardiomyocytes derived from human CD34$^+$ cells, and HLA-ABC and vascular/endothelial—cadherin were used to identify the transformed endothelial cells. The double-positive cells were tested to detect the expression of human and mouse X chromosomes. The results revealed that 73.3% of nuclei derived from HLA-positive and troponin T-positive or Nkx2.5-positive cardiomyocytes contained both human and mouse X chromosomes and that 23.7% contained only human X chromosomes. In contrast, the nuclei of HLA-negative, troponin T-positive cells contained only mouse X chromosomes. Furthermore, 97.3% of endothelial cells derived from CD34$^+$ cells contained human X chromosome only. In conclusion, human CD34$^+$ cells both fused with and transdifferentiated into cardiomyocytes in this mouse model. In addition, human CD34$^+$ cells also transdifferentiated into endothelial cells.

The transdifferentiation of hematopoietic stem cells into a mature hematopoietic fate (e.g., endothelium) in the heart is less controversial (65). In animal models of stem cell therapy in ischemic heart disease, the evidence points toward increased neovascularization (with reduced myocardial ischemia) and consequent improvement in cardiac function (66–68). Bone marrow stem cells may directly contribute to an increase in contractility or, more likely, may passively limit infarct expansion and remodeling. Unfortunately, the limitations of the present animal models leave this question unanswered.

According to current understanding of bone marrow stem cell engraftment, most cells die within the first days after delivery. Arteriogenesis and vasculogenesis are long known to be highly dependent on vascular growth factors. In an elegant study, Kinnaird et al. (69,70) concluded that MSCs contribute to angiogenesis by means of paracrine mechanisms. With this new understanding, one might postulate that the paracrine effects of bone marrow stem cell therapy would result in the recruitment of circulating progenitor cells, the activation of resident cardiac stem cells, or both, triggering a cascade of events resulting in cardiac repair. The important role of resident cardiac stem cells in the process of cardiac repair should also be considered (71). Urbanek et al. (72) were the first to describe evidence of myocyte formation from cardiac stem cells in human cardiac hypertrophy.

Clinical Evidence

In the clinical arena, we recently described the postmortem study of one of our patients who received BMMNCs (73). Eleven months after performing the treatment, we observed no abnormal or disorganized tissue growth, no abnormal vascular growth, and no enhanced inflammatory reactions. Histological and immunohistochemical findings from infarcted areas of the anterolateral ventricular wall (areas that had received bone marrow-cell injections) were reported. The histological findings from the anterolateral wall region were subsequently compared with findings from within the interventricular septum (which had normal perfusion in the central region and no cell therapy) and findings from the previously infarcted inferoposterior ventricular wall (which had extensive scarring and no cell therapy).

Some highly intriguing findings were seen:

1. The cell-treated area with a previous infarction had a higher capillary density than did the nontreated, infarcted areas of the heart (Fig. 5).
2. Proliferation of smooth muscle β-actin-positive pericytes and mural cells was noted exclusively in the cell-treated area.
3. The above-named cells (pericytes and mural cells) expressed specific cardiomyocyte proteins.

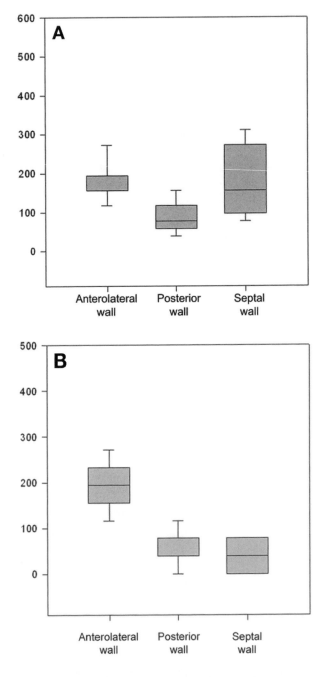

Fig. 5. Number of capillaries per mm^2 in anterolateral, posterior, and septal walls of studied heart. (**A**) Anti-factor VIII-associated antigen counterstained with hematoxylin. (**B**) Anti-smooth muscle-actin antigen counterstained with hematoxylin. (**C**) Capillaries reacted with anti-factor VIII-associated antigen inside fibrotic areas only in anterolateral and posterior walls. ($n = 108$ microscope fields for **A**; 96 microscope fields for **B**; and 40 microscope fields for **C**.) Differences were statistically significant among all groups in pairwise comparisons ($p < 0.05$, Newman-Keuls method) for **A** and **B**. Differences were significantly different ($p < 0.05$) between anterolateral and posterior walls in Mann-Whitney rank-sum test for **C**. (From ref. *73*.)

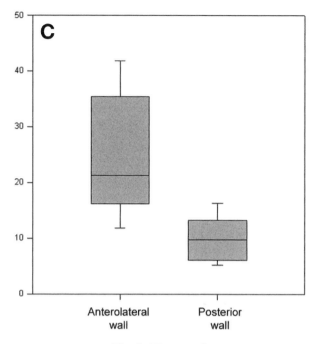

Fig. 5. *(Continued)*

It is well described in the angiogenesis literature that pericytes are essential for achieving a long-lasting physiological angiogenic process. In this postmortem study, the cell-injected wall had marked hyperplasia of pericytes and mural cells. The observed hypertrophic pericytes, although still located in the vascular wall, expressed specific myocardial proteins and were found in distant locations from the vessel walls, suggesting detachment. Migrated pericytes and mural cells were found in adjacent tissue (in the vicinity of cardiomyocytes), either isolated or in small cell clumps. Closer to cardiomyocytes, the expression of myocardial proteins was enhanced, yielding brighter immunostaining throughout the whole cytoplasm. Within the posterior wall, none of the findings was seen, and small blood vessels could only rarely be found. While definitive conclusions regarding autologous BMMNC efficacy are without doubt premature on the basis of one postmortem study, the above findings indeed could be consistent with neoangiogenesis in the cell-treated wall. Those findings, if confirmed in future human studies, are similar to those described in most of the preclinical studies in chronic myocardial ischemia models.

SAFETY OF STEM CELL THERAPY

With regard to left ventricular function, cardiac stem cell therapy is well tolerated overall. No proarrhythmic effects have been observed to date with BMMNC therapy, but there is the possibility of other deleterious effects. Although early concerns about abnormal transdifferentiation and tumorigenesis have subsided, the potential for accelerated atherogenesis remains, given the limited clinical experience and the small number of patients treated. Atherosclerosis is an inflammatory disease triggered and sustained by cytokines, adhesion molecules, and cellular components such as monocytes and macrophages. Another potential deleterious effect of bone marrow stem cell therapy is myocardial calcification. In a recent study, Yoon et al. *(74)* reported that direct transplantation of unselected bone marrow cells into acutely infarcted myocardium may induce significant intramyocardial calcification. It is important to highlight that, in the same study, mononuclear BMMNCs (those widely used in clinical trials) did not elicit the same effect.

Granted, short-term follow-up of the small number of patients treated to date with BMMNCs provides limited data on safety. However, the uniformity of encouraging outcomes for high-risk patients in the completed phase I trials serves to reassure investigators and patients of the safety of the current approaches. Aggressive safety data monitoring is necessary in the ongoing clinical trials.

CONCLUSION AND FUTURE CONSIDERATIONS

Cardiac stem cell therapy is advancing at a fast pace with increasing focus on its utilization in the clinical setting. Autologous mononuclear bone marrow injection is undoubtedly a preliminary strategy for treatment of chronic myocardial ischemia at this point. However it reflects our basic understanding of the field and its vast possibilities with regard to identifying the ideal cell and cell dose. Additionally, interpersonal variability of bone marrow "quality" may significantly influence outcomes, and a new concept of "product quality control" with regard to the bone marrow obtained from patients should be considered when applying this approach to therapy.

Stem cell therapy for chronic myocardial ischemia patients with no option for further revascularization therapy has an enormous therapeutic potential. The future will bring major advances with regard to current strategies and will likely fulfill and exceed current expectations regarding the field of therapeutic myocardial regeneration.

REFERENCES

1. Robbins MA, O'Connell JB. Economic impact of heart failure. In Rose EA, Stevenson LW, eds. Management of End-Stage Heart Disease. Lippincott-Raven, Philadelphia, 1998, pp. 3–13.
2. McNeer JF, Conley MJ, Starmer CF, et al. Complete and incomplete revascularization at aortocoronary bypass surgery: experience with 392 consecutive patients. Am Heart J 1974;88:176–182.
3. Hennebry TA, Saucedo JF. "No-option" patients: a nightmare today, a future with hope. J Inv Cardiol 2004;17:93–94.
4. Laham RJ, Simons M, Sellke F. Gene transfer for angiogenesis in coronary artery disease. Annu Rev Med 2001;52:485–502.
5. Heilmann CA, Attmann T, von Samson P, et al. Transmyocardial laser revascularization combined with vascular endothelial growth factor 121 (VEGF121) gene therapy for chronic myocardial ischemia—do the effects really add up? Eur J Cardiothorac Surg 2003;23:74–80.
6. Perin E, Geng Y, Willerson JT. Adult stem cell therapy in perspective. Circulation 2003;107:935–938.
7. Bruder SP, Jaiswal N, Haynesworth SE. Growth kinetics, self-renewal, and the osteogenic potential of purified human mesenchymal stem cells during extensive subcultivation and following cryopreservation. J Cell Biochem 1997;64:278–294.
8. Bruder SP, Kurth AA, Shea M, Hayes WC, Jaiswal N, Kadiyala S. Bone regeneration by implantation of purified, culture-expanded human mesenchymal stem cells. J Orthop Res 1998;16:155–162.
9. Kadiyala S, Young RG, Thiede MA, Bruder SP. Culture expanded canine mesenchymal stem cells possess osteochondrogenic potential in vivo and in vitro. Cell Transplant 1997;6:125–134.
10. Young RG, Butler DL, Weber W, Caplan AI, Gordon SL, Fink DJ. Use of mesenchymal stem cells in a collagen matrix for Achilles tendon repair. J Orthop Res 1998;16:406–413.
11. Awad HA, Butler DL, Boivin GP, et al. Autologous mesenchymal stem cell-mediated repair of tendon. Tissue Eng 1999;5:267–277.

12. Ferrari G, Cusella-De Angelis G, Coletta M, et al. Muscle regeneration by bone marrow-derived myogenic progenitors. Science 1998;279:1528–1530.
13. Galmiche MC, Koteliansky VE, Briere J, Herve P, Charbord P. Stromal cells from human long-term marrow cultures are mesenchymal cells that differentiate following a vascular smooth muscle differentiation pathway. Blood 1993;82:66–76.
14. Dennis JE, Merriam A, Awadallah A, Yoo JU, Johnstone B, Caplan AI. A quadripotential mesenchymal progenitor cell isolated from the marrow of an adult mouse. J Bone Miner Res 1999;14:700–709.
15. Prockop D.J. Marrow stromal cells as stem cells for nonhematopoietic tissues. Science 1997;276:71–74.
16. Barry FP. Mesenchymal stem cell therapy in joint disease. Novartis Found Symp 2003;249:86–96.
17. Chapel A, Bertho JM, Bensidhoum M, et al. Mesenchymal stem cells home to injured tissues when co-infused with hematopoietic cells to treat a radiation-induced multi-organ failure syndrome. J Gene Med 2003;5:1028–1038.
18. Deng Y, Guo X, Yuan Q, Li S. Efficiency of adenoviral vector mediated CTLA4Ig gene delivery into mesenchymal stem cells. Chin Med J (Engl) 2003;116:1649–1654.
19. Ortiz LA, Gambelli F, McBride C, et al. Mesenchymal stem cell engraftment in lung is enhanced in response to bleomycin exposure and ameliorates its fibrotic effects. Proc Natl Acad Sci USA 2003;100:8407–8411.
20. Castro-Malaspina H, Gay RE, Resnick G, et al. Characterization of human bone marrow fibroblast colony-forming cells (CFU-F) and their progeny. Blood 1980;56:289–301.
21. Majumdar MK, Thiede MA, Mosca JD, Moorman M, Gerson SL. Phenotypic and functional comparison of cultures of marrow-derived mesenchymal stem cells (MSCs) and stromal cells. J Cell Physiol 1998;176:57–66.
22. Dormady SP, Bashayan O, Dougherty R, Zhang XM, Basch RS. Immortalized multipotential mesenchymal cells and the hematopoietic microenvironment. J Hematother Stem Cell Res 2001;10:125–140.
23. Iwami Y, Masuda H, Asahara T. Endothelial progenitor cells: past, state of the art, and future. J Cell Mol Med 2004;8:488–497.
24. Rumpold H, Wolf D, Koeck R, Gunsilius E. Endothelial progenitor cells: a source for therapeutic vasculogenesis? J Cell Mol Med 2004;8:509–518.
25. Shi O, Rafii S, Wu MH, et al. Evidence for circulating bone marrow-derived endothelial cells. Blood 1998;92:362–367.
26. Asahara T, Masuda H, Takahashi T, et al. Bone marrow origin of endothelial progenitor cells responsible for postnatal vasculogenesis in physiological and pathological neovascularization. Circ Res 1999;85:221–228.
27. Quirici N, Soligo D, Caneva L, Servida F, Bossolasco P, Deliliers GL. Differentiation and expansion of endothelial cells from human bone marrow CD1331 cells. Br J Haematol 2001;115:186–194.
28. Murohara T. Therapeutic vasculogenesis using human cord blood-derived endothelial progenitors. Trends Cardiovasc Med 2001;11:303–307.
29. Murohara T, Ikeda H, Duan J, et al. Transplanted cord blood-derived endothelial precursor cells augment postnatal neovascularization. J Clin Invest 2000;105:1527–1536.
30. Hristov M, Erl W, Weber PC. Endothelial progenitor cells: mobilization, differentiation, and homing. Arterioscler Thromb Vasc Biol 2003;23:1185–1189.
31. Harraz M, Jiao C, Hanlon HD, Hartley RS, Schatteman GC. CD34-blood-derived human endothelial cell progenitors. Stem Cells 2001;19:304–312.
32. Kucia M, Dawn B, Hunt G, et al. Cells expressing early cardiac markers reside in the bone marrow and are mobilized into the peripheral blood after myocardial Infarction. Circ Res 2004;95:1191–1199.
33. Deb A, Wang S, Skelding KA. Bone-marrow cardiomyocytes are present in the adult human heart: a study of gender-mismatched bone-marrow transplantation patients. Circulation 2003;107:1247–1249.
34. Schaper W. The Collateral Circulation of the Heart. Elsevier, Amsterdam, 1971.
35. Kornowski R, Fuchs S, Tio FO, et al. Evaluation of the acute and chronic safety of the biosense injection catheter system in porcine hearts. Cathet Cardiovasc Intervent 1999;48:447–453.
36. Fuchs S, Baffour R, Zhou YF, et al.Transendocardial delivery of autologous bone marrow enhances collateral perfusion and regional function in pigs with chronic myocardial ischemia. J Am Coll Cardiol 2001;37:1726–1732.
37. Kamihata H, Matsubara H, Nishiue T, et al. Improvement of collateral perfusion and regional function by implantation of peripheral blood mononuclear cells into ischemic hibernating myocardium. Arterioscler Thromb Vasc Biol 2002;22:1804–1810.
38. Kawamoto A, Tkebuchava T, Yamagichi J, et al . Intramyocardial transplantation of autologous endothelial progenitor cells for therapeutic neovascularization of myocardial ischemia. Circulation 2003;107:461–468.

39. Shintani S, Murohara T, Ikeda H, et al. Mobilization of endothelial progenitor cells in patients with acute myocardial infarction. Circulation 2001;103:2776–2779.
40. Saito T, Kuang JQ, Bittira B, Al-Khaldi A, Chiu RC. Xenotransplant cardiac chimera: immune tolerance of adult stem cells. Ann Thorac Surg 2002;74:19–24.
41. Sarmento-Leite R, Silva GV, Dohman HF, et al. Comparison of left ventricular electromechanical mapping and left ventricular angiography: defining practical standards for analysis of NOGA maps. Tex Heart Inst J 2003;30:19–26.
42. Perin EC, Silva GV, Sarmento-Leite R, et al. Assessing myocardial viability and infarct transmurality with left ventricular electromechanical mapping in patients with stable coronary artery disease: validation by delayed-enhancement magnetic resonance imaging. Circulation 2002;106:957–961.
43. Carmeliet P. Mechanisms of angiogenesis and arteriogenesis. Nat Med 2000;6:389–395.
44. Agbulut O, Vandervelde S, Attar N, et al. Comparison of human skeletal myoblasts and bone marrow-derived CD133+ progenitors for the repair of infarcted myocardium. J Am Coll Cardiol 2004; 44:458–463.
45. Tse HF, Kwong YL, Chan JK, Lo G, Ho CL, Lau CP. Angiogenesis in ischaemic myocardium by intramyocardial autologous bone marrow mononuclear cell implantation. Lancet 2003;361:47–49.
46. Fuchs S, Satler LF, Kornowski R, et al. Catheter-based autologous bone marrow myocardial injection in no-option patients with advanced coronary artery disease: a feasibility study. J Am Coll Cardiol 2003;41:1721–1724.
47. Perin EC, Dohmann HF, Borojevic R, et al. Transendocardial, autologous bone marrow cell transplantation for severe, chronic ischemic heart failure. Circulation 2003;107:2294–2302.
48. Perin EC, Dohmann HF, Borojevic R, et al. Improved exercise capacity and ischemia 6 and 12 months after transendocardial injection of autologous bone marrow mononuclear cells for ischemic cardiomyopathy. Circulation 2004;110(suppl II):213–218.
49. Hamano K, Nishida M, Hirata K, et al. Local implantation of autologous bone marrow cells for therapeutic angiogenesis in patients with ischemic heart disease: clinical trial and preliminary results. Jpn Circ J 2001;65:845–847.
50. Menasche P, Hagege AA, Vilquin JT, et al. Autologous skeletal myoblast transplantation for severe postinfarction left ventricular dysfunction. J Am Coll Cardiol 2003;41:1078–1083.
51. Herreros J, Prosper F, Perez A, et al. Autologous intramyocardial injection of cultured skeletal muscle-derived stem cells in patients with non-acute myocardial infarction. Eur Heart J 2003;24:2012–2020.
52. Siminiak T, Kalawski R, Fiszer D, et al. Autologous skeletal muscle transplantation for the treatment of postinfarction myocardial injury: phase I clinical study with 12 months of follow-up. Am Heart J 2004;148:531–537.
53. Chachques JC, Herreros J, Trainini J, et al. Autologous human serum for cell culture avoids the implantation of cardioverter-defibrillators in cellular cardiomyoplasty. Int J Cardiol 2004;95(suppl I):29–33.
54. Smits PC, Van Geuns RJ, Poldermans D, et al. Catheter-based intramyocardial injection of autologous skeletal myoblasts as a primary treatment of ischemic heart failure. J Am Coll Cardiol 2003;42:2063–2069.
55. Stamm C, Westphal B, Kleine HD, et al. Autologous bone-marrow stem-cell transplantation for myocardial regeneration. Lancet 2003;361:45–46.
56. Stamm C, Kleine HD, Westphal B, et al. CABG and bone marrow stem cell transplantation after myocardial infarction. Thorac Cardiovasc Surg 2004;52:152–158.
57. Assmus B, Honold J, Lehmann R, et al. Transcoronary transplantation of progenitor cells and recovery of left ventricular function in patients with chronic ischemic heart disease: results of a randomized, controlled trial. Circulation 2004;110(suppl III):238.
58. Silva GV, Litowsky S, Assad JA, et al. Mesenchymal Stem cells differentiate into an endothelial phenotype, enhance vascular density and improve heart function in a chronic myocardial ischemia model. Circulation 2005;111(2):150–156.
59. Goodell M. Stem-cell "plasticity": befuddled by muddle. Curr Opin Hematol 2003;10;208–213.
60. Hocht-Zeisberger E, Kahnert H, Kaomei G. Cellular repopulation of myocardial infarction in patients with sex-mismatched heart transplantation. Eur Heart J 2004;25:749–758.
61. Murry CE, Soonpaa MH, Reinecke H, et al. Haematopoietic stem cells do not transdifferentiate into cardiac myocytes in myocardial infarcts. Nature 2004;428:664–668.
62. Losordo DW, Dimmeler S. Therapeutic angiogenesis and vasculogenesis for ischemic disease—part II: cell-based therapies. Circulation 2004;109:2692–2697.
63. Yeh ETH, Zhang S, Wu HD, et al. Transdifferentiation of human peripheral blood CD34+-enriched cell population into cardiomyocytes, endothelial cells, and smooth muscle cells in vivo. Circulation 2003;108:2070–2073.

64. Zhang S, Wang D, Estrov Z. Both cell fusion and transdifferentiation account for the transformation of human peripheral blood CD34-positive cells into cardiomyocytes in vivo. Circulation 2004;110: 3803–3807.

65. Forrester JS, Price MJ, Makkar RR. Stem cell repair of infarcted myocardium: an overview for clinicians. Circulation 2003;108:1139–1145.

66. Tang YL, Zhao Q, Zhang YC, et al. Autologous mesenchymal stem cell transplantation induce VEGF and neovascularization in ischemic myocardium. Regul Pept 2004;117:3–10.

67. Duan HF, Wu CT, Wu DL, et al. Treatment of myocardial ischemia with bone marrow-derived mesenchymal stem cells overexpressing hepatocyte growth factor. Mol Ther 2003;3:467–474.

68. Kudo M, Wang Y, Wani MA, et al. Implantation of bone marrow stem cells reduces the infarction and fibrosis in ischemic mouse heart. J Mol Cell Cardiol 2003,35:1113–1119.

69. Kinnaird T, Stabile E, Burnett MS. Local delivery of marrow-derived stromal cells augments collateral perfusion through paracrine mechanisms. Circulation 2004;109:1543–1549.

70. Kinnaird T, Stabile E, Burnett MS. Marrow-derived stromal cells express genes encoding a broad spectrum of arteriogenic cytokines and promote in vitro and in vivo arteriogenesis through paracrine mechanisms. Circ Res 2004;94:678–685.

71. Anversa P, Sussman MA, Bolli R. Molecular genetic advances in cardiovascular medicine focus on the myocyte. Circulation 2004;109:2832–2838.

72. Urbanek K, Quaini F, Tasca G, et al. Intense myocyte formation from cardiac stem cells in human cardiac hypertrophy. Proc Natl Acad Sci USA 2003;100:10,440–10,445.

73. Dohman HF, Perin EC, Takyia CM, et al. Transendocardial autologous bone marrow mononuclear cell injection in ischemic heart failure: postmortem anatomicopathologic and immunohistochemical findings. Circulation 2005;112:521–526.

74. Yoon YS, Park JS, Tkebuchava T, et al. Unexpected severe calcification after transplantation of bone marrow cells in acute myocardial infarction. Circulation 2004;109:3154–3157.

17

Clinical Angioblast Therapy

Amit N. Patel, MD, MS
and Jorge Genovese, MD, PhD

SUMMARY

Angiogenesis and vasculogenesis are fundamental processes in embryonic development enabling multiorgan characteristics. Through the capillary net, the nutrient diffusion process is successfully achieved in complex cellular organisms. In adults the establishment, maintenance, and renewal of an efficient vascular net are required for the maintenance of normal, viable tissues. This requirement is especially important in the cardiovascular system, where vascular supply efficiency and endothelium normal function are affected in many different pathological entities. Impaired angiogenesis and endothelial dysfunction are the bases of many cardiovascular diseases such as hypertension, coronary artery disease, myocardial infarction, and chronic heart failure.

Two different pathways of vessel development have been described: angiogenesis and vasculogenesis. Vasculogenesis is the process of new vessel development whereby primitive undifferentiated cells (angioblasts) differentiate to endothelial cells, which line a primitive network of embryological blood vessels. Angiogenesis describes the sprouting of differentiated preexisting endothelium into vascular tissue from preexisting capillaries. All blood vessels are lined with endothelial cells that must proliferate to form new vessels, migrate to reach remote targets, and survive in these different environments.

Angioblast/endothelial progenitor cells (EPCs) represent the phenotypic equivalent of embryonic angioblasts because they can be derived from both endothelial and mural cell types. Angioblast/EPCs can be isolated from bone marrow aspirate, peripheral blood, umbilical cord blood, or human adipose tissue. Clinical applications of angioblast/EPCs in cardiovascular disease are oriented to neovascularization induction in ischemic tissues, generation of new vessel nets in regenerative therapies, and endothelization of denuded endothelium, vascular grafts, and tissue engineering devices. The role of angioblast/EPCs directly injected into the myocardium for the treatment of ischemic heart failure will be discussed here.

Key Words: Angioblasts; vasculogenesis; angiogenesis; endothelium; stromal cells; bone marrow progenitor cells.

INTRODUCTION

Angiogenesis and vasculogenesis are fundamental processes in embryonic development enabling multiorgan characteristics. Through the capillary net, the nutrient diffusion process is successfully achieved in complex cellular organisms. In adults the establishment, maintenance, and renewal of an efficient vascular net are required for

From: *Contemporary Cardiology: Stem Cells and Myocardial Regeneration*
Edited by: M. S. Penn © Humana Press Inc., Totowa, NJ

the maintenance of normal, viable tissues. This requirement is especially important in the cardiovascular system, where vascular supply efficiency and endothelium normal function are affected in many different pathological entities. Impaired angiogenesis and endothelial dysfunction are the basis of many cardiovascular diseases, such as hypertension, coronary artery disease (CAD), myocardial infarction (MI), and chronic heart failure (CHF).

The vascular supply with the concomitant endothelium proliferation results from a delicate balance between pro- and antiangiogenic signals. Endothelium hyperproliferation or endothelial dysfunction and cell loss results in different pathological conditions. The adult microvascular system seems to be quiescent without capillary growth. Endothelial cell turnover in the normal healthy adult is low because of the presence of endogenous negative inhibitors suppressing positive signals. The control of this equilibrium is complex, multifactorial, and not yet totally understood. Despite this negative growth control, endothelium is much more than an inert inner cover of the vascular system and a perfect smooth limit between blood and tissues. It is also one of the largest organs in the body, with more than 1×10^{14} endothelial cells involved in the dramatic process of health and disease. The endothelium has a central role in homeostasis control. It is a target organ for many chemical and physical signals and, at the same time, is an active secretor organ that acts as a diffuse gland. Endothelial cells secrete molecules that participate in critical autocrine and paracrine loops. Some endothelial secretions modulate the tone and proliferation of vascular smooth muscle and have anti-inflammatory or antithrombotic effect. Under certain circumstances the endothelium can change its function and structure and specialize for the migration of lymphoid cells or express adhesion molecules for neutrophils (1), becoming a protagonist in the inflammation involved in reparatory or destructive processes. Altered growth control of endothelium is the basis of many diseases with a variety of etiologies, such as diabetes (2–5) or renal failure (6). A characteristic example of a key pathological process that results in altered angiogenesis is tumor proliferation (7,8). It was Judas Folkman's pioneering contribution in cancer research that demonstrated a therapeutic use of angiogenesis modulators (9). Using almost the same signals in the malignant process, changes in basal angiogenesis are required for fundamental physiological processes such as wound healing (10), the female reproduction system cycle, or response to injury or mechanical stress. These findings form the basis for potential therapeutic angiogenesis.

ANGIOGENESIS AND ANGIOBLASTS

Two different pathways of vessel development have been described: angiogenesis and vasculogenesis. Vasculogenesis is the process of new vessel development whereby primitive undifferentiated cells (angioblasts) differentiate to endothelial cells, which line a primitive network of embryological blood vessels. Angiogenesis describes the sprouting of differentiated preexisting endothelium into vascular tissue from preexisting capillaries (11–13). All blood vessels are lined with endothelial cells that must proliferate to form new vessels, migrate to reach remote targets, and survive in these different environments.

It was believed that angiogenesis was the process responsible for neovascularization and vasculogenesis in the adult, but the known mechanism was thought to be limited to only embryonic development. This concept has been refuted by the finding that circulating bone marrow-derived progenitor cells with properties of embryonic angioblasts have been isolated in adults *(14)*. The precursor cell differentiates into mature endothelial cells, which have been termed endothelial progenitor cells or angioblasts (angioblast/EPCs). Postnatal vasculogenesis also occurs, playing a central role in adult neovascularization in normal and pathological conditions *(15–18)*. Adult angioblast/EPCs seeded with human smooth muscle cells form microvessels on porous polyglycolic acid-poly-L-lactic acid (PGA-PLLA) scaffolds *(19)*. This report suggests that angioblast/EPCs may be well suited for creating microvascular networks within tissue-engineered constructs. Angioblast/EPCs control a number of signals, including different growth factors and their receptors, with vascular endothelial growth factor (VEGF) in a central role, as well as other signals that are even more complex, such as mechanical and metabolic stress and the characteristics of the extracellular matrix (ECM).

In the past, the term hemangioblasts was used to define discrete cell masses that develop in chick embryo cultures known for their hematopoietic and endothelial potential *(20,21)*. Today the name hemangioblast is restricted to a single progenitor cell with this function *(22)*. Angioblast/EPCs represent the phenotypic equivalent of embryonic angioblasts because they can be derived from both endothelial and mural cell types *(19)*. The role of bone marrow as source of progenitor endothelial cells was demonstrated in bone marrow transplantation between genetically different dogs. The Dacron graft implanted in the thoracic aorta developed an endothelium that was of donor marrow origin *(23)*. Angioblast/EPCs can be isolated from bone marrow aspirate, peripheral blood, umbilical cord blood, or human adipose tissue *(24–28)*. The relation between angioblast/EPCs and mesoderm is evident, and their presence in other mesenchimatic stroma is predictable. Today, bone marrow is the best studied source of angioblast/EPCs. In bone marrow, cells expressing CD133 and positives for VEGF receptors 1 and 2 (VEGFR-1 and VEGFR-2), Oct-4, and telomerase are part of a heterogeneous population defined as multipotent adult progenitor cells that can also generate other progenitor cells such as mesenchymal stem cells (MSCs) *(29)*. A small portion of those cells, perhaps representing the true angioblast/EPC fraction, will express progenitor and endothelial cell markers such as CD34, vascular-endothelial (VE)-cadherin, and E-selectin *(30)*. These early CD34$^+$ cells secrete VEGF and granulocyte–colony-stimulating factor (G-CSF) via paracrine and autocrine secretion systems. Angioblast/EPCs are understood to be adult cells with the capacity to originate endothelium and constitute a heterogeneous population that includes tissue resident stem cells isolated from the heart *(31)* with a high plasticity in culture. Mobilization of angioblast/EPCs from bone marrow is a highly complex process with many unanswered questions. These cells have the capacity to move from bone marrow, enter into the peripheral circulation (i.e., circulating angioblast/EPCs) (and home to sites of active angiogenesis), where they complete their differentiation and incorporate into the endothelium of new vessels. Angioblast/EPCs recruited in this way participate in the repair of damaged tissues, including the heart *(32–35)*. Circulating angioblast/EPCs, originating in bone marrow, play a significant role in neovascularization of ischemic tissues *(35,36)*, and their injection into the ischemic site induces neovascularization *(37,38)*. Unfortunately, a characteristic of circulating angioblast/EPCs is their low number, and even worse, their number is reduced in some patients with vascular dysfunction. Patients with risk factors for ischemic coronary heart disease have been found with a reduced number of angioblast/EPCs, and these cells showed impaired function and reduced availability to home to the ischemic tissues *(39–41)*. Similar reduction is observed in patients with predisposing atherosclerotic factors *(42)*. The treatment with hydroxymethylglutaryl coenzyme A (HMG-CoA) reductase inhibitors increases the number of circulating angioblast/EPCs *(43,44)*. In a similar mode, estrogen increases bone marrow-derived angioblast/EPC production and diminishes neointima formation *(45)*. A reduced number of angioblast/EPCs is also observed in cardiac transplantation patients with vasculopathy and patients with in-stent restenosis *(46,47)*. The angioblast/EPC number reduction related to aging has not only cardiovascular but systemic effects. Also, the low angioblast/EPC level has a similar role in the pathophysiology of cerebrovascular disease *(48)* and, perhaps, in many other conditions in the elderly. In all these conditions, the potential value of a cell-based regenerative therapy is dramatic, and efforts should be made to obtain sufficient amounts of angioblast/EPCs to perform autologous cell therapy.

Some alternatives to resolve the angioblast/EPC availability limitation are the improvement of isolation and expansion systems, the use of angiogenic factor gene transfer in the affected tissues *(49,50)*, or the use of other sources of angioblast/EPCs. Angioblast/EPC isolation can be improved up to 14-fold using white blood cell reduction filters to obtain material as a starting sample *(51)*. Angioblast/EPC amplification is limited by the time-dependent phenotypic changes observed in culture. In dogs, however, canine angioblast/EPCs can be isolated and successfully cultured from the peripheral blood mononuclear cell fraction (PBMC). The angioblast/EPCs isolated in this manner had a greater growth potential when compared to mature endothelial cells, suggesting that the PBMC fraction is a useful source of angioblast/EPCs for therapy *(52)*. There are other sources of angioblast/EPCs, and these sources appear to be possible alternatives to obtain the major number of cells for the ideal tool for autologous cells therapies for angiogenesis restoration. Human adipose tissue-derived stem cells, for example, are known for their high plasticity and their capacity to improve postnatal neovascularization *(53)*. A recent report describes the isolation and culture of Flk-1[+] cells from human adipose tissue. These cells, cultured in an endothelial cell-specific medium, expressing VE-cadherin, von Willebrand's factor, and a lectin receptor, took up low-density lipoproteins, showing the capacity to incorporate into an endothelial cell tubular network. This method described the ability to yield a large number of Flk-1[+] cells, which are able to differentiate into mature endothelial cells. The proliferative capacity is related to the culture time required to amplify a cell population in vitro. The majority of isolated angioblast/EPCs change their phenotypes in culture in a time-dependent mode and after 4 days express markers of monocyte/macrophage origin. This plasticity should be considered when experiments with angioblast/EPCs will be performed and when it is necessary to define a population that will be assayed.

In vivo, despite the number of circulating angioblast/EPCs, effective mobilization and homing of angioblast/EPCs during an ischemic episode is a critical regulative step of neovascularization. Vascular trauma such as coronary bypass grafting or burn injury induces a rapid but transient mobilization of angioblast/EPCs within a time frame consistent with the release of VEGF, similar to what happens during a myocardial infarct *(54)*, unstable angina *(47)*, or during an acute severe trauma such as a burn *(36,55)*.

CD34[+] cells and angioblast/EPC mobilization occurs in patients with heart failure with a biphasic response: initial elevation with a depression in the advanced phase. The authors correlate this effect with the myelosuppressive role of tumor necrosis factor (TNF)-α *(56)*.

In the murine model of soft tissue ischemia, angioblast/EPCs are recruited to ischemic tissue within 72 hours, and the extent of recruitment is directly proportional to the degree of tissue ischemia. After 7 days, elevated levels of circulating VEGF and the VEGFR-2 cells were observed. At day 21, functional vessels appear, originating from vascular cords derived from the coalescence of proliferate cells clusters (57). A rapid recruitment of angioblast/EPCs is also observed in the myocardium after ischemic preconditioning (58). This early recruitment is a significant parameter when defining the time frame for autologous cells therapies in ischemic episodes. This early demand is an obvious conflict with the paucity of circulating angioblast/EPCs and the difficult in vitro EPC expansion. A preventative collection, expansion, and storage of angioblast/EPCs in patients in clear risk of ischemic episodes, especially those with diminished numbers of angioblast/EPCs, could be useful as an early intervention tool in autologous angiogenic therapy. This strategy could have particular importance for those patients with reduced circulating angioblast/EPCs because this reduction is an independent prediction marker of future cardiovascular events (39,41).

CLINICAL APPLICATIONS OF ANGIOBLAST/EPCs

Clinical applications of angioblast/EPCs in cardiovascular disease are oriented to neovascularization induction in ischemic tissues, generation of new vessel nets in regenerative therapies and endothelization of denuded endothelium (59), vascular grafts, and tissue engineering devices (60). Some of these approaches are discussed in other chapters. The role of angioblast/EPCs directly injected into the myocardium for the treatment of ischemic heart failure will be discussed here.

The positive effects of intramyocardial angioblast/EPC transplantation has been demonstrated in animals (61,62). In humans the most frequent source of cells used to induce angiogenesis has been bone marrow (63–66). There still remains some question as to whether hematopoietic stem cells can transdifferentiate into cardiomyocytes (67), but the beneficial effect of implanted cells on local angiogenesis has been demonstrated (68,69). In this effect, the role of angioblast/EPCs could be fundamental, because bone marrow mononuclear cells contain the cell population that has demonstrated a capacity to home to the ischemic myocardium and participate in neovascularization (32,33, 35–37,54). A recent report of postmortem anatomicopathological and immunohistochemical findings in a heart failure patient treated 11 months prior with transendocardial autologous bone marrow mononuclear cell injections demonstrated objective evidence of perfusion improvement. However, this was a mixture of bone marrow cells, not isolated angioblast/EPCs. Without evidence of abnormal tissue or vascular growth, one of the most significant findings was a higher capillary density in the cell-treated area than in the nontreated areas of heart (70). Although this report is limited to an isolated uncontrolled case, microscopic evidence correlates with the improvement in perfusion assessed in this case and reported by other authors (33,63–65,71). Based on this early angiogenesis work for ischemic heart disease with minimal ventricular dysfunction, our group progressed to evaluate patients with ischemic disease progressively leading to CHF. Our early trials involved the use of bone marrow-derived angioblast/EPCs being directly injected into the myocardium during coronary artery bypass surgery. Patients were selected based on having ischemic heart failure with a least one surgically revascularizable target, usually the left anterior descending artery. Preoperative electrocardiograms, two-dimensional stress echocardiograms, single photon emission computed tomography (SPECT), and a chest X-ray were used to identify regions of nonrevascularizable viable myocardium to be injected. Inclusion criteria were as follows: ischemic heart failure with an ejection fraction of 35% or less on two imaging studies (echocardiogram and multiplanar cardiac catheterization) and a New York Heart Association heart failure functional class III or IV. All patients had prior percutaneous coronary interventions and had optimal medical management of their heart failure. Patients were excluded if they had a current or prior malignancy, any hematological disorder, renal failure requiring dialysis, left ventricular aneurysm, prior cardiac surgery, valvular disease requiring surgery, preoperative steroid therapy, or were within 6 days of an acute coronary event.

Our randomized study was based on 20 patients who received either off-pump coronary artery bypass grafting (OPCAB) or OPCAB plus angioblast/EPC cell therapy. Patients in the OPCAB-only group had a standard sternotomy and OPCAB grafting performed using both apical suction and pressure stabilization of the heart. Patients in the angioblast/EPC therapy group had their bone marrow harvested after a general anesthetic was given. Using this technique, 500–600 mL of bone marrow was harvested. The bone marrow was processed as previously described using a magnetic bead cell isolation system. As the bone marrow was being processed, the OPCAB was performed and the preselected sites of myocardial dyskinesis, akinesis, but not the infarcted regions were injected with the angioblast/EPC preparation using a needle apparatus. The injections were in the following areas: peri-infarcted, viable but dykinetic, or akinetic. There were no injections into the scar itself. The needle apparatus does not have an end hole like most needles; it only has side holes. This reduces the amount of leakage that would be generated during a standard distal end-holed needle. The injection placement was based on prior echocardiogram and SPECT viewing to determine ventricle wall thickness, preventing direct introduction of cells into the ventricle. The cell preparation was delivered as the needle was withdrawn from the myocardium. The injections were spaced up to 1 cm apart to avoid coronary vessels and were 3–5 mm in depth based on echocardiography findings of wall thickness. No direct intracoronary injections were performed. The patients were monitored just as standard postoperative heart surgery patients. The median amount of bone marrow harvested was 550 cc, with a median of 22×10^6 CD34$^+$ cells in the final specimen. The ejection fractions for preoperative, 1-month, 3-month, and 6-month analysis were 31, 36, 36, and 37%, respectively, for the OPCAB-only group, and 29, 42, 45, and 46%, respectively, for the OPCAB + angioblast/EPC group. This demonstrated a significant increase in ejection fraction for the OPCAB + angioblast/EPC group. These improvements where seen on both echocardiography and by SPECT. The only adverse event was related to bone marrow harvest, where the site of harvesting had a hematoma in one patient. There were no other adverse events in either group: neurological, hematological, vascular, death, or infection. The key is that no patients had any postoperative arrhythmias, which are seen with other cell types (66).

This was one of the first prospective randomized blinded approaches to cellular therapy for ischemic heart failure. One of the confounding factors of this study is the adjunctive use of OPCAB, even though the cells were not injected into the same region as the bypass graft. In our more recent trials we are using gated diffusion magnetic resonance imaging. Even though this imaging modality is very important in the evaluation of heart failure patients owing do the fact that multiple parameters, such as anatomy, function, and viability can be assessed, it is limited because it is very expensive and cannot be used in patients with implantable anti-arrhythmic devices. We have evolved the use of angioblast/EPCs to application in patients with nonrevascularizable ischemic heart failure, who are not candidates for surgical revascularization and have not had prior surgery. We had devised a minimally invasive surgical technique to deliver cells into the myocardium. Ongoing randomized trials were expected to be completed in late 2006.

MECHANISMS OF ANGIOBLAST/EPCs: FUNCTION AND REGULATION

In addition to the clinical benefits that have been demonstrated in ischemic heart disease using angioblast/EPCs, the potentials mechanisms of action must be evaluated. Three mechanisms show promise of combined benefits to the ischemic myocardium: transdifferentiation to blood vessels or myocardium, fusion with the native dysfunctional myocytes to augment function and homing, which a may be a systemic or paracrine response for recruiting other cells, and growth factors to help improve oxygen delivery and myocardial function. The paracrine action of bone marrow MSCs implanted after MI in an animal model has been recently reported *(72)*. The grafted MSCs release bFGF, VEGF, and stromal-derived factor (SDF)-1α, induce an efficient vascular regeneration and attenuate the apoptotic pathway. SDF-1α may have an effect on homing circulating angioblast/EPCs; an alternative way through bone marrow implant involves angioblast/EPCs. The detected secretion of angiogenic factors, such as bFGF and VEGF, confirms the notion of paracrine circuits with different cells, including angioblast/EPCs. Furthermore, the increased expression of VEGF is not limited to the injection area, attracting our attention to the potential risk of undesired angiogenesis in nonaffected parts of a specific treated organ or even at a systemic level.

Cytokines and chemokines play a fundamental part in angiogenesis and vasculogenesis and, therefore, are potential therapeutic tools associated with angioblast/EPCs clinical application.

VEGF is the most specific growth factor for vascular endothelium and is required for normal embryonic and adult vasculogenesis and angiogenesis *(73–76)*. It was first discovered in 1983 as a vascular permeability factor and later was well characterized as an endothelial cell mitogen *(77,78)*. VEGF belongs to a gene family that includes placental growth factor (PlGF), VEGF-A, VEGF-B, VEGF-C, VEGF-D, and VEGF-D. There are three VEGF tyrosine kinase receptors identified so far: VEGFR-1 (Flt-1, fms-like tyrosine kinase), VEGFR-2 (Flk1, KDR; kinase insert domain containing receptor), and VEGFR-3 (Ftl-4) *(54,79)*. VEGF-A interacts with both VEGFR-1 and VEGFR-2. VEGF-A induces the recruitment of circulating endothelial precursors (CEPs) in a similar mode than Ang1 but with different kinetics. Ang1 gives a lower but more sustained stimulation. CEP recruitment to the circulation is also dependent on matrix metalloproteinase-9-induced release of soluble kit ligand, which increases cell proliferation, motility, and angioblast/EPC mobilization to the circulation *(80,81)*. VEGF is an endothelial cell-specific mitogen in vitro and an angiogenic inducer in vivo. VEGF also induces vasodilatation of preexisting capillaries through nitric oxide production *(82)* by increasing their permeability and ECM degradation *(83–85)*. Permeability changes will permit proteins extravasations, and these proteins will constitute the preliminary matrix for new vessels. VEGF also induces endothelial fenestration in some vascular beds *(86)*. VEGF is a survival factor for endothelial cells, both in vivo and in vitro, and its antiapoptotic activity was demonstrated in neonatal mice *(87)*. VEGF-C and -D regulate lymphatic angiogenesis *(88,89)*.

PlGF binds VEGFR-1 and VEGFR-2 as a VEGFR-1/VEGFR-2 heterodimer *(90)*. PlGF stimulates the formation of vessels in ischemic heart disease. PlGF also play a critical role in the recruitment and homing of circulating angioblast/EPCs and support recruitment for vasculogenesis at the site of ischemia.

Muscle fibers and skeletal muscle satellite cells *(91,92)* express VEGFR-2, suggesting a specific action of VEGF and P1GF in postischemic cardiac tissue regeneration and a potential application of those growth factors in myoblasts culture and expansion.

Small-scale feasibility and safety clinical trials have been performed to evaluate the use of bone marrow cell transplantation in treatment of myocardial infarction. Some of these trials report little effect on local contractility, but a pronounced improvement was seen in myocardial angiogenesis mediated by AC133[+] cells contained in bone marrow injections *(65)*, while others attribute the detected improvements in treated patients to angiogenesis and cardiomyogenesis *(93)*. Others, more conservative, do not define a mechanism for the observed patient improvement *(94)*. In animal models, angioblast/EPCs have shown a capacity to augment neovascularization of ischemic tissues *(33,61,95,96)*.

An effect of angioblast/EPCs on contractile myocardium activity cannot be discounted either. The ability of circulating angioblast/EPCs from healthy adults and CAD patients to transdifferentiate in vitro into functionally active cardiomyocytes when co-cultivated with rat cardiomyocytes has been reported *(97)*. A similar phenomenon has been described when adipocyte-derived stem cells, already mentioned in this review, are co-cultivated with cardiomyoctyes *(98)*.

Fibroblast growth factor (FGF)-2) but not VEGF upregulates telomerase activity. This suggests that FGF-2 activity could play a functional role in preventing the early onset of senescence and could be implicated in the overproliferation of endothelium *(99,100)*. However, a recent study has reported positive regulation by VEGF of telomerase activity in vitro and in vivo. This result agrees with the mitogenic activity of VEGF and the reduced cell viability, altered differentiation, and impaired regenerative/proliferative responses observed in telomere dysfunction *(101)*.

Erythropoietin stimulates angioblast/EPC proliferation *(102)*, and signals involved in trafficking control of hematopoietic cells such as SDF-1 can mobilize early angioblast/EPCs *(103)*. The regulation of EPC mobilization appeared to be specific for patients with ischemic heart disease *(104)*.

Other cytokines that have been reported to regulate angiogenesis in vivo include epidermal growth factor, transforming growth factor (TGF)-α and -β, platelet-derived growth factor (PDGF-BB), hepatocyte growth factor, interleukin (IL)-1, -6, -8, and -12, interferons, TNF-α, G-CSF *(105)*, and granulocyte-macrophage colony stimulating factor *(106,107)*. Expression of TGF-ββ in transfected smooth muscle cells regulates angioblast/EPC migration and differentiation *(108)*. Furthermore, VEGF induces TGF-β expression in endothelial cells. Alterations in endothelial cells of the aging heart lead to a deregulation in the cardiac myocyte PDGF-B-induced paracrine pathway, which contributes to impaired cardiac angiogenic function. Young, but not old, bone marrow can restore this activity in vitro and in vivo *(109,110)*. Human chorionic gonadotrophin, a hormonal factor of trophoblastic origin, is another angiogenic factor involved in trophoblast invasion, a process to very similar tumor invasion, and placental development *(111,112)*. In addition, the number of circulating angioblast/EPCs increased gradually and paralleled the progression of gestational age. The number of angioblast/EPCs correlates significantly with the level of serum estradiol, suggesting that angioblast/EPCs may play an important role in the regulation and maintenance of the placental development and vascular integrity during pregnancy (113).

Besides chemical signals, physical forces, such as exposure to cold, turbulent blood flow, wall shear stress, capillary wall tension, changes in peripheral resistance, capillary pressure, vessel diameter, and red cell velocity, have all been implicated in angiogenesis. These types of stimuli can cause changes in the endothelial cytoskeleton and the ECM, thus facilitating endothelial cell migration. Increased shear stress is an inducer of different cytokines (114).

Hypoxia is a strong stimulus for angiogenesis and can switch on the expression of several angiogenic factors, including VEGF, nitric oxide synthase (NOS), PDGF, etc., via activating hypoxia-inducible transcription factors (115). This action is not restricted to pathological conditions.

It is well known that regular physical exercise improves endothelial dysfunction and promotes cardiovascular health. It has been recently reported that this type of exercise augments the number of circulating angioblast/EPCs in patients with cardiovascular risk factors and in patients with CAD and is associated with improved vascular function and NOS (116).

Transient stimulus such as high-altitude trekking results in an increase in the number of angioblast/EPCs, which, at sea level, totally reverts in 45 days (117). This mechanism forced us to consider the red-cell compensatory production at altitude. It is demonstrated that a single bout of exercise increases VEGF mRNA (118). In trained subjects this response is attenuated; they show 20% more capillaries in their musculature. Nitric oxide appears to be important in this action because NOS inhibition attenuates the skeletal muscle VEGF mRNA response to exercise (119). In the opposite way, a transient decrease in pulmonary VEGF leads to increased alveolar and bronchial cell apoptosis, air space enlargement, and changes in lung elastic recoil resembling processes characteristic of emphysema (120). Smoking has been reported to reduce the number of circulating angioblast/EPCs, and smoking cessation rapidly increases angioblast/EPC levels in peripheral blood, even in chronic smokers (121).

SUMMARY

The origin, functions, and regulation of angioblast/EPCs have clarified our understanding of adult angiogenesis and vasculogenesis. Information from many disciplines has led to the rapid clinical translation of angioblast/EPCs for the treatment of cardiovascular disease. The early results of direct implantation of cells into the myocardium are very promising and thus far have been safe. However, previous studies have failed to adequately address the fact that the mechanism of action of the cells may be manyfold and may include all of the discussed processes, including transdifferentiation, fusing, and homing. Future studies will need to be performed in which the pathology can be more closely examined. We have started two phase I Food and Drug Administration studies to further evaluate the cells in humans. The first involves implanting angioblast/EPCs into the myocardium at the time of left ventricular assist device implantation as a bridge to cardiac transplantation. This will provide a unique perspective on the specific cellular transformations that occur in ischemic cardiomyopathy, as the entire native heart will be excised at the time of transplantation and be available for evaluation.

The second trial is a double-blinded randomized coronary revascularization study to evaluate if there is a dose-response of angioblast/EPCs. We are only at the beginning of cardiac cell therapy for the treatment of heart failure, but the future is very promising, with new cells and cocktails of cells and growth factors.

REFERENCES

1. Steven A, Lowe J. Blood and lymphatic circulatory system and heart. In:Human Histology, 2nd ed. CV Mosby, Nottingham, UK, 1997, pp. 137–158.
2. Cooper ME, Gilbert RE, Jerums G. Diabetic vascular complications. Clin Exp Pharmacol Physiol 1997;24:770–775.
3. Dahl-Jorgensen K. Diabetic microangiopathy. Acta Paediatr Suppl 1998;425:31–34.
4. Loomans CJM, de Koening EJP, Staal FJT, et al. Endothelial progenitor cell dysfunction. A novel concept in the pathogenesis of vascular complications of type I diabetes. Diabetes 2004;53:195–199.
5. Tepper OM, Galiano RD, Capla JM, et al. Human endothelial progenitor cells from type II diabetes exhibit impaired proliferation, adhesion, and incorporation into vascular structures. Circulation 2002;106:2781–2786.
6. Choi J-H, Kim KL, Huh W, Kim B, Byun J, Suh W, Sung J, Jeon E-S, Oh H-Y, Kim D-K. Decreased number and impaired angiogenic function of endothelial progenitors in patients with chronic renal failure. Arterioscler Thromb Vasc Biol 2004;24:1246–1252.
7. Folkman J. Role of angiogenesis in tumor growth and metastasis. Semin Oncol. 2002;29(6 Suppl 16):15–18.
8. Kyzas PA, Stefanou D, Batistatou A, Agnantis NJ: Hypoxia-induced tumor angiogenic pathway in head and neck cancer: an in vivo study. Cancer Lett 2005;225(2):297–304.
9. Folkman J. Tumor angiogenesis: therapeutic implications 1971. N Engl J Med 285:1182–1186.
10. Suh W, Kim KL, Kim JM. Transplantation of endothelial progenitor cells accelerates dermal wound healing with increased recruitment of monocytes/macrophages and neovascularization. Stem Cells 2005;23(10):1571–1578.
11. Carmeliet P: Mechanism of angiogenesis and arteriogenesis. Nat Med 2000;6:395–398.
12. Quarmby JW, Halliday AW. Angiogenesis: Basic concepts and the application of gene therapy. In: Introduction to Vascular Biology: From Basic Science to Clinical Practice. Cambridge University Press, West Nyack, NY, 2002, pp. 93–129.
13. Grupta K, Zhan J. Angiogenesis: a curse or cure? Postgrad Med J 2005;81:236–242.
14. Asahara T, Murohara T, Sullivan A, et al. Isolation of putative progenitor endothelial cells for angiogenesis. Science 1997;275:964–967.
15. Peichev M, Naiyer AJ, Pereira D, et al. Expression of VEGFR-2 and AC133 by circulating CD34+ cells identifies a population of functional endothelial precursors. Blood 2000;95(3):952–958.
16. Gehling UM, Ergün S, Schumacher U, et al. In vitro differentiation of endothelial cells from AC133-positive progenitor cells. Blood. 2000;95(10):3106–3112.
17. Quirici N, Soligo D, Canela L, et al. Differentiation and expansion of endothelial cells from human bone marrow CD133+cells. Br J Haematol. 2001;115:186–194.
18. Loges S, Fehse B, Brockmann MA, et al. Identification of the adult human hemangioblast. Stem Cells Dev 2004;13(3):229–242.
19. Wu X, Rabkin-Aikawa E, Guleserian KJ, et al. Tissue-engineered microvessels on three-dimensional biodegradable scaffolds using human endothelial progenitor cells. Am J Physiol Heart Circ Physiol 2004;287(2):H480–H487.
20. Murray PDF. The development in vitro of the blood of the early chick embryo. Proc Roy Soc 1932;111:497–521.
21. Choi K. The hemangioblasts: a common progenitor of hematopoietic and endothelial cells. J Hematother Stem Cell Res 2002;11:91–101.
22. Gordon K. The hemangioblasts. Marshak, In: Stem Cell Biology. Cold Spring Harbor Laboratory Press, Woodbury, NY, 2001, p. 346.
23. Shi Q, Rafii S, Wu MH, Wijelath ES, et al. Evidence for circulating bone marrow-derived endothelial cells. Blood 1998;92(2):362–367.
24. Elsheikh E, Uzunel M, He Z, et al. Only a specific subset of human peripheral blood monocytes has endothelial-like functional capacity. Blood 2005;106(7):2347–2355.
25. Pesce M, Orlandi A, Iachininoto MG, et al. Myoendothelial differentiation of human umbilical cord blood-derived stem cells in ischemic limb tissues. Circ Res 2003;93:E51–E62.

26. Schmidta D, Molb A, Neuenschwandera S, et al. Living patches engineered from human umbilical cord derived fibroblasts and endothelial progenitor cells. Eur J Cardiothorac Surg 2005;27:795–800.

27. Kim SY, Park SY, Kim JM, et al. Differentiation of endothelial cells from human umbilical cord blood AC133–CD14+ cells. Ann Hematol 2005;84:417–422.

28. Martinez-Estrada OM, Munoz-Santos Y, Julveb J, et al. Human adipose tissue as a source of Flk-1+ cells: new method of differentiation and expansion. Cardiovasc Res 2005;65:328–333.

29. Hristov M, Weber C. Endotelial progenitor cells: characterization, pathophysiology, and possible clinical relevante. J Cell Mol Med 2004;l8(4):498–508.

30. Rehman J, Li J, Orschell CM, March KL. Peripheral blood "endothelial progenitor cells" bare derived from monocyte/macrophage and secrete angiogenic growth factors Circulation 2003;107:1164–1169.

31. Beltrami AP, Barlucchi L, Torella D, et al. Adult cardiac stem cells are multipotent and support myocardial regeneration. Cell 2003;114(6):763–776.

32. Takahashi T, Kalka C, Masuda H, et al. Ischemia- and cytokine-induced mobilization of bone-marrow-derived endothelial progenitor cells for neovascularization. Nat Med 1999;5:434–438.

33. Kocher AA, Schuster MD, Szabolcs MJ, et al. Neovascularization of ischemic myocardium by human bone-marrow-derived angioblasts prevents cardiomyocyte apoptosis, reduces remodeling and improves cardiac function. Nat Med. 2001;7:430–436.

34. Urbich C, Dimmeler S. Endothelial progenitor cells. Characterization and role in vascular biology. Circ Res 2004;95:343–353.

35. Raffi S, Lyden D. Therapeutic stem and progenitor cell transplantation for organ vascularization and regeneration. Nat Med 2003;9:702–712.

36. Shintani S, Murohara T, Ikeda H, et al. Mobilization of endothelial progenitor cells in patients with acute myocardial infarction Circulation 2001;103:2776–2779.

37. Kalka C, Masuda H, Takahashi T, et al.Vascular endothelial growth factor(165) gene transfer augments circulating endothelial progenitor cells in human subjects Circ Res 2000;86(12):1198–1202.

38. Kawamoto A, Gwon H-C, Iwaguro H, et al. Therapeutic potential of ex vivo expanded endothelial progenitor cells for myocardial ischemia. Circulation 2001;103:634–637.

39. Hill JM, Zalos G, Halcox JP, et al. Circulating endothelial progenitor cells, vascular function and cardiovascular risk. N Engl J Med 2003;348:593–600.

40. Vasa M, Fichtlscherer S, Aicher A, et al. Number and migratory activity of circulating endothelial progenitor cells inversely correlate with risk factors for coronary artery disease. Circ Res 2001;89(1):E1–E7.

41. Schmidt-Lucke C, Rossig L, Fichtlscherer S, et al. Reduced number of circulating endothelial progenitor cells predicts future cardiovascular events: proof of concept for the clinical importance of endogenous vascular repair. Circulation 2005;111(22):2981–2987.

42. Simons M, Bonow RO, Chronos NA, et al. Clinical trials in coronary angiogenesis: issues, problems, consensus: an expert panel summary. Circulation 2002;102:E73–E86.

43. Llevadot J, Murasawa S, Kureishi Y, et al. HMG-CoA reductase inhibitor mobilizes bone marrow-derived endothelial progenitor cells. J Clin Invest 2001;108:339–405.

44. Walter DH, Rittig K, Bahlmann FH, et al. Statin therapy accelerates reendothelialization: a novel effect involving mobilization and incorporation of bone marrow-derived endothelial progenitor cells. Circulation 2002;105:3017–3024.

45. Strehlow K, Werner N, Berweiler J, et al. Estrogen increases bone-marrow derived endothelial progenitor cell production and diminishes neointima formation. Circulation 2003;107:3059–3065.

46. Simper D, Wang S, Deb A, et al. Endothelial progenitor cells are decreased in blood of cardiac allograft patients with vasculopathy and endothelial cells of non cardiac origin are enriched in transplant atherosclerosis. Circulation 2003;107:143–149.

47. George J, Herz I, Goldstein E, et al. Number and adhesive properties of circulating endothelial progenitor cells in patients with in-stent restenosis. Arterioscler Thromb Vasc Biol 2003;23:E57–E60.

48. Ghani U, Shuaib A, Salam A. Endothelial progenitor cells during Cerebrovascular disease. Stroke 2005;36:151–153.

49. Chachques JC, Duarte F, Cattadori B, et al. Angiogenic growth factors and/or cellular therapy for myocardial regeneration: a comparative study. J Thorac Cardiovasc Surg 2004;128(2):245–253.

50. Iwaguro H, Yamaguchi J, Kalka C, et al. Endothelial progenitor cell vascular endothelial growth factor gene transfer for vascular regeneration. Circulation 2000;105(6):732–738.

51. Teleron AA, Carlson B, Young PP. Blood donor white blood cell reduction filters as a source of human peripheral blood-derived endothelial progenitor cells Transfusion 2005;45(1):21–25.

52. Wu H, Riha G.M., Yang H., et al. Differentiation and Proliferation of Endothelial Progenitor Cells from Canine Peripheral Blood Mononuclear Cells. J Surg Res 2005;126:193–198.

53. Miranville A, Heeschen C, Sengenes C, et al. Improvement of postnatal neovascularization by human adipose tissue-derived stem cells. Circulation 2004;110:349–355.
54. Massa M, Rosti V, Ferrario M, et al. Increased circulating hematopoietic and endothelial progenitor cells in the early phase of acute myocardial infarction. Blood 2005;105:199–206.
55. Gill M, Dias S, Hattori K, Rivera ML, et al. Vascular trauma induces rapid but transient mobilization of VEGFR2(+)AC133(+) endothelial precursor cells Circ Res 2001;88(2):167–174.
56. Valgimigli M, Rigolin GM, Fucili A, et al. CD34+ and endothelial progenitor cells in patients with various degrees of congestive heart failure. Circulation 2004;110(10):1209–1212.
57. Tepper OM, Capla JM, Galiano RD, et al. Adult vasculogenesis occurs through in situ recruitment, proliferation, and tubulization of circulating bone marrow-derived cells Blood 2005;105:1068–1077.
58. Li M, Nishimura H, MD, PhD; Iwakura A. Endothelial progenitor cells are rapidly recruited to myocardium and mediate protective effect of ischemic preconditioning via "imported" nitric oxide synthase activity. Circulation 2005;111:1114–1120.
59. Werner N, Junk S, Laufs L, et al. Intravenous transfusion of endothelial progenitor cells reduces neointima formation after vascular injury. Circ Res 2003;93:E17–E24.
60. Griese DP, Ehsan A, Melo LG, et al. Isolation and transplantation of autologous circulating endothelial cells into denuded vessels and prosthetic grafts: implications for cell-based vascular therapy. Circulation 2003;108:2710–2715.
61. Kawamoto A, Asahara T, Losordo DW. Transplantation of endothelial progenitor cells for therapeutic neovascularization Cardiovasc Radiat Med 2002;3(3–4):221–225.
62. Schuster MD, Kocher AA, Seki T, Martens TP. Myocardial neovascularization by bone marrow angioblasts results in cardiomyocyte regeneration. Am J Physiol Heart Circ Physiol 2004; 287(2):H525–H532.
63. Assmus B, Schachinger V, Teupe C, et al. Transplantation of progenitor cells and regeneration enhancement in acute myocardial infarction (TOPCARE-AMI) 2002. Circulation 2002;106:3009–3017.
64. Wollert KC, Meyer GP, Lotz J, Ringes-Lichtenberg S et al.: Intracoronary autologous bone- marrow cell transfer after myocardial infarction: the BOOST randomized clinical trial. Lancet 2004;364: 141–148.
65. Stamm C, Westphal B, Kleine HD et al.: Autologous bone-marrow stem-cell transplantation for myocardial regeneration. Lancet 2003;361:45–46.
66. Patel AN, Geffner L, Viña RF, et al. Surgical treatment for congestive heart failure using autologous adult stem cell transplantation: a prospective randomized study. J Thorac Cardiovasc Surg 2005;130(6):1631–1638.
67. Murry C.E., Soonpaa M.H., Reinecke H, et al. Haematopoietic stem cells do not transdifferentiate into cardiac myocytes in myocardial infarcts. Nature 2000;428:664–668.
68. Fuchs, S., Baffour, R., Zhou, et al. Transendocardial delivery of autologous bone marrow enhances collateral perfusion and reginal function in pigs with chronic experimental myocardial ischemia. J Am Coll Cardiol 2001;37:1726–1732.
69. Liu Y, Guo J, Zhang P, et al. Bone marrow mononuclear cell transplantation into heart elevates the expression of angiogenic factors. Microvasc Res 2004;68(3):156–160.
70. Dohmann FR, Perin EC, et al. Transendocardial autologous bone marrow mononuclear cell injection in ischemic heart failure postmortem anatomicopathologic and immunohistochemical findings. Circulation 2005;112:521–526.
71. Li TS, Hamano K, Hirata K, et al. The safety and feasibility of the local implantation of autologous bone marrow cells for ischemic heart disease J Card Surg 2003;18(Suppl 2):S69–S75.
72. Tang YL, Zhao Q, Qin X, Shen L, et al. Paracrine action enhances the effects of autologous mesenchymal stem cell transplantation on vascular regeneration in rat model of myocardial infarction. Ann Thorac Surg 2005;80(1):229–237.
73. Keck PJ, Hauser SD, Krivi G, et al. Vascular permeability factor, an endothelial cell mitogen related to PDGF. Science 1989;246:1309–1312.
74. Leung DW, Cachianes G, Kuang WJ, et al. Vascular endothelial growth factor is a secreted angiogenic mitogen. Science 1989;246:1306–1309.
75. Carmeliet P, Jain RK. Angiogenesis in cancer and other diseases. Nature 2000;407:249–257.
76. Ferrara N. Role of vascular endothelial growth factor in regulation of physiological angiogenesis. Am J Physiol Cell Physiol 2001;280:C1358–C1366.
77. Senger DR, Galli SJ, Dvorak AM, et al. Tumor cells secrete a vascular permeability factor that promotes accumulation of ascites fluid. Science 1983;219:983–985.

78. Gerber HP, Malik AK, Solar GP, et al. VEGF regulates haematopoietic stem cell survival by an internal autocrine loop mechanism. Nature 2002;417:954–958.
79. Ferrara N. VEGF: an update on biological and therapeutic aspects. Curr Opin Biotechnol 2000;11:617–624.
80. Rabbany SY, Heissig B, Hattori K, et al. Molecular pathways regulating mobilization of marrow-derived stem cells for tissue revascularization. Trends Mol Med 2003;9:109–117.
81. Rafii S, Heissig B, Hattori K. Efficient mobilization and recruitment of marrow-derived endothelial and hematopoietic stem cells by adenoviral vectors expressing angiogenic factors. Gene Ther 2002;9:631–641.
82. Ku DD, Zaleski JK, Liu S, Brock TA. Vascular endothelial growth factor induces EDRF-dependent relaxation in coronary arteries. Am J Physiol 1993;265:H586–H598.
83. Vu TH, Shipley JM, Bergers G, et al. MMP-9/gelatinase B is a key regulator of growth plate angiogenesis and apoptosis of hypertrophic chondrocytes. Cell 1998;93:411–422.
84. Bergers G, Brekken R, McMahon G, et al. Matrix metalloproteinase-9 triggers the angiogenic switch during carcinogenesis. Nat Cell Biol 2000;2:737–774.
85. Auguste P, Lemire S, Larrieu-lahargue F, et al. Molecular mechanism of tumor vascularization. Crit Rev Oncol/Hematol 2005;54:53–61.
86. Roberts WG, Palade GE. Increased microvascular permeability and endothelial fenestration induced by vascular endothelial growth factor. J Cell Sci 1995;108:2369–2379.
87. Gerber HP, McMurtrey A, Kowalski J, et al. Vascular endothelial growth factor regulates endothelial cell survival through the phosphatidylinositol 3'-kinase/Akt signal transduction pathway. Requirement for Flk-1/KDR activation. J Biol Chem 1998;273(46):30,336–30,343.
88. Karkkainen MJ, Makinen T, Alitalo K. Lymphatic endothelium: a new frontier of methastasis research. Nat Cell Biol 2002;4:E2–E5.
89. Al-Rawi MAA, Mansel RE, Jiang WG. Molecular and cellular mechanism of lymphangiogenesis. EJSO 2005;31:117–121.
90. Tammela T, Enholm B, Alitalo K, et al. The biology of vascular endothelial growth factors. Cardiovasc Res 2005;65(3):550–563.
91. Rissanen TT, Vajanto I, Hiltunen MO, et al. Expression of vascular endothelial growth factor and vascular endothelial growth factor receptor-2 (KDR/Flk-1) in ischemic skeletal muscle and its regeneration. Am J Pathol 2002;160(4):1393–1403.
92. Germani A, Di Carlo A, Mangoni A, et al. Vascular endothelial growth factor modulates skeletal myoblast function, Am J Pathol 2003;163(4):1417–1428.
93. Strauer BE, Brehm M, Zeus T. Repair of infarcted myocardium by autologous intracoronary mononuclear bone marrow cell transplantation in humans. Circulation 2002;106(15):1913–1918.
94. Schachinger V, Assmus B, Britten MB, et al. Transplantation of progenitor cells and regeneration enhancement in acute myocardial infarction: final one-year results of the TOPCARE-AMI Trial. J Am Coll Cardiol 2004;44(8):1690–1699.
95. Takahashi T, Kalka C, Masuda H, et al. Ischemia- and cytokine-induced mobilization of bone-marrow-derived endothelial progenitor cells for neovascularization. Nat Med 1999;5:434–438.
96. Asahara T, Kawamoto A. Endothelial progenitor cells for postnatal vasculogenesis Am J Physiol Cell Physiol 2004;287(3):C572–C579.
97. Badorff C, Brandes RP, Popp R, et al.Transdifferentiation of blood-derived human adult endothelial progenitor cells into functionally active cardyomyocytes. Circulation 2003;107(7):1024–1032.
98. Rangappa S, Fen C, Lee EH, et al. Transformation of adult mesenchymal stem cells isolated isolated from the fatty tissue into cardyomyocytes. Ann Thor Surg 2003;75:775–779.
99. Kurz DJ, Hong Y, Trivier E, et al. Fibroblast growth factor-2, but no vascular endothelial growth factor, upregulates telomerase activity in human endothelial cells. Arterioscler Thromb Vasc Biol 2003;23(5):748–754.
100. Trivier E, Kurz DJ, Hong Y, et al. Differential regulation of telomerase in endothelial cells by fibroblast growth factor-2 and vascular endothelial growth factor-a: association with replicative life span. Ann NY Acad Sci 2004;1019:111–115.
101. Zaccagnini G, Gaetano C, Della Pietra L, et al. Telomerase mediates vascular endothelial growth factor-dependent responsiveness in a rat model of hind limb ischemia J Biol Chem 2005;280(15):14,790–14,798.
102. Bahlmann FH, De Groot K, Sapndau JM, et al. Erythropoietin regulates endothelial progenitor cells. Blood 2004;103:921–926.

103. Yamaguchi J, Kusano KF, Masuo O, et al. Stromal cell-derived factor-1 effects on ex vivo expanded endothelial progenitor cell recruitment for ischemic neovascularization. Circulation 2003;107: 1322–1328.

104. Heeschen C, Aicher A, Lehmann R, et al. Erythropoietin is a potent physiologic stimulus for endothelial progenitor cell mobilization. Blood 2003;102:1340–1346.

105. Kong D, Melo LG, Gnecchi M, et al. Cytokine-induced mobilization of circulating endothelial progenitor cells enhances repair of injured arteries. Circulation 2004;110:2039–2046.

106. Cho H-J, Kim H-S, Lee M-M, et al. Mobilized endothelial progenitor cells by granulocyte-macrophage colony-stimulating factor accelerate reendothelialization and reduce vascular inflammation after intravascular radiation. Circulation 2003;108:2918–2925.

107. Hattori K, Heissig B, Wu Y, et al. Placental growth factor reconstitutes hematopoiesis by recruiting VEGFR1(+) stem cells from bone-marrow microenviroment. Nat Med 2002;8:841–849.

108. Zhu C, Ying D, Zhou D, et al. Expression of TGF-beta1 in smooth muscle cells regulates endothelial progenitor cells migration and differentiation. J Surg Res 2005;125:151–156.

109. Edelberg JM, Tang L, Hattori K, et al. Young adult bone marrow-derived endothelial precursor cells restore aging-impaired cardiac angiogenic function. Circ Res 2002;90:E89–E93.

110. Li ZD, Bork JP, Krueger B, et al. VEGF induces proliferation, migration, and TGF-beta1 expression in mouse glomerular endothelial cells via mitogen-activated protein kinase and phosphatidylinositol 3-kinase. Biochem Biophys Res Commun 2005;334(4):1049–1060.

111. Zygmunt M, Herr F, Munstedt K. Angiogenesis and vasculogenesis in pregnancy. Reprod Biol 2003;110:S10–S18.

112. Filicori M, Fazleabas AT, Huhtaniemi I. Novel concepts of human chorionic gonadotropin: reproductive system interactions and potential in the management of infertility. Fertil Steril 2005;84(2):275–284.

113. Sugawara J, Mitsui-Saito M, Hoshiai T, et al. Circulating endothelial progenitor cells during human pregnancy. J Clin Endocrinol Metab 2005;90:1845–1848.

114. Quarmby JW, Halliday AW. Angiogenesis: basic concepts and the114. application of gene therapy. In: Introduction to Vascular Biology : From Basic Science to Clinical Practice. Cambridge University Press, West Nyack, NY, 2002, p. 93.

115. Pugh CW, Ratcliffe PJ. Regulation of angiogenesis by hypoxia: role of the HIF system. Nat Med 2003;9:677–684.

116. Steiner S, Niessner A, Ziegler S, et al. Endurance training increases the number of endothelial progenitor cells in patients with cardiovascular risk and coronary artery disease. Atherosclerosis 2005;181:305–310.

117. Ciulla M, Giorgetti A, Lazzari L, et al. High-altitude trekking in the Himalayas increases the activity of circulating endothelial cells. Am J Hematol 2005;79(1):76–78.

118. Breen EC, Johnson EC, Wagner H, et al. Angiogenic growth factor mRNA responses in muscle to a single bout of exercise. J Appl Physiol 1996;81(1):355–361.

119. Gavin TP, Spector DA, Wagner H, et al. Nitric oxide synthase inhibition attenuates the skeletal muscle VEGF mRNA response to exercise. J Appl Physiol 2000;88(4):1192–1198.

120. Tang K, Rossiter HB, Wagner PD, et al. Lung-targeted VEGF inactivation leads to an emphysema phenotype in mice. J Appl Physiol 2004;97(4):1559–1566.

121. Kondo T, Hayashi M, Takeshita K, et al. Smoking cessation rapidly increases circulating progenitor cells in peripheral blood in chronic smokers. Arterioscler Thromb Vasc Biol 2004;24(8):1442–1447.

18

Use of Skeletal Myoblasts for the Treatment of Chronic Heart Failure

Anthony W. Ashton, MD, David D'Alessandro, MD, and Robert E. Michler, MD

SUMMARY

Recent investigation of cell transplantation has provided new hope for the treatment of heart failure, a historically incurable disease. Although multiple cell types and delivery techniques have been employed, no clear consensus has been reached as to the superiority of any single method. Skeletal myoblasts have several unique properties that make them an attractive cell type for use in the clinical arena. Most importantly they are autologous, readily available, and easily harvested and expanded ex vivo. Furthermore, they can be modified genetically to optimize engraftment. Their successful use in animal studies has justified several clinical trials in the United States and Europe. Autologous engraftment of skeletal myoblasts in patients has been associated with modest improvements in cardiac function. The mechanisms by which these cells might exert their positive effect remain in question, but a direct contribution to contractile function seems unlikely. Enthusiasm for these cells has further been tempered by an apparent arrhythmogenic risk. This chapter explores the use of skeletal myoblasts for the treatment of heart failure. The preclinical and clinical data published to date are reviewed. The ultimate role of these cells in the clinical armamentarium of heart failure treatments will depend on the results of ongoing studies. Regardless of their future, the use of skeletal myoblasts has provided important insights in the burgeoning field of cell therapy for heart failure.

Key Words: Skeletal myoblasts; cellular cardiomyoplasty; chronic heart failure; ejection fraction.

INTRODUCTION

Heart disease remains a leading cause of morbidity and mortality despite continuing advances in various treatment options. With best medical therapy a significant subset of patients are still refractory or respond suboptimally. Chronic heart failure (CHF) is often the clinical sequela of an acute ischemic event. While timeliness and adequacy of reperfusion determine immediate survival after acute myocardial infarction (MI), it is the ensuing changes to left ventricular (LV) shape and function that determine long-term prognosis. Acute MI results in an immediate loss of heart muscle; however, patients that develop CHF as a result display ongoing myocyte loss long after the initial event.

From: *Contemporary Cardiology: Stem Cells and Myocardial Regeneration*
Edited by: M. S. Penn © Humana Press Inc., Totowa, NJ

Ongoing global ventricular remodeling produces ventricular dilatation and concomitant decline in heart function, ultimately leading to CHF and death. Early intervention and therapy are currently unable to reverse or prevent LV dilatation. Alternatively, cell therapy offers a novel approach to regenerate the heart and to restore function.

Cardiac muscle has limited capacity to regenerate once injured *(1–3)*. Cardiac myocyte loss as a result of ischemic or hypertensive heart disease was, until recently, believed to be irreversible because postinfarction repair mechanisms are insufficient to stem myocyte apoptosis or to replace myocyte mass. This is largely thought to be attributable to the generally accepted principle that cardiac myocytes undergo terminal differentiation and irreversibly withdraw from the cell cycle after birth *(3)*. Conversely, skeletal muscle has the capacity for self-repair because of a resident population of proliferative muscle cells, or myoblasts *(4)*. Skeletal myoblasts, once activated, divide and fuse to form new muscle fibers that may restore lost functionality *(5)*. Preclinical data from a variety of animal studies have demonstrated the capacity for skeletal myoblasts to engraft, form myotubes, and enhance cardiac function following transplantation into infarcted, failing myocardium *(6–9)*. More recently, preliminary human studies focusing on patients with ischemic heart disease have demonstrated successful myoblast transplantation into the postinfarction scar *(10–12)*. This chapter will examine the data available on the effectiveness of myoblast transplantation as a treatment for CHF and the impact on/maintenance of cardiac function.

PRECLINICAL STUDIES WITH SKELETAL MYOBLAST TRANSPLANTATION

Unlike cardiac myocytes, skeletal muscle retains an ability to regenerate when injured. It is now well established that the regenerative capacity of skeletal muscle resides in cells known as satellite cells (myoblasts), which were first described in 1961 *(4)*. Successful autologous skeletal myoblast transplantation in a variety of animal models has demonstrated improvement in cardiac function. Although multiple cell types have shown benefit in such models, skeletal myoblasts offer significant advantages for salvaging or restoring myocardial function. Skeletal myoblasts tolerate ischemia well and have proved resilient when used in infarcted regions *(6,13)*. They have a limited spectrum of differentiation, reducing the risk of tumorogenicity *(14)*. Myoblasts, from predominantly fast-twitch skeletal muscle, can selectively differentiate into myofibers expressing fatigue-resistant, slow-twitch myosin heavy-chain isoforms, cardiac sarcoplasmic reticulum, and phospholamban *(13,15)*. The capacity for myoblasts to fuse and differentiate into nonfatigueable myofibers capable of sustaining cardiac function appears to be a response to the physiological milieu into which the myoblasts are placed *(6,13,16)*. This "transdifferentiation" may result from the endogenous innervation of the heart *(17)*, but at minimum requires beating cells *(18)*. Myofibers will contract in vitro and form synchronous contractile elements when in contact with cardiac myocytes *(19)*. Overall, myoblasts are the only cells reported to date to form true myocyte elements once implanted in the myocardium.

In addition, the form of the implanted skeletal myoblasts has a profound effect on the ability to restore function. The two key populations are satellite cells and "side-population" cells. Satellite cells in adult skeletal muscle exist closely juxtaposed against skeletal muscle fibers under the basal lamina and are accepted as dedicated myocyte precursors. Side-population cells are more closely related to bone marrow-derived stem cells because they express Sca1 and CD45. A major difference between the two populations is that satellite cells exclusively differentiate into myocytes after implantation, whereas side-population cells are capable of repopulating many cells types depending upon their environment. After intramuscular transplantation, side-population cells differentiate into both myocytes and satellite cells *(20)*. Although satellite cells may be the more characterized cell type for cellular cardiomyoplasty, these data indicate that side-population cells may offer additional benefits for the regeneration of myocyte number because of their ability to endow the heart with its own potential ongoing pool of myocyte precursors.

Results from preclinical studies using myoblast transplantation in ischemic models of heart failure, where an injury to the myocardium produces LV remodeling, were very promising. Adequate survival and engraftment of myoblasts in infarcted or necrotic myocardium has been documented and is associated with recovery of myocardial contractility and compliance as well as the diastolic pressure–strain relationship in animal models *(6,8)*. The consistent improvement in myocardial performance is independent of the method used to assess function, in vitro (*dP/dt*, force transduction) or in vivo (sonomicrometry, echocardiography, mean aortic pressure, improved LV systolic pressure, and aortic flow), and independent of the species studied *(6,8,16,21,22)*.

The effectiveness of skeletal myoblast transplantation in nonischemic cardiomyopathy models has been less frequently examined, but the results are no less exciting. The models have all allowed the development of failure prior to implantation of skeletal myoblasts and have universally showed improvement in cardiac function. The primary models used have been doxorubicin-induced heart failure *(23)*, salt overload in spontaneously hypertensive rats *(24)*, and hamsters with a sarcodystroglycan deficiency that reproduces all the features of dilated cardiomyopathy in humans *(25,26)*. Local implantation of either isolated skeletal myoblasts or intact myotubes in doxorubicin-induced heart failure improved cardiac function compared with the control treatment (maximum *dP/dt*, 4013.9 ± 96.1 vs 3603.1 ± 102.3 mmHg/second; minimum *dP/dt*, -2313.7 ± 75.1 vs -2057.1 ± 52.4 mmHg/second). A global delivery strategy for myoblasts, via an intracoronary infusion, found similar improvements in maximum and minimum *dP/dt*, associated with a sharper slope of the LV-developed pressure–volume curve and a reduced slope of the end-diastolic pressure–volume relation in myoblast-transplanted hearts *(27)*. Using this approach, myoblasts were indeed globally disseminated and differentiated into multinucleated myotubes that had aligned with the cardiac fiber axis within host myocardium. Thus, coronary delivery of skeletal myoblasts would appear to be the most convenient strategy for heart failure because it avoids the focal accumulation of myocytes associated with a direct injection strategy.

Skeletal myoblast transplantation in cardiomyopathic hamsters showed a significant 24% increase in fractional area change compared to a 6% decrease in controls after 4 weeks *(25)*. Moreover, the cells were able to attenuate ventricular remodeling with no significant change in the development of myocardial fibrosis *(25,26)*. In the hypertensive rats, the treated group showed a significant alleviation of LV dilation and contractile dysfunction, with a 9% decrease in LV end-diastolic dimension and fractional shortening of $38.5 \pm 1.5\%$ vs $32.1 \pm 1.4\%$ 6 weeks after implantation. Moreover, upregulation of the renin–angiotensin and endothelin systems during the transition to heart failure was attenuated by myoblast transplantation. Collectively, these studies show that cellular cardiomyoplasty is an effective therapy to prevent deterioration of ventricular morphology and cardiac function in both ischemic and nonischemic models of cardiomyopathy.

Concerns About the Use of Skeletal Myoblasts for Cellular Cardiomyoplasty

Although the use of skeletal myoblasts has proven successful in many animal models of ischemic heart disease and cardiac failure, they are not without problems. Despite forming myofibers capable of contraction in vivo, recent studies suggest that major structural differences between skeletal and cardiac muscle may limit the use of skeletal myoblasts for cellular cardiomyoplasty. The most substantial problem is that implanted myoblasts appear to remain electromechanically isolated from the host myocardium. The functional unit that integrates and synchronizes cardiac myocyte contraction is the intercalated disk *(28,29)*. This structure is composed of intercellular adhesion molecules, mostly N-cadherin, and structures called gap junctions. These channels permit exchange of small metabolites between the cytoplasm of adjacent cardiac myocytes and provide a low-resistance electrical pathway between cardiac muscle fibers. The dominant gap junction protein in cardiac myocytes is connexin-43 *(28,29)*. Loss of either of these proteins has profound implications for myocyte morphology, and loss of N-cadherin itself can result in a dilated cardiac phenotype *(28,29)*.

Isolated skeletal myoblasts, in co-culture with neonatal cardiac myocytes in vitro, express cardiac-specific proteins (GATA4, Nkx2.5, and ANP) together with cadherin and connexin-43 at the junctions with neighboring cells *(30,31)*. In addition, approx 10% of myotubes contract synchronously with the surrounding cardiac myocytes *(19)*. Taken together, these experiments demonstrate that skeletal myotubes and cardiomyocytes can indeed achieve electromechanical coupling given optimal conditions.

This same level of integration is not observed in vivo. Intracellular recordings of grafted myoblasts in infarcted rat myocardium showed that the contractile activity of newly formed myotubes is hyperexcitable and fully independent of neighboring cardiac myocytes *(32)*. These studies are supported by biochemical analysis of the engrafted cells. The majority of reports indicate absence of N-cadherin and Cx43 expression in the engrafted, differentiated myoblasts at all times examined up to 3 months after implantation *(16,19,33)* despite high expression of both proteins in undifferentiated skeletal myoblasts. A number of potential reasons may explain the discord between the in vitro and in vivo findings. One explanation is that myotubes in vitro are relatively immature and may retain a small, yet functional population of junctional proteins. The expression of these proteins is completely abrogated in engrafted myotubes because the differentiation is more complete in the myocardial environment *(19)*. Another factor may be that skeletal muscle grafts are often separated from the host myocardium by intervening scar tissue *(6,19)*. This would compromise the ability of implanted myoblasts to develop significant cell–cell contacts with the surrounding myocytes, a key criterion identified by the co-culture studies for transdifferentiation. However, because injection of myoblasts into uninjured myocardium results in the same phenotype, this is at best an incomplete explanation. Another contributing factor is the fact that the constant motion of the ventricular wall may exert unfavorable stretch/strain forces on the grafted cells, preventing stable contacts from being formed. Whatever the reason, this phenomenon has led multiple study authors to recognize arrythmogenesis as a major complication of myoblast transplantation *(34)*.

Another basic biochemical difference between the cell types is dihydropyridine receptor (DHPR) expression *(35,36)*. DHPRs determine the mechanism of excitation–contraction coupling in myocytes. In cardiac muscle DHPRs function as fast calcium channels that allow an influx of extracellular calcium, which triggers release of sarcoplasmic calcium stores. Conversely, skeletal muscle DHPRs function as slow calcium channels and voltage sensors that directly control the release of calcium from the sarcoplasmic reticulum. The greatly different electrical properties of the skeletal isoform are inconsistent with the contractile properties of cardiac myocytes and may also add to the genesis of arrhythmias observed upon treatment with skeletal myoblasts.

Without electromechanical integration it is unlikely that any significant force is generated by the intrinsic contractile properties of the implanted cells. This raises questions about the mechanism by which transplanted skeletal myoblasts contribute to recovery of the failing or ischemic myocardium. It is likely that the functional benefits of skeletal myoblast cell transplantation are more related to limitation of adverse postinfarction remodeling and/or paracrine effects on recipient tissue (37). Paracrine mechanisms such as the secretion of hepatocyte growth factor (HGF) (38) or vascular endothelial growth factor (VEGF) (39) could explain the achievement of a better LV function. HGF and VEGF have cardioprotective and antifibrotic effects, and the HGF receptor c-Met is expressed in ischemic myocardium (40,41). Moreover, such a paracrine effect might increase angiogenesis and stem cell recruitment to ameliorate the systolic function. It is well established that capillary density is decreased and capillary morphology altered (luminal swelling, lumen narrowing) in ischemic heart disease. Moreover, these microvascular abnormalities are thought to play an important role in the perpetuation of heart failure (42). Therefore, the observed amelioration of the ejection fraction (EF) could be solely a result of an improvement in angiogenesis and not necessarily the regeneration of cardiomyocyte mass. Indeed, implantation of endothelial precursors appears to have benefits equal to that of skeletal myoblasts; however, their primary effect appears to be to enhanced myocardial perfusion. The use of skeletal myoblasts in cellular cardiomyoplasty has been shown to improve coronary flow reserve (43); however, a formal systematic analysis of the angiogenic density and health of the microvascular endothelium has yet to be performed to qualify this as a bone fide mechanism responsible for the improvement of cardiac function.

Enhancement of Skeletal Myoblast Performance Using Pharmacological Agents

The results of cellular cardiomyoplasty using skeletal myoblasts are impressive, yet the potential to increase the effectiveness of therapy lies in augmenting the survival, efficiency of incorporation, and extent of differentiation of cells after implantation. Aggressive pharmacological intervention is an obvious adjunct therapy that has not been extensively investigated or developed for cellular cardiomyoplasty. Some simple pharmacological compounds have provided encouraging results for this rationale. Pretreatment and co-injection of myoblasts with Tubulyzine, an optimized myoseverin-like molecule, reduces myoblast cell death following transplantation and consequently improved the effectiveness of the treatment (44). Tubulyzine prevented primary myoblasts from apoptosis in vitro and significantly increased the survival of myoblasts in vivo. The result was enhanced integration of skeletal myoblasts into hybrid myofibers.

Moreover, skeletal myoblast implantation appears to work additively with current frontline pharmacological therapy for the treatment of heart failure. Angiotensin-converting enzyme inhibition and skeletal myoblast transplant separately gave approximately the same the extent of improvement in EF in ischemic rat hearts; however, the combination increased EF far beyond the effects observed with either alone ($43.9 \pm 1.4\%$ vs 19.8 ± 0.7 in controls) (45). In addition, the resultant arrhythmia that manifests in many experimental models of cellular cardiomyoplasty with myoblasts can be managed effectively by pharmacological means. Treatment of ventricular tachycardia after myoblast transplant can be terminated by nitrendipine, an L-type calcium channel blocker, but not by the Na channel blocker lidocaine (46). Moreover, amiodarone, a combined α/β-adrenergic receptor blocker, can attenuate arrhythmia when given prior to cell transplantation (10).

Combination therapy with recombinant angiogenic growth factors also appears to be another fruitful area to exploit. In addition to their potential to revascularize the myocardium, these factors have multiple effects on the myoblasts themselves. Muscle cell migration plays an important role in the incorporation of transplanted myoblasts, and pharmacological manipulation of the efficiency of myoblast migration may improve their participation in cardiac regeneration. Chemokinetic cytokines, such as insulin growth factor (IGF)-1 or basic fibroblast growth factor (bFGF), enhance myoblast migration in vitro. The co-injection of these chemokinetic factors with myoblasts improved their migration in vivo through upregulation of matrix metalloprotease-9 and urokinase plasminogen activator, two extracellular proteolytic enzymes that degrade matrix proteins and facilitate migration through matrix-rich scar tissue (47,48). Thus, IGF and FGF-2 appear to be better candidates than other pro-angiogenic cytokines such as VEGF. Although VEGF enhances myoblast migration and prevents apoptosis in differentiating myoblasts both in vitro and in vivo (41). VEGF co-injection does not always enhance cardiac function. In a sheep model of ischemic heart failure, simultaneous injection of both VEGF and myoblasts did not greatly potentiate the effects of the myoblasts alone (49). Similar improvements in the limitation of LV dilation and regional fractional area change were observed despite the number of capillaries in the peri-infarct region of the VEGF/myoblast group being 50% more than in the myoblast-only group. These results suggest that IGF-1 or bFGF may be useful in developing new approaches that will increase the efficacy of skeletal myoblast use in cellular cardiomyoplasty. Although many compounds are untested in the complex environment of cardiac failure, this strategy is likely to have profound effects on the biochemical and physiological responses of skeletal myoblasts during implantation.

Genetic Modifications of Skeletal Myoblasts and Their Effect on Graft Performance

Some of the most important questions remaining in the field of cellular cardiomyoplasty are some of the most fundamental. Identification of the molecular regulators affecting key aspects of myoblast response to implantation, such as cell survival, integration, differentiation, and functional efficiency are still in their infancy. As new mechanisms are identified, however, the cell type that offers the greatest advantages for translational medicine is the skeletal myoblast. Satellite cells need to be propagated ex vivo before transplant into diseased myocardium, providing a unique opportunity for genetic augmentation. The ability of skeletal myoblasts to express and secrete foreign proteins after implantation is already well established (50). The effectiveness of genetic manipulation of skeletal myoblasts, however, is dependent on two criteria: an efficient gene transfer system that integrates the gene(s) of interest into the myoblast genome and appropriate promoters that will coordinately regulate gene expression with the differentiation of myoblasts in the diseased myocardium. The obvious choice for the vector of infection is some form of virus. Retroviral vectors are now the gold standard in experimental and clinical gene transfer studies and have excellent rates of infection in skeletal myoblasts—approx 70% on average (51). However, how to regulate gene expression is not so simple. Reinecke et al. (52) found that overexpression using constitutive viral promoters caused significant death upon differentiation and resulted in a lack of target gene expression in transfected myoblasts after grafting, possibly resulting from promoter silencing. Alternatively, the use of muscle creatine kinase promoter, active only upon myocyte differentiation, resulted in high levels of protein expression in differentiated myotubes without significant cell death. These results stress that the temporal and spatial expression of the cargo is crucial to the success of this strategy.

The first application of such a powerful technology could be to sustain the newly implanted myoblasts immediately after implantation. Survival and proliferation of skeletal myoblasts within the cardiac environment are crucial to the therapeutic efficacy of myoblast transplantation. Unfortunately, the kinetics of cell death in the implanted skeletal myoblast population are swift and profound. Implantation of [^{14}C]thymidine-labeled myoblasts into mouse hearts has shown that 58% of cells are lost within 10 minutes of implantation. This steadily increases to 85% loss after 24 hours and 92% loss by 3 days (53,54). The same authors later showed that acute inflammation after transplantation was the cause of cell death, although ischemia is also implicated (55). These studies suggest that the initial oxidative stress and subsequent inflammatory response are important mechanisms contributing to acute graft attrition.

Attractive approaches have been developed to improve myoblast survival after transplantations. Zhang et al. (55) showed that cell death can be limited by engineering the transplantable cells to activate the cytoprotective Akt pathway. Moreover, heat shock prior to transplantation (56,57) endows robust protection of myoblasts from death, indicating that overexpression of heat-shock protein (HSP)70 is another likely candidate for genetic augmentation to increase survival of grafted myoblasts. Finally, overexpression of interleukin (IL)-1 receptor antagonist in skeletal myoblasts prior to implantation protected cells from the acute inflammatory response and enhanced the recovery of myocardial function (58). Other candidate genes to increase survival might also include antiapoptotic Bcl family members, such as Bcl-2 or Bcl-XL, or novel apoptosis suppressors specific to striated muscle, whose expression is lost during disease. One such candidate would be the protein ARC (apoptosis repressor with CARD domain), recently identified as a master inhibitor of apoptosis initiated by either the death receptor or mitochondrial pathways, as it robustly inhibits cell death resulting from free radicals such as superoxide (59,60).

As yet there is little in vivo evidence to suggest that skeletal myoblasts are capable of forming gap junctions with native cardiac myocytes. Differentiation along a myocyte linage in primary myoblasts ablates expression of Cx43 and N-cadherin (19). Thus, genetically engineering myoblasts to express these proteins during their expansion in vitro prior to implantation may enhance their integration as a coherent part of the host myocardium. Genetic modification of myoblasts to express Cx43 uniformly increases coupling between cardiac myocytes and myoblasts in vitro. This enhanced communication has been observed to decrease arrhythmogenicity in co-cultures, enhance the rate of myotube formation, and result in the formation of synchronously beating networks, where cardiomyocytes capture and pace skeletal muscle cells via intercalated disk-like structures containing gap junctions (46,61,62). The implantation of skeletal myoblasts, engineered to express Cx43 only in fully differentiated myotubes, resulted in close apposition to host cardiomyocytes and possibly electrical coupling (63). These data indicate that augmentation of skeletal myoblasts with cardiac junctional proteins may permit electrical coupling of skeletal and cardiac muscle and circumvent the arrythmogenic side effects observed during cellular cardiomyoplasty with skeletal myoblasts.

However, expression of Cx43 without N-cadherin results in disarray of the gap junctions and poor intercellular communication *(28,29)*. This indicates that the expression of both proteins needs to be restored simultaneously for optimal integration and that other genes that regulate the expression of both proteins, such as the cardiotropic hormone relaxin *(64)*, may be better candidates to enhance the integration of implanted myoblasts with host myocytes.

The genetic manipulation of skeletal myoblasts has been shown to halt the progression from compensatory hypertrophy to CHF in animal models *(24)*. Skeletal myoblasts transferred with the *cardiotrophin-1* gene, a member of the IL-6 superfamily, were injected into the myocardial free wall of hypertensive rats already experiencing hypertrophy. Cardiotrophin-1 engineered myoblasts were more effective at alleviating LV dilation and contractile dysfunction than were unaltered myoblasts. Cardiotrophin-1 was not determined to enhance myoblast integration or differentiation; however, it may have improved function as a result of a combination of reducing myoctye loss and stabilizing the hypertrophic response, because cardiotrophin-1 is a pro-survival agent and hypertrophic stimulus.

Mutations in multiple genes, including lysosymal integral membrane proteins *(65)* and lamin A/C *(66)*, cause autosomal-dominant dilated cardiomyopathy. Other mutations, such as those in the sarcodystroglycan complex, reduce the proliferative capacity and differentiation potential of isolated myoblasts and restrict their ability to integrate with a potential host myocardium *(67)*. The ability to augment the properties of skeletal myoblasts ex vivo raises the possibility of correcting genetic anomalies and restoring full function to the cells that will form the basis of the new myocardium.

Finally, to ensure graft viability and prevent further scar formation, myocyte replacement should be coupled with concurrent myocardial revascularization. An obvious candidate gene for is hypoxia-inducible factor *(HIF)*-1α, a master gene that controls the expression of a wide array of angiogenic factors. Ejection fraction in rats receiving myoblasts expressing HIF-1α increased dramatically (by 27%) compared to values prior to transplantation and those in other control groups *(68)*. The improvement in EF was accompanied by a significantly greater degree of angiogenesis, cell engraftment, and cell survival.

VEGF is another promising gene to mediate the simultaneous recruitment of vessels to the repairing graft. Human myoblasts transduced with *VEGF-165* gene produce six times more capillaries in porcine myocardium than untransduced cells *(69)*, demonstrating the efficiency of the technique; however, cellular cardiomyoplasty using VEGF-tranduced myoblasts has provided mixed results. Myocardial VEGF expression from implanted VEGF-engineered myoblasts remains elevated for 2 weeks before declining to baseline *(70)*. This transient expression of VEGF resulted in enhanced angiogenesis, reduced infarct size, and improved cardiac function *(70)*. The findings were supported by another group using VEGF-transduced human myoblasts in a porcine model of chronic infarction *(71)*. Moreover, although delivery of VEGF using direct adenoviral injection and engineered myoblasts gave equivalent neovascularization response in an infarction model in rats, only cell-based delivery resulted in increased cardiac function *(72)*. The improved function correlated with less apoptosis in the border zone in those animals that received the VEGF-165 expressing skeletal myoblasts.

Conversely, one study using myoblasts where VEGF expression was driven by a retroviral promoter had a disastrous outcome *(73)*. All the mice in the VEGF group died by 14 days, compared with no deaths in a group treated with myoblasts engineered to express the β-galactosidase gene. Histochemistry documented intramural vascular tumors resembling hemangiomas surrounding injected myoblasts in the VEGF myoblast-injected myocardium. This led the authors to conclude that myoblast delivery of VEGF was not suitable for cellular myoplasty and underscores the importance of temporal/spatial regulation of genes in the pursuit to refine cellular myoplasty in order to enhance outcome.

PHASE I HUMAN TRIALS OF AUTOLOGOUS SKELETAL MYOBLASTS

Driven by the promising results achieved in animal models of heart failure, human autologous skeletal myoblast transplantation has been undertaken in both Europe and the United States. Menasché et al. *(11)* reported the first clinical application of replacement cell therapy for the treatment of CHF in June 2000. Although multiple cell types have been investigated in preclinical studies, skeletal myoblasts were chosen because they have several advantages in the clinical arena in addition to those outlined earlier. These cells are easily harvested from small amounts of the patients' own skeletal muscle and expand readily in culture, overcoming the shortages of donor tissue *(13)*. The use of autologous cells avoids the ethical issues constraining stem cells and obviates the need for immunosuppression. Since Menasché's first report, several prospective clinical trials have been initiated in the United States and Europe to investigate the safety and effectiveness of skeletal myoblasts for the treatment of patients with advanced heart failure. The following discussion will briefly outline the phase I clinical trials that have been reported to date.

As part of the first phase I trial in Europe, Menasché et al. reported on 10 patients who underwent cell grafting at the time of surgical coronary revascularization *(12)*. Inclusion criteria were EF of 35% or less, presence of nonviable postinfarction scarring, and indication for coronary artery bypass surgery (CABG). Patients had an average of 800 million cells injected at the time of surgery. These investigators showed that at an average follow-up of 10.9 months, the average New York Heart Association (NYHA) functional class improved from 2.7 ± 0.2 to 1.6 ± 0.1. Objectively, the group's average left ventricular ejection fraction (LVEF) improved from $24 \pm 1\%$ to $32 \pm 1\%$, and blinded echocardiographic assessment of regional wall function demonstrated improvement in 63% of implanted scars. These encouraging results, however, were tempered by a disturbing number of ventricular arrhythmias necessitating automatic implanted cardiac defibrillator (AICD) implantation in four patients. Moreover, the improvements in postoperative wall motion attributable to the grafted cells was difficult to interpret in the setting of concomitant CABG, a procedure known to improve cardiac function in patients with ischemic heart failure. Despite these limitations, the investigators demonstrated the feasibility and relative safety of this technique, justifying further investigation.

Herreros and colleagues *(10)*, using a similar study design, reported comparable findings. This European phase I study enrolled 12 patients with a mean follow-up of 6.5 months. Inclusion criteria were remote history (>4 weeks) of myocardial infarction (MI), presence of akinetic or dyskinetic nonviable scar, indication for CABG, and LVEF greater than 25%. Eleven patients were treated with a mean of $211 \pm 107 \times 10^6$ cells. Follow-up positron emission tomography (PET) imaging was done at 3 months and echocardiography at 40 days and 3 months. Postoperative LVEF improved form $35.5 \pm 2.3\%$ to $53.5 \pm 4.98\%$ at 3 mo. Furthermore, in the 7 patients in whom ^{18}F-FDG

PET imaging was performed, both pre- and postoperatively, glucose uptake was significantly increased in both the whole myocardium and the infarct areas. Importantly, only one of the treated patients experienced ventricular arrhythmias during the follow-up period, and this patient underwent a concomitant anuerysmectomy at the time of surgery. The authors speculate that a major complication is altered immunogenicity in the implanted cells by prolonged ex vivo culture conditions, and the use of autologous serum in the cellular preparation prevents the immunological inflammatory reaction that triggers arrhythmias.

The findings of a third clinical trial were reported by Siminiak et al. Inclusion criteria for this study were prior history of MI (minimum of 3 months before surgery), suitable anatomy for CABG, EF between 25 and 40% with one or more dyskinetic segments on echocardiography, and lack of myocardial viability on dobutamine echocardiography. The investigators documented improved LVEFs in all nine surviving patients. Although the first two treated patients did suffer ventricular arrhythmias, the addition of amiodarone prevented further episodes in these and subsequent patients.

The result of the first US Food and Drug Administration phase 1 multi-institutional human clinical trial was recently updated *(74)*. Twenty-four patients with a history of previous MI and LVEF of less than 40% were enrolled in the CABG arm. In a second arm, six patients underwent left ventricular assist device (LVAD) implantation as a bridge to heart transplantation, and patients donated their hearts for testing at the time of heart transplant. Patients were transplanted with between 10 and 300 million cells. Echocardiography demonstrated an average improvement in LVEF from 25 to 34% at 1 year and further improved to 36% at 2 years. PET imaging showed new areas of viability within infarcted scars. Ventricular arrhythmias were not a significant problem in this group.

In all the aforementioned clinical trials, myoblast transplantation was performed in conjunction with surgical revascularization. The benefit attributable to the transplanted cells is thus impossible to ascertain. More recently initiated trials are perhaps better designed to evaluate the effectiveness of these cells in the clinical setting.

Smits and colleagues *(75)* designed and reported on the first study to evaluate percutaneous transplantation of autologous myoblasts as stand-alone therapy. They reported on the safety and feasibility of their approach in five patients with 6 months of follow-up. Inclusion criteria included remote (>4 weeks) history of MI, LVEF between 20 and 45%, and presence of myocardial scar. They evaluated change in EF by LV angiography, demonstrating an increase in the group mean from $36 \pm 11\%$ to $45 \pm 8\%$ by 6 months. Ventricular arrhythmias were only problematic in one patient in their series, in whom a prophylactic AICD was eventually implanted.

Recently, Siminiak and others reported their initial findings in a phase I clinical trial in which myoblasts were administered as sole therapy in post-MI patients using a percutaneous delivery system *(76)*. Designed to evaluate feasibility and safety, these investigators enrolled 10 patients and reported on 6-month follow-up. Inclusion criteria were remote history of MI (minimum of 3 months), LVEF between 25 and 40%, presence of one to three akinetic or dyskinetic segments on echocardiography, and lack of viability as assessed by dobutamine echocardiography. Patients were treated prophylactically with amiodarone beginning the day prior to the procedure. Ventricular arrhythmia was experienced in only one patient in whom amiodarone was not given because of allergy. This patient was successfully treated with a previously implanted AICD. Amiodarone therapy was discontinued after 2–3 weeks in all patients, and subsequent Holter monitoring revealed no sustained ventricular arrhythmias. Although they found only modest improvements in LVEF (3–8% improvement in six of nine patients treated), there was symptomatic improvement in all nine patients treated, with all nine improving to NYHA class I by 6 months. In contrast, the one patient who was not successfully grafted showed no change in either his LVEF or his NYHA class by 6 months.

Most recently, Ince et al. reported their findings in a similar study but with matched controls (77). Six patients were treated with $210 \times 10^6 \pm 150 \times 10^6$ cells and compared to controls at 6 months. The study group's mean LVEF increased from $24.3 \pm 6.7\%$ to $33.2 \pm 10.2\%$. In contrast, the control group's remained unchanged ($24.7 \pm 4.6\%$ vs $22.2 \pm 6.2\%$). These investigators found similar improvements with respect to exercise capacity and NYHA functional class. Although far from conclusive, these reports suggest that skeletal myoblast transplantation may be beneficial in the absence of surgical revascularization. They further validate minimally invasive techniques that could significantly broaden the applicability of this burgeoning technology.

Histopathological analysis of transplanted skeletal myoblasts in humans is limited to date. Menasché and colleagues (12,78) reported on one patient who died of a stroke 17.5 months after surgery. On postmortem examination, myotubes were found embedded in the scar tissue. No gap junctions or other evidence of cardiomyogenic differentiation was appreciated. They further quantified the percentages of cells staining positive for slow myosin heavy-chain isoforms, demonstrating more than half of the surviving cells staining positive, with 33% of cells coexpressing fast and slow isoforms. This is in contrast to native skeletal muscle populations, in which only 0.6% expresses both isoforms.

Pagani and colleagues reported on the outcomes in four patients who received cellular grafts at the time of LVAD implantation (79). In three patients in whom a dose of 300×10^6 cells was transplanted, surviving autologous skeletal muscle cells were identified by trichrome staining. The majority of skeletal myofibers were aligned in parallel with the resident myocardial fibers. Additionally, these investigators noted expression of slow-twitch myosin isoforms, evidence of myoblast differentiation. This study did not investigate the presence of gap junctions in the grafted cells. The authors estimate that the survival of transplanted myoblasts was less than 1% of the total cells grafted based on histological analysis. Furthermore, they noted surviving cells in the epicardial fat, presumably resulting from postinjection leakage of transplanted cells. These findings further support the viability and possible functionality of these transplanted myoblasts but suggest limitations to their ultimate ability to differentiate into functional cardiomyocytes.

Cell transplantation for the treatment of heart failure is a promising field, but many questions remain to be answered. The aggregate findings of multiple studies suggest a modest beneficial effect from the autologous transplantation of skeletal myoblasts in patients who suffer from heart failure. The mechanisms through which these cells exert their effect remain elusive. The notion that these cells provide a significant contractile force in the absence of gap junctions seems simplistic. Alternative explanations include a potential role in limiting postinfarction remodeling to possible paracrine effects on host tissue (37). Future studies will need to better evaluate the safety and efficacy of a wider range of cell numbers and delivery techniques. Furthermore, issues about the optimal timing of delivery will need to be addressed. We might expect that through continuing collaborative efforts combining insights derived from animal studies and well-designed clinical trials, skeletal myoblasts will be a useful and effective part of a clinical armamentarium to treat heart failure.

REFERENCES

1. Soonpaa MH, Field LJ. Assessment of cardiomyocyte DNA synthesis during hypertrophy in adult mice. Am J Physiol 1994;266:H1439–1445.
2. Soonpaa MH, Field LJ. Assessment of cardiomyocyte DNA synthesis in normal and injured adult mouse hearts. Am J Physiol 1997;272:H220–H226.
3. Soonpaa MH, Field LJ. Survey of studies examining mammalian cardiomyocyte DNA synthesis. Circ Res 1998;83:15–26.
4. Mauro A. Satellite cell of skeletal muscle fibers. J Biophys Biochem Cytol 1961;9:493–495.
5. Bischoff R. Regeneration of single skeletal muscle fibers in vitro. Anat Rec 1975;182:215–235.
6. Taylor DA, Atkins BZ, Hungspreugs P, et al. Regenerating functional myocardium: improved performance after skeletal myoblast transplantation. Nat Med 1998;4:929–933.
7. Pouzet B, Vilquin JT, Hagege AA, et al. Factors affecting functional outcome after autologous skeletal myoblast transplantation. Ann Thorac Surg 2001;71:844–851.
8. Atkins BZ, Hueman MT, Meuchel JM, Cottman MJ, Hutcheson KA, Taylor DA. Myogenic cell transplantation improves in vivo regional performance in infarcted rabbit myocardium. J Heart Lung Transplant 1999;18:1173–1180.
9. Jain M, DerSimonian H, Brenner DA, et al. Cell therapy attenuates deleterious ventricular remodeling and improves cardiac performance after myocardial infarction. Circulation 2001;103:1920–1927.
10. Herreros J, Prosper F, Perez A, et al. Autologous intramyocardial injection of cultured skeletal muscle-derived stem cells in patients with non-acute myocardial infarction. Eur Heart J 2003;24: 2012–2020.
11. Menasche P, Hagege AA, Scorsin M, et al. Myoblast transplantation for heart failure. Lancet 2001;357:279–280.
12. Menasche P, Hagege AA, Vilquin JT, et al. Autologous skeletal myoblast transplantation for severe postinfarction left ventricular dysfunction. J Am Coll Cardiol 2003;41:1078–1083.
13. Tang YL. Cellular therapy with autologous skeletal myoblasts for ischemic heart disease and heart failure. Methods Mol Med 2005;112:193–204.
14. Tremblay JP, Roy B, Goulet M. Human myoblast transplantation: a simple assay for tumorigenicity. Neuromuscul Disord 1991;1:341–343.
15. Koh GY, Klug MG, Soonpaa MH, Field LJ. Differentiation and long-term survival of C2C12 myoblast grafts in heart. J Clin Invest 1993;92:1548–1554.
16. Murry CE, Wiseman RW, Schwartz SM, Hauschka SD. Skeletal myoblast transplantation for repair of myocardial necrosis. J Clin Invest 1996;98:2512–2523.
17. Erzen I, Primc M, Janmot C, Cvetko E, Sketelj J, d'Albis A. Myosin heavy chain profiles in regenerated fast and slow muscles innervated by the same motor nerve become nearly identical. Histochem J 1999;31:277–283.
18. Muller P, Beltrami AP, Cesselli D, Pfeiffer P, Kazakov A, Bohm M. Myocardial regeneration by endogenous adult progenitor cells. J Mol Cell Cardiol 2005;39:377–387.
19. Reinecke H, MacDonald GH, Hauschka SD, Murry CE. Electromechanical coupling between skeletal and cardiac muscle. Implications for infarct repair. J Cell Biol 2000;149:731–740.
20. Asakura A, Seale P, Girgis-Gabardo A, Rudnicki MA. Myogenic specification of side population cells in skeletal muscle. J Cell Biol 2002;159:123–134.
21. Chiu RC, Zibaitis A, Kao RL. Cellular cardiomyoplasty: myocardial regeneration with satellite cell implantation. Ann Thorac Surg 1995;60:12–18.
22. Huwer H, Winning J, Vollmar B, et al. Long-term cell survival and hemodynamic improvements after neonatal cardiomyocyte and satellite cell transplantation into healed myocardial cryoinfarcted lesions in rats. Cell Transplant 2003;12:757–767.
23. Suzuki K, Murtuza B, Heslop L, et al. Single fibers of skeletal muscle as a novel graft for cell transplantation to the heart. J Thorac Cardiovasc Surg 2002;123:984–992.
24. Toh R, Kawashima S, Kawai M, et al. Transplantation of cardiotrophin-1-expressing myoblasts to the left ventricular wall alleviates the transition from compensatory hypertrophy to congestive heart failure in Dahl salt-sensitive hypertensive rats. J Am Coll Cardiol 2004;43:2337–2347.
25. Pouly J, Hagege AA, Vilquin JT, et al. Does the functional efficacy of skeletal myoblast transplantation extend to nonischemic cardiomyopathy? Circulation 2004;110:1626–1631.
26. Ohno N, Fedak PW, Weisel RD, Mickle DA, Fujii T, Li RK. Transplantation of cryopreserved muscle cells in dilated cardiomyopathy: effects on left ventricular geometry and function. J Thorac Cardiovasc Surg 2003;126:1537–1548.

27. Suzuki K, Murtuza B, Suzuki N, Smolenski RT, Yacoub MH. Intracoronary infusion of skeletal myoblasts improves cardiac function in doxorubicin-induced heart failure. Circulation 2001;104:1213–1217.
28. Ferreira-Cornwell MC, Luo Y, Narula N, Lenox JM, Lieberman M, Radice GL. Remodeling the intercalated disc leads to cardiomyopathy in mice misexpressing cadherins in the heart. J Cell Sci 2002;115:1623–1634.
29. Perriard JC, Hirschy A, Ehler E. Dilated cardiomyopathy: a disease of the intercalated disc? Trends Cardiovasc Med 2003;13:30–38.
30. Iijima Y, Nagai T, Mizukami M, et al. Beating is necessary for transdifferentiation of skeletal muscle-derived cells into cardiomyocytes. FASEB J 2003;10:1096–1111.
31. Formigli L, Francini F, Tani A, et al. Morphofunctional integration between skeletal myoblasts and adult cardiomyocytes in coculture is favored by direct cell-cell contacts and relaxin treatment. Am J Physiol Cell Physiol 2005;288:C795–C804.
32. Leobon B, Garcin I, Menasche P, Vilquin JT, Audinat E, Charpak S. Myoblasts transplanted into rat infarcted myocardium are functionally isolated from their host. Proc Natl Acad Sci USA 2003;100:7808–7811.
33. Reinecke H, Poppa V, Murry CE. Skeletal muscle stem cells do not transdifferentiate into cardiomyocytes after cardiac grafting. J Mol Cell Cardiol 2002;34:241–249.
34. Menasche P. Myoblast transplantation: feasibility, safety and efficacy. Ann Med 2002;34:314–315.
35. Mikami A, Imoto K, Tanabe T, et al. Primary structure and functional expression of the cardiac dihydropyridine-sensitive calcium channel. Nature 1989;340:230–233.
36. Garcia J, Tanabe T, Beam KG. Relationship of calcium transients to calcium currents and charge movements in myotubes expressing skeletal and cardiac dihydropyridine receptors. J Gen Physiol 1994;103:125–147.
37. Menasche P. Skeletal myoblast for cell therapy. Coron Artery Dis 2005;16:105–110.
38. Tatsumi R, Hattori A, Ikeuchi Y, Anderson JE, Allen RE. Release of hepatocyte growth factor from mechanically stretched skeletal muscle satellite cells and role of pH and nitric oxide. Mol Biol Cell 2002;13:2909–2918.
39. Yau TM, Li G, Weisel RD, et al. Vascular endothelial growth factor transgene expression in cell-transplanted hearts. J Thorac Cardiovasc Surg 2004;127:1180–1187.
40. Nakamura T, Mizuno S, Matsumoto K, Sawa Y, Matsuda H. Myocardial protection from ischemia/reperfusion injury by endogenous and exogenous HGF. J Clin Invest 2000;106:1511–1519.
41. Germani A, Di Carlo A, Mangoni A, et al. Vascular endothelial growth factor modulates skeletal myoblast function. Am J Pathol 2003;163:1417–1428.
42. Liu PP, Mak S, Stewart DJ. Potential role of the microvasculature in progression of heart failure. Am J Cardiol 1999;84:23L–26L.
43. Assmus B, Schachinger V, Teupe C, et al. Transplantation of Progenitor Cells and Regeneration Enhancement in Acute Myocardial Infarction (TOPCARE-AMI). Circulation 2002;106:3009–3017.
44. El Fahime E, Bouchentouf M, Benabdallah BF, et al. Tubulyzine, a novel tri-substituted triazine, prevents the early cell death of transplanted myogenic cells and improves transplantation success. Biochem Cell Biol 2003;81:81–90.
45. Pouzet B, Ghostine S, Vilquin JT, et al. Is skeletal myoblast transplantation clinically relevant in the era of angiotensin-converting enzyme inhibitors? Circulation 2001;104:1223–1228.
46. Abraham MR, Henrikson CA, Tung L, et al. Antiarrhythmic engineering of skeletal myoblasts for cardiac transplantation. Circ Res 2005;97:159–167.
47. El Fahime E, Mills P, Lafreniere JF, Torrente Y, Tremblay JP. The urokinase plasminogen activator: an interesting way to improve myoblast migration following their transplantation. Exp Cell Res 2002;280:169–178.
48. Lafreniere JF, Mills P, Tremblay JP, Fahime EE. Growth factors improve the in vivo migration of human skeletal myoblasts by modulating their endogenous proteolytic activity. Transplantation 2004;77:1741–1747.
49. Chachques JC, Duarte F, Cattadori B, et al. Angiogenic growth factors and/or cellular therapy for myocardial regeneration: a comparative study. J Thorac Cardiovasc Surg 2004;128:245–253.
50. Powell C, Shansky J, Del Tatto M, et al. Tissue-engineered human bioartificial muscles expressing a foreign recombinant protein for gene therapy. Hum Gene Ther 1999;10:565–577.
51. El Oakley RM, Ooi OC, Bongso A, Yacoub MH. Myocyte transplantation for myocardial repair: a few good cells can mend a broken heart. Ann Thorac Surg 2001;71:1724–1733.
52. Reinecke H, Minami E, Virag JI, Murry CE. Gene transfer of connexin43 into skeletal muscle. Hum Gene Ther 2004;15:627–636.

53. Suzuki K, Murtuza B, Beauchamp JR, et al. Dynamics and mediators of acute graft attrition after myoblast transplantation to the heart. FASEB J 2004;18:1153–1155.

54. Suzuki K, Murtuza B, Beauchamp JR, et al. Role of interleukin-1beta in acute inflammation and graft death after cell transplantation to the heart. Circulation 2004;110:11219–11224.

55. Zhang M, Methot D, Poppa V, Fujio Y, Walsh K, Murry CE. Cardiomyocyte grafting for cardiac repair: graft cell death and anti-death strategies. J Mol Cell Cardiol 2001;33:907–921.

56. Su CY, Chong KY, Chen J, Ryter S, Khardori R, Lai CC. A physiologically relevant hyperthermia selectively activates constitutive hsp70 in H9c2 cardiac myoblasts and confers oxidative protection. J Mol Cell Cardiol 1999;31:845–855.

57. Suzuki K, Murtuza B, Sammut IA, et al. Heat shock protein 72 enhances manganese superoxide dismutase activity during myocardial ischemia-reperfusion injury, associated with mitochondrial protection and apoptosis reduction. Circulation 2002;106:1270–1276.

58. Suzuki K, Murtuza B, Smolenski RT, et al. Overexpression of interleukin-1 receptor antagonist provides cardioprotection against ischemia-reperfusion injury associated with reduction in apoptosis. Circulation 2001;104:1308–1313.

59. Nam YJ, Mani K, Ashton AW, et al. Inhibition of both the extrinsic and intrinsic death pathways through nonhomotypic death-fold interactions. Mol Cell 2004;15:901–912.

60. Neuss M, Monticone R, Lundberg MS, Chesley AT, Fleck E, Crow MT. The apoptotic regulatory protein ARC (apoptosis repressor with caspase recruitment domain) prevents oxidant stress-mediated cell death by preserving mitochondrial function. J Biol Chem 2001;276:33,915–33,922.

61. Suzuki K, Brand NJ, Allen S, et al. Overexpression of connexin 43 in skeletal myoblasts: relevance to cell transplantation to the heart. J Thorac Cardiovasc Surg 2001;122:759–766.

62. Murry CE, Whitney ML, Reinecke H. Muscle cell grafting for the treatment and prevention of heart failure. J Card Fail 2002;8:S532–S541.

63. Reinecke H, Minami E, Virag JI, Murry CE. Gene transfer of connexin43 into skeletal muscle. Hum Gene Ther 2004;15:627–636.

64. Formigli L, Francini F, Chiappini L, Zecchi-Orlandini S, Bani D. Relaxin favors the morphofunctional integration between skeletal myoblasts and adult cardiomyocytes in coculture. Ann NY Acad Sci 2005;1041:444–445.

65. Mohapatra B, Jimenez S, Lin JH, et al. Mutations in the muscle LIM protein and alpha-actinin-2 genes in dilated cardiomyopathy and endocardial fibroelastosis. Mol Genet Metab 2003;80:207–215.

66. Ostlund C, Bonne G, Schwartz K, Worman HJ. Properties of lamin A mutants found in Emery-Dreifuss muscular dystrophy, cardiomyopathy and Dunnigan-type partial lipodystrophy. J Cell Sci 2001;114:4435–4445.

67. Ng SK, Lewis KE. Characteristics of myoblasts isolated from golden Syrian and dystrophic (strain CHF-146) hamsters. Can J Biochem Cell Biol 1985;63:730–736.

68. Azarnoush K, Maurel A, Sebbah L, et al. Enhancement of the functional benefits of skeletal myoblast transplantation by means of coadministration of hypoxia-inducible factor 1alpha. J Thorac Cardiovasc Surg 2005;130:173–179.

69. Law PK, Haider K, Fang G, et al. Human VEGF165-myoblasts produce concomitant angiogenesis/myogenesis in the regenerative heart. Mol Cell Biochem 2004;263:173–178.

70. Suzuki K, Murtuza B, Smolenski RT, et al. Cell transplantation for the treatment of acute myocardial infarction using vascular endothelial growth factor-expressing skeletal myoblasts. Circulation 2001;104:1207–1212.

71. Haider H, Ye L, Jiang S, et al. Angiomyogenesis for cardiac repair using human myoblasts as carriers of human vascular endothelial growth factor. J Mol Med 2004;82:539–549.

72. Askari A, Unzek S, Goldman CK, et al. Cellular, but not direct, adenoviral delivery of vascular endothelial growth factor results in improved left ventricular function and neovascularization in dilated ischemic cardiomyopathy. J Am Coll Cardiol 2004;43:1908–1914.

73. Lee RJ, Springer ML, Blanco-Bose WE, Shaw R, Ursell PC, Blau HM. VEGF gene delivery to myocardium: deleterious effects of unregulated expression. Circulation 2000;102:898–901.

74. Dib N, Michler RE, Pagani FD, et al. Safety and feasibility of autologous myoblast transplantation in patients with ischemic cardiomyopathy: 4 year follow-up. Circulation 2005;112(12):1748–1755.

75. Smits PC, van Geuns RJ, Poldermans D, et al. Catheter-based intramyocardial injection of autologous skeletal myoblasts as a primary treatment of ischemic heart failure: clinical experience with six-month follow-up. J Am Coll Cardiol 2003;42:2063–2069.

76. Siminiak T, Fiszer D, Jerzykowska O, et al. Percutaneous trans-coronary-venous transplantation of autologous skeletal myoblasts in the treatment of post-infarction myocardial contractility impairment: the POZNAN trial. Eur Heart J 2005;26:1188–1195.

77. Ince H, Petzsch M, Rehders TC, Kische S, Chatterjee T, Nienaber CA. [Percutaneous transplantation of autologous myoblasts in ischemic cardiomyopathy]. Herz 2005;30:223–231.
78. Hagege AA, Carrion C, Menasche P, et al. Viability and differentiation of autologous skeletal myoblast grafts in ischaemic cardiomyopathy. Lancet 2003;361:491–492.
79. Pagani FD, DerSimonian H, Zawadzka A, et al. Autologous skeletal myoblasts transplanted to ischemia-damaged myocardium in humans. Histological analysis of cell survival and differentiation. J Am Coll Cardiol 2003;41:879–888.

B ACUTE MYOCARDIAL INFARCTION

19

Bone Marrow and Angioblast Transplantation

Marc S. Penn, MD, PhD, Samuel Unzek, MD, Niladri Mal, MD, and Kai Wang, MD, PhD

SUMMARY

Clinical trials using autologous hematopoietic or whole bone marrow preparations in patients in the peri-infarct period are ongoing. These trials are attempting to improve myocardial function. Although it has been demonstrated in animal models that these stem cells do not differentiate into cardiac myocytes, there is now clear evidence in animal models and clinical human trials that their use is likely beneficial when delivered soon after acute myocardial infarction. It should be noted that all of these trials have been performed in days to less than 2 weeks from myocardial injury. The end product of myocardial injury translates into heart failure, an entity that may be minimized by this type of therapy. One comes to the conclusion that the data are promising, but there are still many questions to be answered, for example: What type of cell(s) should be transplanted, and what should be their mode of delivery, optimal time of transplant, etc.

Key Words: Hematopoietic stem cells; mesenchymal stem cells; myocardial infarction; ejection fraction.

Hematopoietic stem cells (HSCs) comprise 1–2% of the adult bone marrow. HSC transplantation is able to permanently reconstitute the entire hematopoietic system. HSCs maintain the ability to differentiate into lineages of blood-forming cells, some of which are able to differentiate into cells contained in myocardial tissue (e.g., endothelial cells) *(1,2)*. In addition to the CD34[+] HSCs used to reconstitute hematopoietic cells to treat hematopoietic ailments, CD45[+], CD117[+] (or c-kit[+]), CD133[+], and CD14[+] markers also characterize subpopulations of HSCs. The original impetus for taking these cell populations to the clinic was the concept that the CD34[+]- and CD117[+]-derived bone marrow stem cell population had plasticity *(3,4)*. The assumption was that the plasticity of this population permits environmental signals generated by the myocardium to encourage transdifferentiation of these cells into cardiac myocytes or endothelial cells postengraftment *(1,2)*. Unfortunately, emerging data indicate that these cell types do not differentiate into cardiac myocytes *(5,6)*. However, even if these bone marrow-derived cells do not differentiate into cardiac myocytes, there is good evidence that suggests that this bone marrow-derived stem cell population homes to *(7)* and supports the newly

From: *Contemporary Cardiology: Stem Cells and Myocardial Regeneration*
Edited by: M. S. Penn © Humana Press Inc., Totowa, NJ

injured myocardium and improves left ventricular function *(3)*. Thus, while controversy still exists regarding whether the early experiments of Orlic and colleagues actually resulted in regeneration of cardiac myocytes, it is critical to note that no controversy exists as to whether myocardial function was improved in these studies by the delivery of hematopoietic stem cells to the heart at the time of myocardial infarction (MI).

Mononuclear preparations from bone marrow aspirates contain not only HSCs, but also multiple other stem cell types, the most distinct perhaps being the mesenchymal stem cell (MSC) *(8)*. In bone marrow transplant trials, MSCs have been shown to support HSC engraftment, suggesting that MSCs work in symphony with HSCs to revascularize the myocardium *(9)*. These cells are known to express multiple cytokines, which may alter the repair response of freshly injured myocardium *(10)*, and have been shown by some *(11,12)* but not all groups *(13,14)*.

STEM CELL TRANSPLANTATION IN ACUTE MI

Early Trials

A number of issues remain unresolved regarding the delivery of stem cells to myocardial tissue. Perhaps the most obvious is the mode of delivery, via either direct intramyocardial injection at the time of surgery, percutaneous direct myocardial injection into the endocardium, or percutaneous via intracoronary infusion. Amazingly, the original rodent studies were published in May 2001, and the first studies investigating the safety of these different approaches in different clinical populations were published beginning the very next year (Table 1). The first of these was a phase I trial in 10 patients within days of MI, suggesting that intracoronary delivery of bone marrow-derived mononuclear cells resulted in improved left ventricular (LV) contractility and improved perfusion of the infarct zone 3 months later *(15)*. Expanding on these data, it has been demonstrated that intracoronary infusion of either bone marrow-derived mononuclear cells or peripheral blood-derived endothelial progenitor cells (endothelial characteristics defined as Dil-acetylated low-density lipoprotein uptake, lectin binding, and the expression of typical endothelial marker proteins, including CD105, vascular endothelial growth factor receptor [VEGFR]2, von Willebrand factor, CD31, and CD146) within days of MI resulted in improved regional LV function and viability within the infarct zone *(16)*.

One year follow-up of the Transplantation of Progenitor Cells and Regeneration Enhancement in Acute Myocardial Infarction trial including additional patients *(17)* showed no adverse events with stem cell therapy, including no increase in subsequent MI or ventricular arrhythmia. Importantly, they demonstrated that the level of increase in ejection fraction (EF) was directly related to the degree of LV dysfunction at the time of cell therapy. Linear regression revealed that there was an absolute 20% increase in EF for patients who started with an EF of 20%; however, the increase in EF was only 5% in patients with an initial EF of 60%.

Randomized Trials

The first randomized stem cell trial for patients with acute MI was the Benefits of Oxygen Saturation Targeting (BOOST) trial *(18)*. In the BOOST trial, all patients were emergently reperfused by primary percutaneous coronary intervention and received optimal medical care. One half of the patients were randomized to receive intracoronary infusion of a mononuclear preparation of cells from the marrow space of the iliac

Table 1
Hematopoietic or Bone Marrow-Derived Stem Cell Studies in Patients With Acute Myocardial Infarction

Study (ref.)	No. patients/ placebo control	Cell type	Delivery method	Time after infarct (a)	Baseline LV function (%)	Comments
Strauer (15)	10/No	Mononuclear BM-derived cells	Intracoronary	5–9	57	An improvement in LV cavity dimensions and systolic function as well as improved myocardial perfusion were seen at 3 m follow-up. No acute procedure related complications or long term complications were seen.
Assmus (16)	20/No	BM-derived mononuclear cells	Intracoronary	4.3 ± 1.5	52	Improved EF, regional contractile function and increased myocardial viability were seen within the infarct zone at 4 mo follow-up. No acute procedure-related complications or long-term complications were seen.
Fuchs (25)	10/No	BM-derived stem cells	Transendocardial	N/A	N/A	Study on patients with myocardial ischemia without option for percutaneous or surgical revascularization. CCS Angina Class before vs 3 mo after: 3.1 ± 0.3 vs 2.0 ± 0.94.
Chen (24)	69/Yes	BM-derived MSC	Intracoronary	18.4 ± 1.5	49–53	Improvement in perfusion cardiac function and decreased LV dilation. No increase in restenosis noted.
BOOST (18)	60/Yes	BM-derived mononuclear cells	Intracoronary	4.8	50–51	Six months after MI, increase in EF (6.7%) in patients received BM cells compared to 0.6% in optimal medical management.

(Continued)

Table 1 (*Continued*)

Study (ref.)	No. patients/ placebo control	Cell type	Delivery method	Time after infarct (a)	Baseline LV function (%)	Comments
OPCARE-MI (17)	59/No	BM-derived mononuclear cells or peripheral blood derived progenitor cells	Intracoronary	4.9 ± 1.5	49–51	Improved EF and decreased LV end-systolic volume at 4 mo after stem cell therapy. No arrhythmias out to 12 m after cell therapy. No difference between BM-derived or peripheral blood-derived cells.
ASTAMI (20)	100/Yes	BM-derived mononuclear cells	Intracoronary	5–8	46	Noted chest pain and/or EKG changes with infusion. No improvement 6 mo after cell stem cell infusion.
REPAIR-AMI (19)	204/Yes	BM-derived mononuclear cells	Intrcoronary	4	47–48	Modest improvement in EF 4 mo after stem cell infusion 5.5% with stem cells vs 3.0% for placebo. For EF <49% at baseline, improvement was 7.5% with stem cells vs 2.5% for placebo.
Janssens (21)	66/Yes	BM-derived	Intracoronary	4	46–49	First randomized, placebo controlled blinded study for cell therapy at thetime of AMI. No benefit seen.

LV, left ventricular; BM, bone marrow; EF, ejection fraction; MSC, mesenchymal stem cell; AMI, acute myocardial infarction.

Table 2

Baseline and Follow-up Ejection Fraction Measurements in Control and Active Arms
of Randomized Hematopoietic Stem Cell or Bone Marrow-Derived Mononuclear Cell Trials
in Patients with Actue Myocardial Infarction

Trial (ref.)	Baseline EF (%)		Follow-up (mo)	Follow-up EF (%)		Difference control/active
	Control	Active		Control	Active	
Boost (18)	51.3	50	6	52	56.7	0.7/6.7
ASTAMI (20)	46	46	6	48.1	49.1	2.1/3.1
REPAIR-AMI (19)	47	48	4	50	54	3.0/5.5
Janssens (21)	46.9	48.5	4	49.1	51.8	2.2/3.4

EF, ejection fraction.

crest. The intracoronary infusion occurred between 4 and 5 days after MI. This study demonstrated that cell infusion did not result in an increase in troponin levels. Six months after cell infusion, patients in the active arm of the BOOST trialdemonstrated on average a 6.7% increase in EF, without significant changes in LV end-systolic or -diastolic volumes. Patients in the control arm exhibited only a 0.6% increase in EF. This unusually small increment in cardiac function with optimal medical therapy (Table 2) resulted in the improvement seen, with cell therapy being statistically significant.

The results seen in the BOOST population have recently been reproduced by those seen in the Reinfusion of Enriched Progenitor Cells and Infarct Remodeling in Acute Myocardial Infarction (REPAIR-AMI) trial (19). In the REPAIR-AMI trial, patients with acute MI received intracoronary infusion of bone marrow-derived cells 4 days after primary percutaneous coronary intervention. The absolute benefit seen in the REPAIR-AMI trial was smaller than that seen in the BOOST trial (6 vs 2.5%); both reached statistical significance. Of more concern is the fact that, on average, the entry LV function was less in the REPAIR-AMI trial than in the BOOST trial (Table 2). If our current understanding and our hope for future therapy were correct, we would have predicted the opposite: the sicker the heart, the better the improvement.

Whether this therapy has a real future is further complicated by the recent release of the Autologous Stem Cell Transplantation in Acute Myocardial Infarction (ASTAMI) trial results (20) and those of Janssen and colleagues (21). The ASTAMI trial was an open-label study in patients with acute ST-elevation anterior wall MI. This is the first study to limit enrollment to patients with anterior wall MI, arguably the patient population that is at greatest risk for developing chronic heart failure (CHF) and, thus, the one on whom we should be focusing the most. The ASTAMI trial showed no benefit with infusion of autologous bone marrow-derived mononuclear cells. Although this was a well-designed and -executed study, some concern could be raised regarding the timing of stem cell infusion. It is unclear whether stem cells will home to the heart 5–8 days after MI because of the possible lack of stem cell homing factor expression that long after MI (7,22).

The study by Janssen et al. is the first randomized, placebo-controlled, blinded study of stem cell therapy in patients with acute MI (21). All patients underwent bone marrow biopsy and infusion into the infarct-related coronary artery. However, 50% of the patients received saline instead of their own cells. Although a heroic and ideal study design, one might have hoped that, considering the invasive nature of the control arm, only a patient population at high risk for the development of CHF would have been eligible. That said, the right coronary artery was the infarct-related artery in one-third of the patients, and the baseline ejection fraction at the time of enrollment for the complete study population was approx 47% by magnetic resonance imaging (MRI).

Performing a blinded, placebo-controlled study was critical to the field because questions have arisen as to whether the improvement in EF seen in other studies was a result of the procedure involved in delivering the stem cells, or the stem cells themselves. In most trials in which stem cells are infused, there is transient and repeated cessation of blood flow in the infarct-related vessel at the time of stem cell infusion. Concerns have been raised that this technique could induce preconditioning-like responses in the myocardium, resulting in improved LV remodeling. Transient ischemia could also prolong stem cell homing signals within the myocardium, resulting in a prolonged healing response (7,23). Unfortunately, in this well-done study no improvement in cardiac function was observed 4 months after MI. Importantly, the investigators did note a significant increase in the likelihood of improved contractility in segments with increasing transmural involvement in those patients who received bone marrow-derived cells compared to controls. They also observed a greater reduction in infarct size as measured as late enhancement volume by MRI at 4 months after MI. Whether these types of changes will result in long-term benefit is unknown but is critical if these therapies are to ultimately be considered useful.

Mesenchymal Stem Cells

There are limited clinical data for the specific use of MSCs in acute MI. The largest experience to date is that of Chen and colleagues (24). In this study bone marrow was harvested 8 days after MI, and MSCs were expanded in culture for 7–10 days in order to obtain a sufficient number of cells. On average, 18 days after acute MI the cells or saline were delivered via an intracoronary infusion into the infarct-related vessel. Baseline ejection of the population at the time of intracoronary infusion was 49 ± 9%. Three months later, a significant improvement in cardiac function was observed in those patients who received bone marrow-derived MSCs (67% ± 11%) compared to saline (53% ± 8%). Whether MSCs are a better cell type than a whole bone marrow preparation or hematopoietic stem cells is still uncertain. Furthermore, it is likely that prior to broad adoption of MSCs, the issue of whether allogeneic MSCs can be implemented needs to be fully addressed.

SUMMARY

A significant amount of data has been amassed regarding the feasibility, safety, and efficacy of autologous intracoronary stem cell infusion within days of an acute MI. Some premature conclusions may be drawn. First, the strategy is feasible; second, the strategy appears safe, without any untoward events noted in the patients who receive intracoronary stem cell therapy; third, there appears to be no concern about an increase in MI or arrhythmia in patients who receive hematopoietic stem cell or whole bone marrow preparations. Although this favors going forward with this strategy, the issue of efficacy is still uncertain. Disappointingly, investigators to date have in general taken all patients, without any regard for the degree of LV dysfunction. Thus, most patients studied to date would have been at relatively low risk for the development of death or CHF.

The potential power and hope of stem cell therapy was first demonstrated in animal models with large MIs. The benefits were profound (1,3). To date we have not seen this profound benefit in clinical populations. Whether this is because we have not focused our clinical trials to date in high-risk patients or whether the strategy will not translate well to clinical populations is unknown. We now realize that the likelihood of true myocardial regeneration with this strategy is unlikely *(5,6)*. Whether and how this field moves forward is unclear. No doubt larger clinical trials with strategies implemented to date that demonstrate modest benefits will be undertaken. However, perhaps a focus on patients at high risk for morbidity and mortality following acute MI needs to be undertaken, in collaboration with our colleagues at the bench who are trying to unravel and optimize the biology at play.

REFERENCES

1. Orlic D, Kajstura J, Chimenti S, et al. Bone marrow cells regenerate infarcted myocardium. Nature 2001;410:701–705.
2. Orlic D, Kajstura J, Chimenti S, et al. Mobilized bone marrow cells repair the infarcted heart, improving function and survival. Proc Natl Acad Sci USA 2001;98:10,344–10,349.
3. Kocher AA, Schuster MD, Szabolcs MJ, et al. Neovascularization of ischemic myocardium by human bone-marrow-derived angioblasts prevents cardiomyocyte apoptosis, reduces remodeling and improves cardiac function. Nat Med 2001;7:430–436.
4. Orlic D, Fischer R, Nishikawa S, Nienhuis AW, Bodine DM. Purification and characterization of heterogeneous pluripotent hematopoietic stem cell populations expressing high levels of c-kit receptor. Blood 1993;82:762–770.
5. Murry CE, Soonpaa MH, Reinecke H, et al. Haematopoietic stem cells do not transdifferentiate into cardiac myocytes in myocardial infarcts. Nature 2004;428:664–668.
6. Balsam LB, Wagers AJ, Christensen JL, Kofidis T, Weissman IL, Robbins RC. Haematopoietic stem cells adopt mature haematopoietic fates in ischaemic myocardium. Nature 2004;428:668–673.
7. Askari A, Unzek S, Popovic ZB, et al. Effect of stromal-cell-derived factor-1 on stem cell homing and tissue regeneration in ischemic cardiomyopathy. Lancet 2003;362:697–703.
8. Haynesworth SE, Baber MA, Caplan AI. Cell surface antigens on human marrow-derived mesenchymal cells are detected by monoclonal antibodies. Bone 1992;13:69–80.
9. Koc ON, Gerson SL, Cooper BW, et al. Rapid hematopoietic recovery after coinfusion of autologous-blood stem cells and culture-expanded marrow mesenchymal stem cells in advanced breast cancer patients receiving high-dose chemotherapy. J Clin Oncol 2000;18:307–316.
10. Haynesworth SE, Baber MA, Caplan AI. Cytokine expression by human marrow-derived mesenchymal progenitor cells in vitro: effects of dexamethasone and IL-1 alpha. J Cell Physiol 1996;166:585–592.
11. Mangi AA, Noiseux N, Kong D, et al. Mesenchymal stem cells modified with Akt prevent remodeling and restore performance of infarcted hearts. Nat Med 2003;9:1195–1201.
12. Toma C, Pittenger MF, Cahill KS, Byrne BJ, Kessler PD. Human mesenchymal stem cells differentiate to a cardiomyocyte phenotype in the adult murine heart. Circulation 2002;105:93–98.
13. Guarita-Souza LC, Carvalho KA, Rebelatto C, et al. Cell transplantation: differential effects of myoblasts and mesenchymal stem cells. Int J Cardiol in press.
14. Fazel S, Chen L, Weisel RD, et al. Cell transplantation preserves cardiac function after infarction by infarct stabilization: augmentation by stem cell factor. J Thorac Cardiovasc Surg 2005;130:1310.
15. Strauer BE, Brehm M, Zeus T, et al. Repair of infarcted myocardium by autologous intracoronary mononuclear bone marrow cell transplantation in humans. Circulation 2002;106:1913–1918.
16. Assmus B, Schachinger V, Teupe C, et al. Transplantation of progenitor cells and regeneration enhancement in acute myocardial infarction (TOPCARE-AMI). Circulation 2002;106:3009–3017.
17. Schachinger V, Assmus B, Britten MB, et al. Transplantation of progenitor cells and regeneration enhancement in acute myocardial infarction: final one-year results of the TOPCARE-AMI Trial. J Am Coll Cardiol 2004;44:1690–1699.
18. Wollert KC, Meyer GP, Lotz J, et al. Intracoronary autologous bone-marrow cell transfer after myocardial infarction: the BOOST randomised controlled clinical trial. Lancet 2004;364:141–148.
19. Schachinger V, Tonn T, Dimmeler S, Zeiher AM. Bone-marrow-derived progenitor cell therapy in need of proof of concept: design of the REPAIR-AMI trial. Nat Clin Pract Cardiovasc Med 2006; Suppl 1:S23–S28.

20. Lunde K, Solheim S, Aakhus S, et al. and ASTAMI investigators. Autologous stem cell transplantation in acute myocardial infarction: the ASTAMI randomized controlled trial intracoronary transplantation of autologous mononuclear bone marrow cells, study design and safety aspects. Second Cardiovasc J 2005;39:150–158.

21. Janssen S, Dubois C, Bogaert J, et al. Autologous bone marrow-derived stem cell transfer in patients with ST-segment elevation myocardial infarction. A double-blind, randomised, controlled study. Lancet 2006;367:113–121.

22. Hofmann M, Wollert KC, Meyer GP, et al. Monitoring of bone marrow cell homing into the infarcted human myocardium. Circulation 2005;111:2198–2202.

23. Ceradini DJ, Kulkarni AR, Callaghan MJ, et al. Progenitor cell trafficking is regulated by hypoxic gradients through HIF-1 induction of SDF-1. Nat Med 2004;10:858–864.

24. Chen SL, Fang WW, Qian J, et al. Improvement of cardiac function after transplantation of autologous bone marrow mesenchymal stem cells in patients with acute myocardial infarction. Clin Med J (Engl) 2004;117:1443–1448.

25. Fuchs S, Satler LF, Kornowski R, et al. Catheter-based autologous bone marrow myocardial injection in no-option patients with advanced coronary artery disease: a feasibility study. J Am Coll Cardiol 2003;41:1721–1724.

20

Strategies for Cytokine Modification and Stem Cell Mobilization for Acute Myocardial Infarction

Stephen G. Ellis, MD and Brian J. Bolwell, MD

SUMMARY

Previous dogma held that an acute myocardial infarction (MI) resulted in absolute death of the involved myocardium and could only be modulated by reperfusion therapy. Recent data demonstrating the presence of a natural repair process stimulated by the release of chemokines in response to injury have challenged that belief. Unfortunately, this natural repair mechanism occurs at a rate that precludes any meaningful recovery of myocardial tissue and function. The feasibility of myocardial repair/regeneration has been demonstrated through delivery of either exogenously expanded stem cells or endogenously mobilized stem cells expanded by growth factors (i.e., granulocyte–colony-stimulating factor). Although data regarding the use of various growth factors in order to attenuate the extent of damage or facilitate repair of injured myocardium remain limited, the early experiences have suggested safety. From these data, one may envision a potential therapeutic strategy that augments the naturally occurring repair process early following a MI through mobilization of stem cells that will minimize damage and limit the dysfunction for a substantial proportion of patients.

Key Words: Stem cells, mobilization, growth factors, myocardial repair/regeneration, acute MI.

CLINICAL BACKGROUND AND PATHOPHYSIOLOGY

Following injury to most organs, local and systemic reparative processes are activated, generally leading to partial or complete restoration of function *(1–4)*. In the case of ischemic injury to the heart, in addition to local processes, transient elaboration of cytokines leads to homing of cells normally circulating or resident in the bone marrow *(5)*. A simplified schematic of pathways, cytokines, and cell markers is provided in Fig. 1. Unfortunately, the number of recruited cells is meager, their paracrine effects are difficult to measure, and the overall clinical benefit is modest *(6,7)*.

Although the number is actually falling slightly, nearly 1 million patients present to US hospitals annually with ST-elevation myocardial infarction (MI). Reperfusion therapy has dramatically improved the prognosis for many, but those with appreciable heart muscle dysfunction manifest by Killip class III–IV symptoms (chronic heart failure

From: *Contemporary Cardiology: Stem Cells and Myocardial Regeneration*
Edited by: M. S. Penn © Humana Press Inc., Totowa, NJ

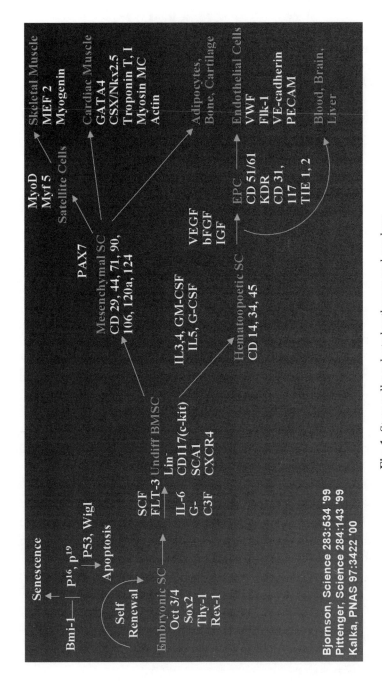

Fig. 1. Stem cells: selected pathways and markers.

or cardiogenic shock) at or early after presentation are left with a 30–50% 30-day mortality rate *(8–11)*. Principal functional gain is seen when reperfusion is achieved within 4 hours of infarct onset *(7,11)*. It is the patient with large infarction and/or delayed reperfusion in particular for whom stem cell or other novel forms of repairative/protective therapy is most well-suited.

Approaches to "stem cell therapy" in this setting have developed along two general lines—intracoronary injection of relatively crude purifications of bone marrow aspirates *(12–14)* and attempts to enhance the normal mobilization and homing processes. This chapter will focus on the latter approach.

Without the stimulous of tissue damage, stem cell contribution to maintenance and repair cardiac function is very modest *(15,16)*. To study the role of stem cells in tissue damage, Jackson and colleagues utilized a mouse model of infarction and Rosa 26 (*LacZ*-positive) repopulation of bone marrow following irradiation to allow tracking of bone marrow-derived cells. They demonstrated that 3 weeks after coronary artery occlusion, approx 3% of cardiac endothelial cells and 0.02% of myocytes appeared to be bone marrow-derived *(6)*.

To study the consequences of a more robust stem cell effect, Kocher injected 2×10^6 granulocyte–colony-stimulating factor (G-CSF)-mobilized human $CD34^+$ cells (90% $CD45^+$, 70% $CD117^+$, 1% $CD14^+$) into the tail veins of athymic nude rats 48 h after infarction and reported the effects 2 weeks later. Recombinant human G-CSF (Neupogen) has been in clinical use to treat neutropenias and to augment blood progenitor cell collection for more than a decade. Given subcutaneously, it leads to a 30-fold increase in circulating $CD34^+$ cells within 4–5 days *(17)*. Cytometric characterization of mobilized cells is shown in Fig. 2 *(18)*. Histopathological evidence of neoangiogenesis, less apoptosis, more than 50% smaller infarcts, and better left ventricular (LV) function was seen compared with sham-treated animals *(18)*. Similar results were reported by Schuster *(19)*. Interestingly, mobilized and engrafted cell survival appeared to be extremely modest *(20)*. Although initial interpretation of benefit focused on the possibility of milieu-based transdifferentiation into cardiomyocytes *(21,22)*, more recent data suggest that neoangiogenesis and paracrine effects predominate *(18)*.

These observations led to the seminal study of Anversa and Orlic, wherein utilizing a mouse infarct model after splenectomy to minimize sequestration of mobilized cells, G-CSF and another mobilizer, stem cell factor (SCF), were given for 5 days prior to MI. Four weeks after MI they reported histopathological evidence of transdifferentiation into cardiomyocyte-like cells at the infarct border zone, in conjunction with dramatic improvement in LV function and survival to 30 days compared with sham-treated animals *(21)*. Also in a mouse model, but more clinically relevant in that the therapy was given after infarction, Fujita and colleagues reported similar results with G-CSF, but cautioned that another stimulating factor, granulocyte macrophage (GM)-CSF, was associated with increased early mortality as a result of myocardial rupture *(23)*. Minatoguchi used postinfarction G-CSF in a rabbit model and found a significant reduction in scar area at 3 months as well as confocal microscopic suggestion of bone marrow-derived cardiomyocytes *(24)*. Alteration of postinfarction healing (increase in transforming growth factor-β, pro-collagen types I and III) has also been reported with G-CSF in small animal models *(25)*, and G-CSF has also been reported to have direct effects on the survival of ischemic cardiomyocytes via activation of the Jak/Stat3 pathway *(26)*. Anversa, however, has not been able to replicate such results in large animal models *(27)*.

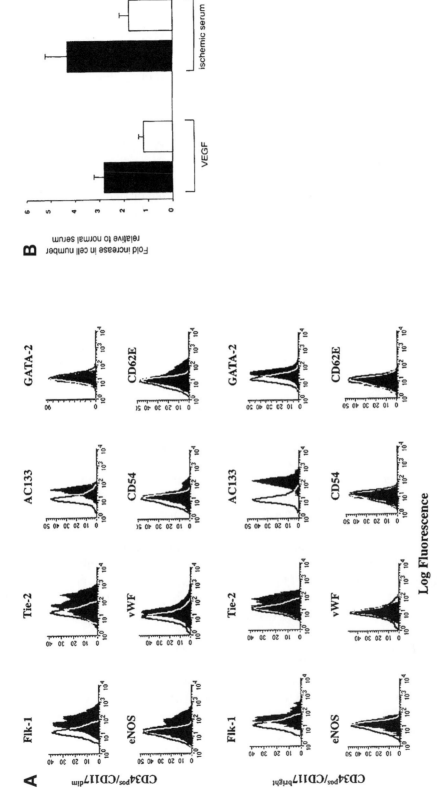

Fig. 2. G-CSF mobilizes into the circulation a human bone marrow-derived population that differentiates into endothelial cells. (**A**) Four-parameter flow cytometric phenotypic characterization of living (defined by 7-AAD straining), G-CSF–mobilized cells derived from adult human bone marrow. For each marker used, shaded areas represent background log fluorescence relative to isotype control antibody. (**B**) Proliferative responses to various stimuli of single-donor CD34+ human cells sorted on the basis of bright and dim CD117 expression and co-expression of intracellular GATA-2 protein. Graph shows 96-hour proliferative responses ■, CD117 Bright/GATA-2Hi; □, CD117Dim/GATA-2Lo ($p < 0.01$ for both comparisons).

BEYOND G-CSF

Treatment with G-CSF remains the gold standard for hematopoietic stem cell mobilization for patients undergoing autologous hematopoietic cell transplantation. It is also known that there is a surge in CD34$^+$ cells into the peripheral blood as patients recover from certain cytotoxic chemotherapeutic agents, including cyclophosphamide and etoposide *(28–30)*. SCF interacts synergistically with G-CSF to mobilize stem cells, but SCF has yet to gain Food and Drug Administration (FDA) approval in the United States. A newer agent, AMD 3100, a CXCR-4 inhibitor, has shown great promise as a new and novel mobilizing agent.

STEM CELL FACTOR

SCF is a ligand for the receptor encoded by the c-*kit* proto-oncogene, which is expressed on a variety of cells, including hematopoietic cells and mast cells *(31–34)*. The c-kit ligand plays a major physiological role in stem cell development.

In the 1990s, several clinical trials were conducted investigating the use of SCF, usually in conjunction with G-CSF, as a stem cell-mobilizing agent. A summary of clinical trials studying large numbers of patients is shown in Table 1. Several themes are apparent. First, SCF combined with G-CSF is an effective mobilizing regimen. SCF plus G-CSF generally mobilizes more CD34$^+$ cells than does G-CSF alone. The usual treatment schedule is to receive SCF plus G-CSF for 5–9 days, with stem cell collection beginning on the fifth day of therapy. SCF plus G-CSF results in moderately increased numbers of CD34$^+$ cells collected over every leukapheresis day.

Early studies of SCF noted a small but defined incidence of allergic reactions, which were occasionally severe *(34–38)*. Local reactions at injection sites were also seen. Subsequent studies generally used a three-drug pretreatment regimen of ranitidine, albuterol, and either diphenhydramine or cetirizine to decrease mast cell-mediated side effects of the drug. Even with this extensive premedication, approx 10% of patients still experience severe allergic reactions *(38)*.

In summary, although SCF is synergistic with G-CSF and results in moderately increased numbers of CD34$^+$ cells collected, local toxicities at injection sites are common, and some allergic toxicities, which may be severe, have been described. SCF is not an FDA-approved drug in the United States at the present time.

AMD 3100

AMD 3100 is a selective antagonist of CXCR-4, the cognate receptor for stromal-derived factor I (SDF-I), which is expressed on CD34$^+$ hematopoietic progenitor cells *(39,40)*. AMD 3100 was first studied for its selective inhibition of HIV type I and II replication through binding to the CXCR-4 receptor, used by HIV for entry into CD4$^+$ cells *(41–43)*. As these studies progressed, it was noted that the HIV type I co-receptor CXCR-4 is preferentially expressed on the more immature CD34$^+$ hematopoietic stem cells *(44–46)*. Clinical trials were then designed to evaluate the pharmacokinetics and safety of AMD 3100 as a potential anti-HIV agent. However, Hendricks et al. described the use of AMD 3100 in human volunteers and noted a dramatic rise in peripheral white blood cell count 6–10 hours after receiving a dose of AMD 3100 *(47)*. As additional preclinical data noted that SDF-I and CXCR-4 may represent a new mechanism for

Table 1
Clinical Trials of SCF as a Mobilizing Agent

Author	Ref.	Year	Comment
Glaspy	8	1997	215 BC pts received G-CSF + SCF or G-CSF alone. G-CSF + SCF mobilized more CS34$^+$ cells. Allergic reactions described.
Facon	9	1999	102 MM pts received Cy + G-CSF or Cy + SCF + G-CSF. SCF group had 3-fold greater chance of reaching5 × 10^6 CD34$^+$ cells/kg in one leukopheresis. Mild to moderate injection site reactions common.
Weaver	10	1998	48 pts with OC received Cy + G-CSF alone or Cy + G-CSF + SCF. SCF + G-CSF mobilized more CD34$^+$ cells. Local reactions common; one patient developed anaphylactoid reaction.
Stiff	11	2000	102 heavily pretreated NHL or HD pts received SCF + G-CSF or G-CSF alone. Combination group mobilized more CD34$^+$ cells. Premedication with antihistamines and albuterol in all patients, but 10% still had "severe mast cell mediated reactions."

SCF, stem cell factor; Cy, cyclophosphamide; BC, breast cancer; OC, ovarian cancer; NHL, non-Hodgkin's lymphoma; HD, Hodgkin's disease; MM, multiple myeloma.

CD34$^+$ mobilization *(48–50)*, trials began to investigate AMD 3100 with and without G-CSF as a mobilizing agent in the clinical setting.

Liles et al. described the use of AMD 3100 in healthy volunteers and found a dose–response effect of AMD 3100 on CD34$^+$ cell mobilization into the peripheral blood *(51)*. The mobilization was rapid, with elevations of CD34$^+$ cells detected 3 hours after receiving a subcutaneous dose of AMD 3100, peaking at 9–10 hours after dosing. All adverse effects were mild and transient. The mobilization was detectable with a single dose of AMD 3100. A subsequent study of human volunteers combined AMD 3100 with recombinant human G-CSF for stem cell mobilization. Stem cell mobilization with AMD 3100 alone was similar to G-CSF alone. However, the combination of G-CSF and AMD 3100 resulted in a dramatic increase in circulating CD34$^+$ cells, again peaking approx 10 hours after AMD 3100 injection. Toxicities were mild and transient *(52)*.

One study of AMD 3100 for clinical CD34$^+$ mobilization prior to autologous stem cell transplant included 13 patients with hematological malignancies (7 with multiple myeloma and 6 with non-Hodgkin's lymphoma) who received AMD 3100 alone for stem cell mobilization. AMD 3100 resulted in a rapid and statistically significant increase in both total white blood cell count and peripheral blood CD34$^+$ cell counts *(53)*.

Taken together, these data have resulted in a multi-institutional, randomized, double-blind, placebo-controlled comparative trial of AMD 3100 plus G-CSF vs G-CSF plus placebo to mobilize CD34⁺ cells in both non-Hodgkin's lymphoma patients and multiple myeloma patients. These studies have just begun and should require approx 1 year for patient accrual. Investigators await these results with great interest as it appears that AMD 3100 is an effective, fast, and relatively nontoxic mobilizing agent with a novel mechanism of action.

EARLY CLINICAL TRIALS

Based on these preclinical data, several very small randomized and registry experiences have been undertaken in humans, providing glimpses of both potential benefit and risk. Kang and colleagues were the first to report preliminary data, in the form of the Myoblast Autologous Grafting in Ischemic Cardiomyopathy (MAGIC) trial *(54)*. Twenty-seven patients at least 48 hours after acute MI who were stable for at least 24 hours after percutaneous coronary intervention were randomized between intracoronary infusion of G-CSF mobilized peripheral blood stem cells, administration of 10 μg/kg/d G-CSF alone, or placebo. Intracoronary cell infusion limited infarct size, improved ejection fraction, and enhanced exercise time. Implanted bare metal stents in both the intracoronary cell therapy and G-CSF groups frequently developed restenosis, however (five of seven in the intracoronary infusion group and two of three in the G-CSF-alone group). Subsequently, both Nienaber and Ellis separately reported results from small-scale randomized trials randomizing patients between G-CSF and placebo, in conjunction with standard therapy for acute MI *(55,56)*. Nienabèr's study required ST elevation in at least three electrocardiogram leads and percutaneous coronary intervention within 24 hours of infarct onset, whereas our study required LV ejection fraction (EF) less than 40% and percutaneous coronary intervention 4–48 hours within infarct onset. Nienaber's study utilized G-CSF at a dose of 10 μg/kg per day, randomized 30 patients, and demonstrated a statistically significant improvement in EF between baseline and 6 months (52–56%, $p < 0.05$) and restenosis in only 13% of patients. Our study involved dose escalation from 5 to 10 μg/kg per day in 18 patients, and to date we have only reported on the low-dose results. No adverse events were noted, and the number of patients randomized was too small to adequately assess changes in LV function. In a nonrandomized study of 13 patients, De Lezo and colleagues reported a statistically significant relationship between peak CD34 level and gain in ejection fraction at 3 mo, but splenic rupture 8 d after G-CSF in one patient *(57)* (very rarely noted when G-CSF is utilized for approved indications). Potentially more troubling still are unconfirmed reports of an excess in acute coronary syndrome events when G-CSF is experimentally used in the chronic setting to try to induce angiogenesis *(58)*.

REFERENCES

1. Sell S. Heterogeneity and plasticity of hepatocyte lineage cells. Hepatology 2001;33:738–750.
2. Cohen IK, Diegelmann RF, Lindblad WJ, eds. Wound Healing: Biochemical and Clinical Aspects. Saunders, Philadelphia, 1992.
3. Veizovic T, Beech JS, Stroemer P, Watson WP, Hodges H. Resolution of stroke deficits following contralateral grafts of conditionally immortal neuroepithelial stem cells. Stroke 2001;32: 1012–1019.
4. Asahara T, Masuda H, Takahashi T, et al. Bone marrow origin of endothelial progenitor cells responsible for postnatal vasculogenesis in physiological and pathological neovascularization. Circ Res 1999;85:221–228.

5. Askari AT, Unzek S, Popovic ZB, et al. Effect of stromal-cell-derived factor 1 on stem-cell homing and tissue regeneration in ischaemic cardiomyopathy. Lancet 2003;362:697–703.
6. Jackson K, Majka SM, Wang H, et al. Regeneration of ischemic cardiac muscle and vascular endothelium by adult stem cells. J Clin Invest 2001;107(11):1395–1402.
7. Sheiban I, Fragasso G, Lu C, Tonni S, Trevi GP, Chierchia SL. Influence of treatment delay on long-term left ventricular function in patients with acute myocardial infarction successfully treated with primary angioplasty. Am Heart J 2001;141:603–609.
8. Gruppo Italiano per lo Studio della Streptochinasi nell'Infarto Miocardico (GISSI). Effectiveness of intravenous thrombolytic treatment in acute myocardial infarction. Lancet 1986;327:397–402.
9. Assessment of the safety and efficacy of a new thrombolytic (ASSENT-2) investigators. Single-bolus tenecteplase compared with front-loaded alteplase in acute myocardial infarction: the ASSENT-2 double-blind randomized trial. Lancet 1999;354:716–722.
10. GUSTO IIb Angioplasty Substudy Investigators (Ellis SG, principal investigator). A clinical trial comparing primary coronary angioplasty with tissue plasminogen activator for acute myocardial infarction. N Engl J Med 1997;336:1621–1628.
11. Hochman JS, Buller CE, Sleeper LA, et al. Cardiogenic shock complicating acute myocardial infarction—etiologies, management and outcome: a report from the SHOCK Trial Registry. Should we emergently revascularize occluded coronaries for cardiogenic shock? J Am Coll Cardiol 2000; 36:1063–1070.
12. Wollert KC, Meyer GP, Lotz J, et al. Intracoronary autologous bone-marrow cell transfer after myocardial infarction: the BOOST randomized controlled clinical trial. Lancet 2004;364: 141–148.
13. Schachinger V, Assmus B, Britten MB, et al. Transplantation of progenitor cells and regeneration enhancement in acute myocardial infarction: final one-year results of the TOPCARE-AMI Trial. J Am Coll Cardiol 2004;44(8):1690–1699.
14. Kawada H, Fujita J, Kinjo K, et al. Non-hematopoetic mesenchymal stem cells can be mobilized and differentiated into cardiomyocytes after myocardial infarction. Blood 2004;104:12:3581–3587.
15. Wagers AJ, Sherwood RI, Christensen JL, Weissman IL. Little evidence for developmental plasticity of adult hematopoietic stem cells. Science 2002;297:2256–2259.
16. Quaini F, Urbanek K, Beltrami AP, et al. Chimerism of the transplanted heart. N Engl J Med 2002;346:5–15.
17. Bishop MR, Tarantolo SR, Jackson JD, et al. Allogeneic-blood stem-cell collection following mobilization with low-dose granulocyte colony-stimulating factor. J Clin Oncol 1997;15: 1601–1607.
18. Kocher AA, Schuster MD, Szabolcs MJ, et al. Neovascularization of ischemic myocardium by human bone-marrow-derived angioblasts prevents cardiomyocyte apoptosis, reduces remodeling and improves cardiac function. Nat Med 2001;7:430–436.
19. Schuster MD, Kocher AA, Seki T, et al. Myocardial neovascularization by bone marrow angioblasts results in cardiomyocyte regeneration. Am J Physiol Heart Circ Physiol 2004;287:H525–H532.
20. Murry CE, Soonpaa MH, Reinecke H, et al. Haematopoietic stem cells do not transdifferentiate into cardiac myocytes in myocardial infarcts. Nature 2004;428.
21. Orlic D, Kajstura J, Chimenti S, et al. Mobilized bone marrow cells repair the infracted heart, improving function and survival. PNAS 2001;98(18):10,344–10,349.
22. Rangappa S, Entwistle JWC, Wechsler AS, Kresh JY. Cardiomyocytes can induce human mesenchymal stem cells to express cardiac phenotype and genotype. Circulation 2002;106(19):II-235.
23. Fujita J, Suzuki Y, Ando K, et al. G-CSF improves post-infarction heart failure by mobilizing bone marrow stem cells, but GM-CSF increases the mortality by deteriorating heart function in mice. Circulation 2002;106(19):11–15.
24. Minatoguchi S, Takemura G, Chen XH, et al. Acceleration of the healing process and myocardial regeneration may be important as a mechanism of improvement of cardiac function and remodeling by postinfarction granulocyte colony-stimulating factor treatment. Circulation 2004;109:2572–2580.
25. Sugano Y, Anzai T, Yoshikawa T, et al. Granulocyte colony-stimulating factor attenuates early ventricular expansion after experimental myocardial infarction. Cardiovasc Res 2005;65:446–456.
26. Harada M, Qin Y, Takano H, et al. G-CSF prevents cardiac remodeling after myocardial infarction by activating the Jak-Stat pathway in cardiomyocytes. Nat Med 2005;11:305–311.
27. Orlic D, Arai AE, Sheikh FH, et al. Cytokine mobilized CD34+ cells do not benefit rhesus monkey following induced myocardial infarction. Blood 2002;100,(11):28a.

28. Möhle R, Pförsich M, Fruehauf S, Witt B, Krämer A, Haas R. G-CSF post-chemotherapy mobilizes more CD34+ cells with use during steady-state hematopoiesis. Bone Marrow Transplant 1994;14:827–832.

29. Meisenberg B, Brehm T, Schmeckel A, Miller W, McMillan R. A combination of low-dose cyclophosphamide and colony-stimulating factors is more cost-effective than granulocyte-colony-stimulating factors alone in mobilizing peripheral blood stem and progenitor cells. Transfusion 1998;38:209–215.

30. Copelan E, Ceselski S, Essone S, et al. Mobilization of peripheral-blood progenitor cells with high-dose etoposide and granulocyte colony-stimulating factor in patients with breast cancer, non-Hodgkin's lymphoma, and Hodgkin's disease. J Clin Oncol 1997;15:759–765.

31. Zsebo K, Wypych J, McNiece I, et al. Identification, purification, and biological characterization of hematopoietic stem cell factor from buffalo rat liver-conditioned medium. Cell 1990;63:195–201.

32. Anderson D, Lyman S, Baird A, et al. Molecular cloning of mast cell growth factor, a hematopoietin that is active in both membrane bound and soluble forms. Cell 1990;63:235–243.

33. Martin F, Suggs S, Langley K, et al. Primary structure and functional expression of rat and human stem factor DNAs. Cell 1990;63:203–211.

34. Zsebo K, Willimas D, Geissler E, et al. Stem cell factor is encoded at the SI locus of the mouse and is the ligand for the c-kit tyrosine kinase receptor. Cell 1990;63:213–224.

35. Glaspy JA, Shpall EJ, LeMaistre CF, et al. Peripheral blood progenitor cell mobilization using stem cell factor in combination with G-CSF in breast cancer patients. Blood 1997;90:2939–2951.

36. Facon T, Harousseau J, Maloisel F, et al. Stem cell factor in combination with G-CSF after chemotherapy improves peripheral blood progenitor cell yield and reduces apheresis requirements in multiple myeloma patients: a randomized, controlled trial. Blood 1999;94:1218–1225.

37. Weaver A, Chang J, Wrigley E, et al. Randomized comparison of progenitor-cell mobilization using chemotherapy, stem-cell factor, and G-CSF or chemotherapy plus G-CSF alone in patients with ovarian cancer. J Clin Oncol 1998;16:2601–2612.

38. Stiff P, Gingrich R, Luger S, et al. A randomized phase 2 study of PBPC mobilization by stem cell factor and G-CSF in heavily pretreated patients with Hodgkin's disease or non-Hodgkin's lymphoma. Bone Marrow Transplant 2000;26:471–481.

39. Möhle R, Bautz F, Fafii S, et al. The chemokine receptor CXCR-4 is expressed on CD34+ hematopoietic progenitors and leukemic c ells and mediates transendothelial migration induced by stromal cell-derived factor-1. Blood 1998;91:4523–4530.

40. Aiuti A, Tavian M, Cipponi A, et al. Expression of CXCR4, the receptor for stromal cell-derived factor-1 on fetal and adult human lympho-hematopoietic progenitors. Eur J Immunol 1999;29:1823–1831.

41. Schols D, Esté J, Henson G, De Clercq E. Cibyclams, a class of potent anti-HIV agents, are targeted at the HIV coreceptor Fusin/CXCR-4. Antiviral Res 1997;35:147–156.

42. Labrosse B, Brelot A, Heveker N, et al. Determinants for sensitivity of human immunodeficiency virus coreceptor CXCR4 to the bicyclam AMD3100. J Virol 1998;72:6381–6388.

43. Egberink H, De Clercq E, Van Vliet A, et al. Bicyclams, selective antagonists of the Human chemokine receptor CXCR4, potently inhibit feline immunodeficiency virus replication. J Virol 1999;73:6346–6352.

44. Viardot A, Kronenwett R, Deichmann M, Haas R. The human immunodeficiency virus (HIV)-type 1 coreceptor CXCR-4 (fusin) is preferentially expressed on the more immature CD34+ hematopoietic stem cells. Ann Hematol 1998;77:193–197.

45. Rosu-Myles M, Gallacher L, Murdoch B, et al. The human hematopoietic stem cell compartment is heterogeneous for CXCR4 expression. PNAS 2000;97:14,626–14,631.

46. Lataillade J, Clay D, Dupuy C, et al. Chemokine SDF-1 enhances circulating CD34+ cell proliferation in synergy with cytokines: possible role in progenitor survival. Blood 2000;95:756–768.

47. Hendrix C, Flexner C, MacFarland R, et al. Pharmacokinetics and safety of AMD 3100, a novel antagonist of the CXCR-4 chemokine receptor, in human volunteers. Antimicrobial agents and chemotherapy 2000;44:1667–1673.

48. Aiuti A, Webb I, Bleul C, Springer T, Gutierrez-Ramos JC. The chemokine SDF-1 is a chemoattractant for human CD34+ hematopoietic progenitor cells and provides a new mechanism to explain the mobilization of CD34+ progenitors to peripheral blood. J Exp Med 1997;185:111–120.

49. Lévesque J, Hendy J, Takamatsu Y, Simmons P, Bendall L. Disruption of the CXCR4/CXCL12 chemotactic interaction during hematopoietic stem cell mobilization induced by GCSD or cyclophosphamide. J Clin Invest 2003;110:187–196.

50. Lapidot T, Petit I. Current understanding of stem cell mobilization: The roles of chemokines, proteolytic enzymes, adhesion molecules, cytokines, and stromal cells. Exper Hematol 2002;30:973–981.

51. Liles W, Broxmeyer H, Rodger E, et al. Mobilization of hematopoietic progenitor cells in healthy volunteers by AMD3100, a CXCR4 antagonist. Blood 2003;102:2728–2730.

52. Liles W, Rodger E, Broxmeyer H, et al. Augmented mobilization and collection of CD34+ hematopoietic cells from normal human volunteers stimulated with granulocyte-colony-stimulating factor by single-dose administration of AMD3100, a CXCR4 antagonist. Transfusion 2005;45:295–300.

53. Devine S, Flomenberg N, Vesole D, et al. Rapid mobilization of CD34+ cells following administration of the CXCR4 antagonist AMD3100 to patients with multiple myeloma and non-Hodgkin's lymphoma. J Clin Oncol 2004;22:1095–1102.

54. Kang HJ, Kim HS, Zhang SY, et al. Effects of intracoronary infusion of peripheral blood stem-cells mobilized with granulocyte-colony stimulating factor on left ventricular systolic function and restenosis after coronary stenting in myocardial infarction: the MAGIC cell randomized clinical trial. Lancet 2004;363:751–756.

55. O'Neill WW, Dixon SR, Grines CL. The year in interventional cardiology. J Am Coll Cardiol 2005;45(7):1117–1134.

56. Ellis SG, Penn M, Bolwell B, Brezina K, McConnell G. Randomized trial of G-CSF for patients with large acute myocardial infarction: preliminary results of phase 1 study. Am J Cardiol 2004;94(6):86E.

57. DeLezo JS, Pan M, Medina A, et al. Rapamycin-eluting stents for the treatment of bifurcated coronary lesions: a randomized comparison of a simple versus complex strategy. Am Heart J 2004;148(5):857–864.

58. Hill JM, Syed MA, Arai AE, et al. Outcomes and risks of granulocyte colony-stimulating factor in patients with coronary artery disease. J Am Coll Cardiol 2005;46(9):1643–1648.

V SUMMARY/FUTURE CHALLENGES

21 Summary and Future Challenges

Marc S. Penn, MD, PhD

SUMMARY

We are on the verge of an extraordinary and exciting time in cardiovascular medicine. Until recently, it was believed that tissue damaged during a myocardial infarction was permanently lost. We now understand that there is a stem cell-based repair process that attempts to repair the injured myocardium. Unfortunately, this is a clinically inefficient process because of the short period during which the molecular signals are expressed, too few stem cells and/or the wrong cell type entering the injured tissue, or the lack of coordinating and/or differentiation signals expressed in the injured tissue. Importantly, we are now actively developing strategies that we believe could not only recover cardiac function but regenerate myocardial tissue as well. Further development and clinical fruition of these strategies for the treatment and/or prevention of chronic heart failure will require a high level of collaboration between the basic scientist and clinician and a great deal of rigorous work on both sides. The combination of the increasing prevalence of congestive heart failure, the economic burden of caring for these patients and the morbidity and mortality associated with the diagnosis, the potential human and societal benefits of unlocking the potential of stem cell therapy as a treatment is extraordinary.

Key Words: Regenerative medicine; congestive heart failure; gene therapy; clinical trials.

FUTURE CHALLENGES

If only because of the aging population, the need for regenerative strategies in general is great. This need is compounded because we have made great strides in the treatment of acute illnesses, leading patients to live in circumstances in which in the past they might have died, but with significant morbidity owing to decreased end-organ function. In the case of coronary artery disease and acute myocardial infarction (MI), the needs are exacerbated because of the rapidly increasing number of patients with chronic heart failure (CHF) worldwide.

Although great optimism has been generated by early preclinical studies that suggested the potential of myocardial regeneration using stem cells, clearly a number of critical clinical and scientific issues need to be addressed before these therapies will become either optimized or part of routine clinical practice to either prevent or treat CHF following MI. That said, the field continues to mature; no longer are case reports sensationalized in the media, and we have already progressed through noncontrolled phase I trials to randomized controlled trials for the administration of bone marrow-derived mononuclear cells to patient with acute MI. Perhaps now more than ever it continues to

From: *Contemporary Cardiology: Stem Cells and Myocardial Regeneration*
Edited by: M. S. Penn © Humana Press Inc., Totowa, NJ

be crucial that the public be accurately informed and have realistic expectations. Given the pervasiveness of the disease, the pressure/interest from patients and special interest groups is significant.

We have already learned a great deal from those investigators who have performed either feasibility and/or placebo-controlled studies for patients in the peri-infarct period or with CHF *(1–10)*. The majority of these studies implemented hematopoietic stem cells or preparations of whole bone marrow harvests. As discussed in other chapters, although these strategies for patients with acute MI have been show to be feasible and safe, studies with the most rigorous trial designs, either as a result of being blinded *(10)* or limiting patients to those with anterior wall MI *(9)*, have failed to demonstrate significant benefit. Although there is real hope for these cell types in patients with ischemic cardiomyopathy and CHF *(4,6)*, this strategy awaits blinded randomized trial results.

Along with hematopoietic stem cells and whole bone marrow mononuclear preparations, autologous skeletal myoblasts are being actively studied in clinical trials *(11–14)*. Skeletal myoblasts are not a stem cell type and do not differentiate into endogenous cells normally found in the heart. However, they do offer some hope for improving cardiac function when transplanted into patients with ischemic cardiomyopathy. Concerns still exist regarding the potential for skeletal myoblasts to increase the arrhythmogenic risk in patients *(11,12,15,16)*. Whether skeletal myoblasts will ultimately serve as a platform for gene delivery *(15,17,18)* or as a stand-alone cell population for the treatment of CHF is unclear. What is clear is that until one of the many stem cell types discussed earlier in this book is rigorously studied in clinical populations, skeletal myoblast therapy will likely be a viable option.

With respect to stem cell therapy for acute MI and/or CHF, many issues need to be addressed.

BASIC BIOLOGY

To ascertain which population of stem cells can differentiate into cardiac myocytes:

- The appropriate source or identity of a stem cell population that can be expanded sufficiently to allow for clinical application as well as predictably differentiate into a cardiac myocyte still remains to be identified.
- We need to identify the molecular pathways critical for stem cell differentiation into cardiac myocytes *(19)* and determine how to deliver those factors to injured myocardial tissue *(17,20)*. It is likely that this goal will be best achieved through the use of embryonic stem cells *(21)*.

The benefits of stem cell therapy for patients with acute MI require that a sufficient number of cells be available within days of the MI. Optimally, this would be obtained via an allogeneic source of appropriate stem cells for myocardial regeneration: Many of the cell types currently of interest will require a significant amount of time (weeks) in order to obtain a sufficient number of cells for each person. Therefore, an easily expanded and reliable source of allogeneic stem cells will likely be required *(22,23)*, and we need to determine how closely major histocompatibility complex class I and II matching is required to yield benefit without requiring immunosuppression.

Stem Cell Delivery Systems

Multiple catheter systems are being developed to deliver stem cells to myocardial tissue. Each of these approaches and systems requires validation. Similarly, depending

on the ability of the injected stem cell to migrate and respond to the local miroenviron-
ment, we will need to determine if myocardial mapping (e.g., NOGA system *[6]*) will
be required to optimize therapy.

The issues of timing of therapy and the dose of cells need to be studied and optimized for each stem cell population of interest.

Arrhythmogenic Effects

Early clinical studies with skeletal myoblasts have demonstrated that skeletal
myoblast transplantation may increase the arrhythmogenic risk in patients already at
significant risk *(11,12)*. These findings suggest that there could be adverse effects
following cell therapy. We need to identify the factors that make one cell type pro-
arrhythmogenic and others less arrhythmogenic. Once we understand that, we can further define the parameters that identify an optimal stem cell for myocardial
regeneration.

CLINICAL TRIALS

Clinical trials to date have focused on autologous stem cell sources. As the biology
of stem cell transplantation is better understood, studies implementing allogeneic
sources of stem cells will need to be under taken. General use immunosuppression in
such a large clinical population such as that with CHF seems impractical.

One of the more important decisions with regard to clinical trials at this stage is
whether patients enrolled in cell therapy trials for CHF should have to have implantable
cardioverter defibrillators (ICDs) in place. The reason is twofold:

- If there is an increased arrhythmogenic risk with cell therapy, then ICD implantation
  would protect these patients.
- If there is not an increased risk of arrhythmogenic risk, then ICD interrogation of these
  patients will offer data that will be important for future patients and clinical trials.

Given the recent results from ICD trials in patients with ischemic cardiomyopathy,
virtually all patients who fit the entry criteria for stem cell therapy at a time remote
from MI would qualify for an ICD. The real issue is overseas trials, where ICDs are not
as readily accessible.

As clinical trials mature from feasibility studies to outcomes, the issue of endpoints for
these trials may become a significant issue. Although clearly the eventual goal, it is not
clear that early stem cell strategies will prolong life. Unlike a pharmacological treatment
where the main mechanism of action is well defined and comparative trials look for dose
effects *(24)* or subtle differences in preparations *(25)*, different stem cell populations
could have profound and mechanistically distinct effects. Therefore, agreement on short-
term functional measures will greatly enhance development of the field. The study by
Perin and colleagues *(6)* in which they quantified both functional measures by treadmill
testing and left ventricular parameters by echocardiography should serve as a prototype.

A great problem facing the field of stem cell therapy for the treatment of myocardial
infarction is not knowing the effects of different stem populations on the underlying
atherosclerosis that ultimately caused the heart failure. Based on the current state of
knowledge, it is theoretically possible that stem cells will decrease, have no effect, or
increase the risk of plaque rupture and MI. To date, based on the hundreds of patients
that have been treated with whole bone marrow preparations or hematopoietic stem
cells, there is no indication for increased MI at 6–12 months.

CELL-BASED GENE THERAPY

There are several basic biological and clinical issues facing stem cell therapy before it can be clearly efficacious and widely available. However, one treatment strategy that may be directly benefiting from the cell therapy investigations performed to date is gene therapy for CHF and/or chronic ischemia. One of the difficulties with early gene therapy strategies was the difficult decision as to whether to inject plasmid DNA *(26,27)* or viral vectors *(28)* encoding the gene of interest. Plasmid DNA results in low transfection efficiency, but no significant systemic or local inflammatory reaction, whereas viral vectors, in particular adenoviral vectors, result in high tissue levels of expression, but carry the risk of system can local inflammation that have been associated with morbidity and mortality in clinical trials. Neither plasmid DNA nor viral vectors allow for cell-type specific transfection.

The relative acceptance of the concept of cell therapy for CHF and/or chronic ischemia has opened up the possibility of delivering engineered/manipulated cells *(15,17,18,20,29)*. The advantages of this approach are several, including (1) cell type-specific gene expression, (2) ex vivo use of high-efficiency viral vectors for cell transfection avoiding system exposure, and (3) ability to develop/deliver cells engineered to respond to local environmental cues such as hypoxia and/or oral drug therapy. An additional advantage is that cell-based gene therapy may require fewer cells to obtain benefit than cell-only therapy. Thus, before we fully understand the fundamental issues of stem cell therapy, we may be able to offer patients significant benefit through cell-based gene therapy, since many of the genes of interest have been identified previously.

CONCLUSIONS

The simple conclusion is that we are on the verge of an extraordinary and exciting time in cardiovascular medicine. Until recently it was believed that tissue damaged during an MI was permanently lost. We now understand that there is a stem cell-based repair process that attempts to repair the injured myocardium. Unfortunately, this is a clinically inefficient process because of either the short period during which the molecular signals are expressed, too few stem cells and/or the wrong cell type entering the injured tissue, or the lack of coordinating and/or differentiation signals expressed in the injured tissue. We are now actively developing strategies that we believe could not only recover cardiac function but regenerate myocardial tissue as well. Further development and clinical fruition of these strategies for the treatment and/or prevention of CHF will require a high level of collaboration between the basic scientist and clinician and a great deal of rigorous work on both sides. The combination of the increasing prevalence of CHF, the economic burden of caring for these patients and the morbidity and mortality associated with the diagnosis, and the potential human and societal benefits of unlocking the potential of stem cell therapy as a treatment is extraordinary.

REFERENCES

1. Strauer BE, Brehm M, Zeus T, et al. Repair of infarcted myocardium by autologous intracoronary mononuclear bone marrow cell transplantation in humans. Circulation 2002;106:1913–1918.
2. Assmus B, Schachinger V, Teupe C, et al. Transplantation of progenitor cells and regeneration enhancement in acute myocardial infarction (TOPCARE-AMI). Circulation 2002;106:3009–3017.
3. Stamm C, Westphal B, Kleine HD, et al. Autologous bone-marrow stem-cell transplantation for myocardial regeneration. Lancet 2003;361:45–46.
4. Tse HF, Kwong YL, Chan JK, Lo G, Ho CL, Lau CP. Angiogenesis in ischaemic myocardium by intramyocardial autologous bone marrow mononuclear cell implantation. Lancet 2003;361:47–49.

5. Seiler C, Pohl T, Wustmann K, et al. Promotion of collateral growth by granulocyte-macrophage colony-stimulating factor in patients with coronary artery disease: a randomized, double-blind, placebo-controlled study. Circulation 2001;104:2012–2017.

6. Perin EC, Dohmann HF, Borojevic R, et al. Transendocardial, autologous bone marrow cell transplantation for severe, chronic ischemic heart failure. Circulation 2003.

7. Schachinger V, Assmus B, Britten MB, et al. Transplantation of progenitor cells and regeneration enhancement in acute myocardial infarction: final one-year results of the TOPCARE-AMI Trial. J Am Coll Cardiol 2004;44:1690–1699.

8. Schachinger V, Tonn T, Dimmeler S, Zeiher AM. Bone-marrow-derived progenitor cell therapy in need of proof of concept: design of the REPAIR-AMI trial. Nat Clin Pract Cardiovasc Med 2006; Suppl 1:S23–S28.

9. Lunde K, Solheim S, Aakhus S, et al. and ASTAMI investigators, Autologous stem cell transplantation in acute myocardial infarction: the ASTAMI randomized controlled trial. Intracoronary transplantation of autologous mononuclear bone marrow cells, study design and safety aspects. Scand Cardiovasc J 2005;39:150–158.

10. Janssens S, Dubois C, Bogaert J, et al. Autologous bone marrow-derived stem cell transfer in patients with ST-segment elevation myocardial infarction: a double-blind, randomised, controlled study. Lancet 2006;367:113–121.

11. Dib N, Michler RE, Pagani FD, et al. Safety and feasibility of autologous myoblast transplantation in patients with ischemic cardiomyopathy: four-year follow-up. Circulation 2005;112:1748–1755.

12. Menasche P, Hagege AA, Vilquin JT, et al. Autologous skeletal myoblast transplantation for severe postinfarction left ventricular dysfunction. J Am Coll Cardiol 2003;41:1078–1083.

13. Smits PC, van Geuns RJ, Poldermans D, et al. Catheter-based intramyocardial injection of autologous skeletal myoblasts as a primary treatment of ischemic heart failure: clinical experience with six-month follow-up. J Am Coll Cardiol 2003;42:2063–2069.

14. Siminiak T, Fiszer D, Jerzykowska O, et al. Percutaneous trans-coronary-venous transplantation of autologous skeletal myoblasts in the treatment of post-infarction myocardial contractility impairment: the POZNAN trial. Eur Heart J 2005;26:1188–1195.

15. Deglurkar I, Mal N, Mill W, et al. Cell-based gene therapy to re-establish stem cell homing improves cardiac function in ischemic cardiomyopathy. Amer Assoc Thor Surg 2005 annual meeting.

16. Mills WR, Mal N, Kiedrowski M, et al. Stem cell therapy enhances electrical viability in myocardial infarction. AHA Scientific Sessions 2005.

17. Askari A, Unzek S, Goldman CK, et al. Cellular, but not direct adenoviral delivery of VEGF results in improved LV function and neovascularization in dilated ischemic cardiomyopathy. J Am Coll Cardiol 2004;43:1908–1914.

18. Suzuki K, Murtuza B, Smolenski RT, et al. Cell transplantation for the treatment of acute myocardial infarction using vascular endothelial growth factor-expressing skeletal myoblasts. Circulation 2001;104:I207–I212.

19. Kofidis T, de Bruin JL, Yamane T, et al. Stimulation of paracrine pathways with growth factors enhances embryonic stem cell engraftment and host-specific differentiation in the heart after ischemic myocardial injury. Circulation 2005;111:2486–2493.

20. Bian J, Kiedrowski M, Mal N, Forudi F, Penn MS. Engineered cell therapy for sustained local myocardial delivery of non-secreted proteins. Cell Transplant 2006;15:67–74.

21. Kehat I, Kenyagin-Karsenti D, Snir M, et al. Human embryonic stem cells can differentiate into myocytes with structural and functional properties of cardiomyocytes. J Clin Invest 2001;108:407–414.

22. Dai W, Hale SL, Martin BJ, et al. Allogeneic mesenchymal stem cell transplantation in postinfarcted rat myocardium: short- and long-term effects. Circulation 2005;112:214–223.

23. Amado LC, Saliaris AP, Schuleri KH, et al. Cardiac repair with intramyocardial injection of allogeneic mesenchymal stem cells after myocardial infarction. Proc Natl Acad Sci USA 2005; 102:11,474–11,479.

24. Nissen SE, Tuzcu EM, Schoenhagen P, et al. Statin therapy, LDL cholesterol, C-reactive protein, and coronary artery disease. N Engl J Med 2005;352:29–38.

25. Poole-Wilson PA, Swedberg K, Cleland JG, et al. Comparison of carvedilol and metoprolol on clinical outcomes in patients with chronic heart failure in the Carvedilol or Metoprolol European Trial (COMET): randomised controlled trial. Lancet 2003;362:7–13.

26. Freedman SB, Vale P, Kalka C, et al. Plasma vascular endothelial growth factor (VEGF) levels after intramuscular and intramyocardial gene transfer of VEGF-1 plasmid DNA. Hum Gene Ther 2002;13:1595–1603.

27. Losordo DW, Vale PR, Hendel RC, et al. Phase 1/2 placebo-controlled, double-blind, dose-escalating trial of myocardial vascular endothelial growth factor 2 gene transfer by catheter delivery in patients with chronic myocardial ischemia. Circulation 2002;105:2012–2018.
28. Rosengart TK, Lee LY, Patel SR, et al. Angiogenesis gene therapy: phase I assessment of direct intramyocardial administration of an adenovirus vector expressing VEGF121 cDNA to individuals with clinically significant severe coronary artery disease. Circulation 1999;100:468–474.
29. Askari A, Unzek S, Popovic ZB, et al. Effect of stromal-cell-derived factor-1 on stem cell homing and tissue regeneration in ischemic cardiomyopathy. Lancet 2003;362:697–703.

INDEX